Cardiology

FIFTH EDITION

D0840670

Cardiology
FIFTH EDITION

Joel W. Heger, M.D.
USC School of Medicine
USC University Hospital
Los Angeles, California

James T. Niemann, M.D.
UCLA School of Medicine
Harbor General Hospital
Torrance, California

J. Michael Criley, M.D.
UCLA School of Medicine
Harbor General Hospital
Torrance, California

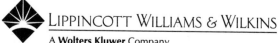

LIPPINCOTT WILLIAMS & WILKINS
A **Wolters Kluwer** Company
Philadelphia · Baltimore · New York · London
Buenos Aires · Hong Kong · Sydney · Tokyo

Acquisitions Editor: Ruth W. Weinberg
Developmental Editor: Lisa R. Kairis
Production Editor: Emily Lerman
Manufacturing Manager: Colin J. Warnock
Cover Designer: Christine Jenny
Compositor: Maryland Composition
Printer: R.R. Donnelley, Crawfordsville

© 2004 by LIPPINCOTT WILLIAMS & WILKINS
530 Walnut Street
Philadelphia, PA 19106 USA
LWW.com

All rights reserved. This book is protected by copyright. No part of this book
may be reproduced in any form or by any means, including photocopying, or
utilized by any information storage and retrieval system without written
permission from the copyright owner, except for brief quotations embodied in
critical articles and reviews. Materials appearing in this book prepared by
individuals as part of their official duties as U.S. government employees are not
covered by the above-mentioned copyright.

Printed in the USA

Library of Congress Cataloging-in-Publication Data

Heger, Joel W.
    Cardiology / Joel W. Heger, James T. Niemann, J. Michael Criley.—5th ed.
        p. ; cm.
    Rev. ed. of: Cardiology / Joel W. Heger . . . [et al.]. 4th ed. c1998.
Includes bibliographical references and index.
ISBN 0-7817-4498-9 (alk. paper)
    1. Heart—Diseases. 2. Cardiology. I. Niemann, James T. II. Criley, J.
Michael. III. Cardiology. IV. Title.
    [DNLM: 1. Heart Diseases—Handbooks. 2.
Cardiology—methods—Handbooks, WG 39 H462ca 2004]
RC681.H445 2004
616.1′2—dc21

                                                                    2003056492

Care has been taken to confirm the accuracy of the information presented and
to describe generally accepted practices. However, the authors and publisher
are not responsible for errors or omissions or for any consequences from
application of the information in this book and make no warranty, expressed or
implied, with respect to the currency, completeness, or accuracy of the contents
of the publication. Application of this information in a particular situation
remains the professional responsibility of the practitioner.

The authors and publisher have exerted every effort to ensure that drug
selection and dosage set forth in this text are in accordance with current
recommendations and practice at the time of publication. However, in view of
ongoing research, changes in government regulations, and the constant flow of
information relating to drug therapy and drug reactions, the reader is urged to
check the package insert for each drug for any change in indications and dosage
and for added warnings and precautions. This is particularly important when the
recommended agent is a new or infrequently employed drug.

Some drugs and medical devices presented in this publication have Food
and Drug Administration (FDA) clearance for limited use in restricted research
settings. It is the responsibility of the health care provider to ascertain the FDA
status of each drug or device planned for use in their clinical practice.

10 9 8 7 6 5 4 3 2 1

To my father, Jack W. Heger—
the world's best father and friend.

To my children, Andrew, Erik, and Christian,
whom I love unconditionally and with
all my heart.

Joel W. Heger, M.D.

Contents

Preface

This present text has been extensively changed from its predecessor, *Cardiology for the House Officer, Fourth Edition*. The authors hope to provide the reader with straightforward, current information with an emphasis on understanding the pathophysiology of the various disease states. We have focused on the fundamentals of diagnosis and treatment, and tried to impart the clinical pearls and pitfalls in patient management. In this edition, we have included a chapter on unstable angina and non–ST-segment elevation myocardial infarction. All diagnosis and treatment recommendations are based on the current guidelines published by the American Heart Association and the American College of Cardiology, and we have added an evidence-based approach, utilizing the latest clinical trial information.

JWH
JTN
JMC

Acknowledgments

The authors acknowledge the doctors who have helped with previous editions, including Keith Bowman, M.D., Richard Haskell, M.D., Mayer Rashtian, M.D., Fernando Roth, M.D., and Milton Smith, M.D. We are also grateful to the many house officers and medical students who have made excellent suggestions and recommendations over the past twenty-five years. We recognize the various institutions where this book has been field tested, including Harbor UCLA Medical Center, LAC-USC Medical Center, USC University Hospital, Huntington Memorial Hospital, and Arcadia Methodist Hospital.

A special thanks to all of our support staff, friends, and families who have given of their time and effort.

The authors gratefully acknowledge the invaluable assistance of David Criley, Blaufuss Multimedia, LLC, for the preparation of the artwork in Chapters 4, 11, and 12.

Cardiology

FIFTH EDITION

BASIC ELECTROCARDIOLOGY

This chapter reviews common causes of abnormalities of atrial and ventricular depolarization and repolarization, which may be recognized on the electrocardiogram (ECG). Arrhythmias commonly encountered in the clinical setting will be discussed in Chapter 2.

It is beyond the scope of this text to provide a comprehensive presentation of basic electrocardiography and vectorcardiography. Discussions of electrophysiologic mechanisms underlying changes in the surface ECG are minimized in the following discussions, and it is assumed that the reader has a basic understanding of ECG vector analysis (e.g., calculating mean axes). Emphasis has been placed on the differential diagnosis of QRS, ST, and T wave changes and providing the reader with readily available ECG criteria for the diagnosis of commonly encountered ECG abnormalities. Comprehensive discussions of basic electrocardiography may be found in a number of texts (1–3).

NORMAL ELECTROCARDIOGRAM

The ECG is the surface representation of cardiac electrical activity. During myocardial depolarization and repolarization, deflections or waves are inscribed on the ECG. By convention, positive forces (electrical forces directed toward an ECG lead) produce upright deflections, and negative forces (forces directed away from an ECG lead) are represented by downward deflections. The distances between deflections and waves are called segments and intervals, respectively.

P WAVE

- P wave represents atrial depolarization.
- P wave duration (width) is a measure of the time required for depolarization to spread through the atria to the atrioventricular (AV) node. In the normal adult, maximum P wave duration is 0.10 seconds.
- Mean frontal plane P wave axis (vector) normally is directed inferiorly and leftward (15 to 75 degrees), and an upright deflection should be recorded in ECG leads I, II, and aVF. A negative deflection is seen in aVR. The P wave may be upright, isoelectric (flat), or inverted in III and aVL.
- Normal P wave amplitude is 0.5 to 2.5 mm (0.05 to 0.25 mV).

PR INTERVAL

- Represents the time required for a supraventricular impulse to depolarize the atria, traverse the AV node, and enter the ventricular conduction system
- Measured from the beginning of the P wave to the initial deflection of the QRS complex (Q or R wave) in the frontal plane lead with the longest PR interval
- Normal PR interval is 0.12 to 0.20 seconds in adults in sinus rhythm. The PR interval normally shortens as heart rate increases

and lengthens at slower heart rates. First-degree AV block is said to be present if the PR interval is more than 0.20 seconds. A PR interval of less than 0.12 seconds may be seen as a normal variant, in hypocalcemia, with ventricular preexcitation, and in ectopic junctional or low atrial rhythms.

QRS COMPLEX

- Represents ventricular depolarization
- Q wave—the first downward or negative deflection after the P wave and/or preceding the first upright deflection
- R wave—the first positive deflection after a P wave
- S wave—a negative deflection following an R wave
- QS wave—a single downward deflection not preceded or followed by an upright deflection
- R′ wave—a second positive deflection after the R wave
- Uppercase and lowercase letters frequently are used to signify approximate voltages or amplitudes of R waves
- QRS interval (duration)—an indication of intraventricular conduction time. This measurement should be made in the frontal plane lead in which it is widest. The normal QRS duration in the adult is less than 0.12 seconds.
- Mean frontal plane QRS vector in the normal adult is -30 to +110 degrees

ST SEGMENT

- An isoelectric segment following ventricular depolarization and preceding ventricular repolarization
- Measured from the end of the QRS complex to the beginning of the T wave
- In contrast to the PR and QRS intervals, changes in the length of the ST segment are not as important as its deviation from baseline or the isoelectric point. The interval from the end of the T wave to the beginning of the P wave (TP interval) usually is taken as the isoelectric reference point. Elevation or depression of the ST segment by ±1 mm (0.1 mV) from the isoelectric baseline is considered "abnormal."

T WAVE

- ECG representation of ventricular repolarization
- T wave vector normally directed inferiorly and leftward
- T wave vector normally "tracks" with the QRS vector. If the QRS is predominantly negative in a frontal plane lead, an inverted T wave usually is seen and is not necessarily abnormal.
- An inverted (negative) T wave in V1 is considered normal. Inverted T waves in V2 and V3 may be normal in patients younger than 30 years of age and in patients with "funnel chest" or "straight back" body habitus.

QT INTERVAL

- Measured from the beginning of the QRS complex to the end of the T wave and represents duration of electrical systole. Mechanical systole usually begins during inscription of the QRS complex.
- This interval varies with heart rate. The normal QT interval, corrected for heart rate, is usually less than 0.44 to 0.46 seconds and is calculated by dividing the measured QT interval (in seconds)

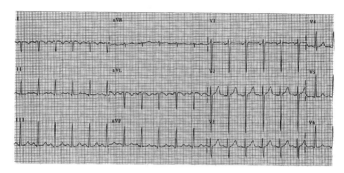

Fig. 1.1. Reversed electrocardiogram leads.

by the square root of the R-R interval (in seconds). The QT interval should be measured in the lead with the most clearly defined T wave.

U WAVE

- A deflection following the T wave; electrophysiologic origin uncertain
- U wave vector tracks with the T wave vector (i.e., polarity or direction similar)
- Amplitude greatest in precordial leads V2–V4

MISPLACED ELECTROCARDIOGRAM LEADS

Figure 1.1 is an ECG tracing obtained from the same patient as in Fig. 1.2. Note the difference in the axes of the P wave, QRS complex, and T wave recorded in the standard limb leads. This is a common technician error caused by reversing the right and left arm ECG leads (Fig. 1.1). In switching the right and left arm leads, the frontal plane P, QRS, and T wave axes have been shifted rightward. Such frontal plane vector changes also may be seen in dextrocardia. However, in this example, the presence of a normal precordial (V1–V6) ECG eliminates dextrocardia as a differential possibility. With dextrocardia, horizontal plane QRS forces should be directed anteriorly

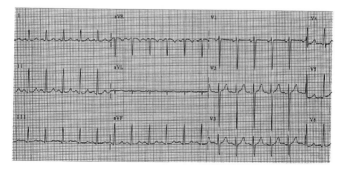

Fig. 1.2. Correct lead placement.

and to the right, with decreasing R wave amplitude over the left precordium.

EARLY REPOLARIZATION

Normal variant ST segment elevation may be noted in the precordial and limb leads. "Early repolarization" is the descriptive term applied to this ECG pattern (Fig. 1.3) (4). Whether accelerated subepicardial repolarization is actually responsible for the ECG variant is uncertain. ST segment elevation is most prominent in the lateral precordial leads (V4–V6). The T waves in these leads are characteristically broadbased, tall (usually more than 5 mm), and upright. The limb leads also may show some degree of ST elevation but rarely greater than 2 mm. The early repolarization variant has been reported in all age groups and is more common in males.

This variant may be confused with the ST segment changes noted during acute pericarditis (5). There are no universally accepted ECG criteria that accurately or absolutely distinguish between the two when a single ECG is examined. However, it has been suggested that the ratio of the ST segment amplitude (in millimeters) to the T wave amplitude (in millimeters) in lead V6 using the PR segment as the baseline helps to distinguish the benign variant (6). In early repolarization, the ST/T ratio in V6 is generally less than 0.25. A ratio of more than 0.25 usually is seen in acute pericarditis.

PERICARDITIS

The ECG may be of considerable value in the diagnosis of pericarditis, especially if serial tracings are obtained (7). Evolutionary changes (stages) may be noted over several days.

Stage 1 (Acute Phase)

See Fig. 1.4.

- There is an ST segment elevation in the precordial leads, especially V5 and V6, and in leads I and II.
- An isoelectric or depressed ST segment commonly is seen in V1.
- PR segment depression may be noted in leads II, aVF, and V4–V6.

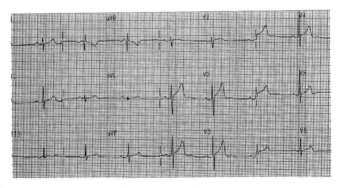

Fig. 1.3. Early repolarization.

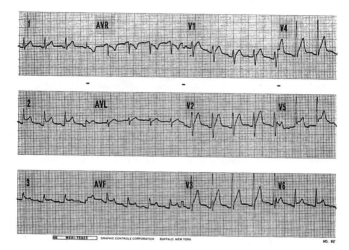

Fig. 1.4. Pericarditis (acute phase).

Stage 2

- ST segment begins returning to baseline (isoelectric line).
- T wave amplitude decreases.

Stage 3

- ST segment is isoelectric.
- T waves are inverted in those leads previously showing ST segment elevation.

Stage 4

- Resolution of T wave changes.

Additional ECG abnormalities may be noted during pericarditis (see Chapter 14) and include arrhythmias, low-voltage QRS complexes (less than 5-mm R wave amplitude in limb leads), and electrical alternans.

ELECTROCARDIOGRAM IN CHAMBER ENLARGEMENT

Atrial Enlargement

Atrial enlargement may result from the following:

- Valvular heart disease (e.g., mitral stenosis)
- Pulmonary hypertension
- Congenital heart disease (e.g., tricuspid atresia)
- Ventricular hypertrophy (e.g., systemic hypertension)

The initial portion of the P wave results from right atrial depolarization, and the terminal portion results from left atrial depolarization. The normal mean P vector is the sum of the vectors generated by both atria and is directed leftward and inferiorly. Atrial enlargement may alter the P wave amplitude, duration, or vector orientation.

An accurate ECG diagnosis of atrial enlargement is not always

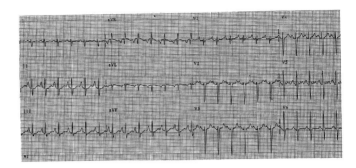

Fig. 1.5.   Right atrial enlargement.

possible. There is considerable normal variation in P wave amplitude, duration, and morphology. Tachycardia alone may increase P wave amplitude. Although it is not always possible to diagnose left atrial enlargement (LAE) or right atrial enlargement (RAE) electrocardiographically, the following criteria may be helpful.

Right Atrial Enlargement
See Fig. 1.5.

- P wave amplitude of more than 2.5 mm in lead II
- Frontal plane P wave vector shifted rightward (more than +75 degrees)
- Rarely noted as an isolated finding (i.e., most frequently associated with ECG criteria for right ventricular hypertrophy)

Left Atrial Enlargement
See Fig. 1.6.

- P wave duration of more than 0.11 seconds and P wave usually notched in lead II
- Frontal plane P wave vector shifted leftward (0 to -30 degrees) (terminal part of P wave may be negative in lead III and aVF)
- Biphasic P wave in lead V1 with wide, deep terminal component (more than 0.04 seconds in duration and 1 mm in depth)

Left Ventricular Hypertrophy
Left ventricular hypertrophy (LVH) manifests itself primarily as an increase in voltage (height of R wave) in those ECG leads that reflect left ventricular potentials (Fig. 1.7). The increase in voltage is the result of an increase in muscle mass and surface area and/or the proximity of the dilated heart to the sensing ECG electrode (heart closer to chest wall). The mean QRS vector tends to be rotated leftward and posteriorly. LVH does not change the sequence of ventricular depolarization, but it may delay it (delayed onset of intrinsicoid deflection). Repolarization may be altered—the left precordial leads may show depressed ST segments and inverted T waves—resulting in a left ventricular strain pattern. The ECG diagnosis of LVH is based on voltage changes, ST-T wave alterations, axis deviations, and conduction delay (QRS duration of more than 0.08 seconds but

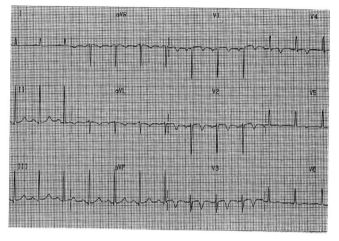

Fig. 1.6. Left atrial enlargement.

less than 0.12 seconds). Many ECG criteria have been advanced, all of which have varying degrees of sensitivity and specificity.

Common Electrocardiogram Voltage Criteria for Left Ventricular Hypertrophy in the Adult

- Sum of S wave in V1 or V2 and R wave in V5 or V6 is more than 35 mm, or
- Sum of highest R and deepest S waves in precordial leads is more than 45 mm, or
- R wave in V6 of more than 18 mm, or
- R wave in aVL of more than 12 mm, or
- Sum of R wave in I and S wave in III is more than 16 mm, or
- R wave in I of more than 14 mm

Limb lead criteria are less sensitive but highly specific.

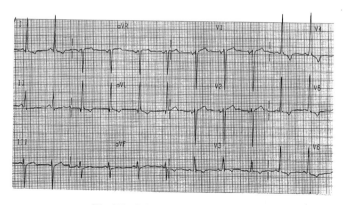

Fig. 1.7. Left ventricular hypertrophy.

Point Score System for Diagnosis of Left Ventricular Hypertrophy

Because LVH may affect the amplitude, axis, and duration of the QRS complex, as well as produce ST segment and T wave changes (downsloping ST segment depression and asymmetric T wave inversion in V4–V6—strain pattern), a point score system (Estes criteria) was developed to improve diagnostic specificity (Table 1.1) (8). This historic and commonly referenced point score system is less sensitive than QRS voltage criteria. With the current trend toward improved or high sensitivity to prompt the physician to seek more definitive or specific confirmation (echocardiography), the contemporary value of the noted criteria is questionable. The authors do not use this point system.

Right Ventricular Hypertrophy

The ECG diagnosis of right ventricular hypertrophy (RVH) is less sensitive and less specific than that of LVH, and the ECG frequently is normal in the presence of RVH. The following ECG abnormalities are suggestive of RVH:

- Right axis deviation (more than + 110 degrees in an adult) in the absence of right bundle branch block (RBBB), left posterior inferior fascicular block, or anterolateral or inferior myocardial infarction
- Dominant R wave (more than 7 mm) in lead V1 [also may be seen in RBBB, posterior myocardial infarction, and Wolff-Parkinson-White (WPW) syndrome and as a normal variant]
- R/S ratio in lead V1 of more than 1.0
- R/S ratio in V5 or VG6 of less than 1.0
- RSR pattern in lead V1 with a QRS duration of less than 0.12 seconds

Table 1.1.   Point score system (Estes criteria)

Criteria	Points
1. Amplitude of QRS	3
R in V5 or V6 >30 mm	
S in V1 or V2 >30 mm	
Largest R or S in limb leads >20 mm	
If any one of the above present	
2. ST-T strain pattern	
In the absence of digitalis therapy	3
Digitalis therapy	1
3. Left atrial enlargement present	3
4. Left axis deviation ($\leq 30°$)	2
5. QRS duration >0.9 sec	1
6. Intrisicoid QRS deflection of >0.05 sec in V5 or V6	1
5 or more points = definite left ventricular hypertrophy	
4 or more points = probable left ventricular hypertrophy	

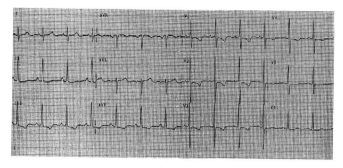

Fig. 1.8. Right ventricular hypertrophy.

The diagnosis of RVH is supported by the presence of RAE and/or right ventricular strain pattern (ST segment depression and T wave inversion in V1–V3) (Fig. 1.8). The ECG diagnosis of RVH may be obscured if an RBBB also is present.

Combined Left Ventricular Hypertrophy and Right Ventricular Hypertrophy

The value of the ECG in the diagnosis of combined ventricular hypertrophy is limited. In many instances, the ECG will demonstrate alterations suggesting hypertrophy of only one of the ventricles.

Electrocardiogram Criteria Suggestive of Combined Ventricular Hypertrophy

- Voltage changes in the precordial leads "diagnostic" of both LVH and RVH
- Voltage criteria for LVH plus:
  - Right axis deviation (more than +110 degrees), or
  - R/S ratio in V1 of more than 1.0, or
  - More than 7 mm R wave in V1, or
  - Deep S wave in V6, or
  - RAE and a vertical mean QRS axis
- Voltage criteria for RVH plus:
  - R/S ratio in V2–V4 and/or in two or more limb leads of nearly 1.0 (Katz-Wachtel sign), or
  - Large R waves in V5 or V6 with strain pattern and LAE

The ECG shown in Fig. 1.9 demonstrates evidence of LVH (V6 R wave more than 18 mm and LAE-precordial leads are recorded at 1/2 standard). However, there is also RAE, and a right ventricular strain pattern is evident in the anterior precordial leads. The frontal plane QRS axis is 90 degrees—a more rightward axis would be expected with LVH alone. The tracing is compatible with biatrial and biventricular hypertrophy.

RIGHT BUNDLE BRANCH BLOCK

RBBB usually is associated with organic heart disease (ischemic, rheumatic, congenital) (Fig. 1.10). In RBBB, the sequence of ventricular activation is abnormal, resulting in a terminal QRS vector that

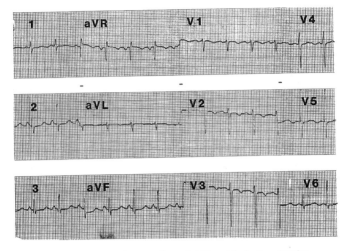

Fig. 1.9. Left ventricular hypertrophy and right ventricular hypertrophy (precordial leads ½ standard).

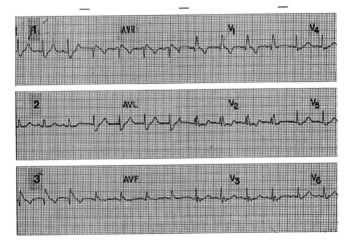

Fig. 1.10. Right bundle branch block.

is directed rightward and anteriorly (large R wave in V1, S wave in V6). The cardiac vector is not altered significantly during the first 0.06 seconds of ventricular depolarization. The left ventricle is depolarized in a normal fashion, septal activation occurs from left to right, and the mean frontal plane QRS vector (axis) is usually normal. The site of block within the right bundle branch may be proximal or more peripheral.

Electrocardiogram Criteria for the Diagnosis of Right Bundle Branch Block
- QRS duration of more than 0.12 seconds in limb leads
- Triphasic QRS complexes (RSR′ pattern) in the anterior precordial leads (V1–V3); the ST segment often is depressed, and the T wave is inverted in these leads.
- Wide S wave (0.25 seconds in duration) in lateral precordial leads (V5, V6) and lead I
- Normal time of onset of the intrinsicoid deflection in lead V6

Associated RVH should be suspected if the secondary R wave in V1 is greater than 15 mm in amplitude or if there is right axis deviation of the mean frontal plane QRS vector.

LEFT BUNDLE BRANCH BLOCK
Left bundle branch block (LBBB) is almost always an indicator of organic heart disease (Fig. 1.11). In LBBB, the entire sequence of ventricular activation is abnormal, the primary abnormality being a change in the direction of the initial QRS vector. Initial depolarization and the mean QRS vector are directed leftward and posteriorly. Septal activation occurs from right to left. There is also a change in the direction of repolarization—ST and T vectors rotate away from the mean QRS vector, resulting in ST segment depression and T wave inversion in the lateral precordial leads, lead I, and lead aVL.

The main left bundle branch divides into two major divisions (fascicles) soon after entering the interventricular septum—the left anterior superior fascicle and the left posterior inferior fascicle. Thus,

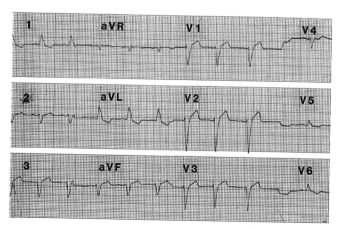

Fig. 1.11. Left bundle branch block (precordial leads ½ standard).

LBBB may result from a lesion in the main left bundle, from simultaneous block in some portion of the anterior and posterior fascicles, or from peripheral block. The site(s) of block cannot be distinguished electrocardiographically.

Electrocardiographic Criteria for the Diagnosis of Left Bundle Branch Block

- QRS duration is more than 0.12 seconds.
- Large, broad, notched, or slurred R waves in the lateral precordial leads, lead I, and lead aVL are present. Q waves and S waves are characteristically absent, the ST segment is depressed, and the T wave is inverted in these leads.
- A small R wave precedes a deep S wave in leads II, III, and aVF.
- In most instances, left axis deviation (LAD; less than −30 degrees) is present. However, LBBB may be seen without LAD.
- Initial R waves followed by deep S waves are present in the anterior precordial leads (V1–V3). The ST segment may be elevated in these leads.
- Onset of the intrinsicoid deflection is delayed in V6, but is normal in V1.

From the description of the characteristic ECG findings, it should be apparent that a diagnosis of LVH or acute infarction is difficult in the presence of LBBB.

FASCICULAR BLOCKS

The main left bundle can be considered to divide into two major divisions or fascicles soon after entering the interventricular septum—the left anterior superior fascicle and the left posterior inferior fascicle. Conduction delay in either fascicle (or hemiblock) will alter the sequence of left ventricular depolarization and produce distinctive ECG changes. Left anterior superior hemiblock, either alone or in association with AV nodal or right bundle branch conduction disturbance(s), is far more common than left posterior inferior hemiblock. This disparity may be the result of the following: (a) the greater length and smaller diameter of the anterior fascicle, (b) the location of the anterior superior fascicle within the turbulent outflow tract of the left ventricle, and/or (c) the single blood supply (left anterior descending coronary artery) of the anterior fascicle compared to the dual blood supply of the posterior fascicle (left anterior descending and right coronary artery).

Left Anterior Superior Hemiblock

If the anterior fascicle is blocked, the wave of depolarization will travel through the fibers of the posterior fascicle and then spread to the portions of the left ventricular myocardium normally activated by the anterior fascicle (Fig. 1.12). The sequence of left ventricular depolarization, thus, proceeds in an inferior to superior direction. Left anterior superior hemiblock may be caused by coronary artery disease, valvular heart disease, congenital heart disease, cardiomyopathy, and myocarditis.

Electrocardiogram Criteria for the Diagnosis of Left Anterior Superior Hemiblock

- Left axis deviation (mean frontal plane QRS axis of ≤ −45 degrees)
- QRS duration usually ≤0.10 seconds

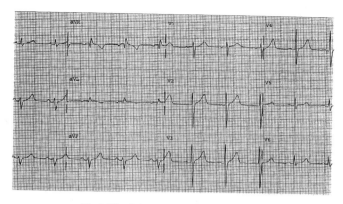

Fig. 1.12. Left anterior superior hemiblock.

- Small R waves in leads II, III, and aVF and small Q waves in leads I and aVF
- Deep S waves in II, III, and aVF
- Exclusion of other causes of LAD: body habitus, inferior myocardial infarction, hyperkalemia, ventricular preexcitation, etc.

LEFT POSTERIOR INFERIOR HEMIBLOCK

Ventricular activation proceeds in a superior to inferior direction. The mean frontal plane QRS axis will be directed inferiorly and rightward. Left posterior inferior hemiblock is far less common than left anterior superior hemiblock, rarely occurs in the absence of associated AV nodal or right bundle branch conduction disturbances, and almost invariably indicates organic heart disease (Fig. 1.13).

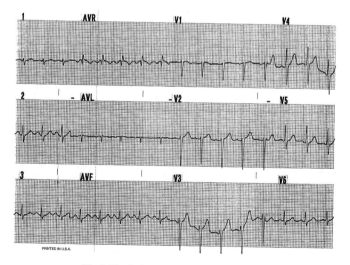

Fig. 1.13. Left posterior inferior hemiblock.

Electrocardiogram Criteria for the Diagnosis of Left Posterior Inferior Hemiblock
- Right axis deviation (mean frontal plane QRS axis of $\geq +110$ degrees)
- QRS duration of ≤ 0.10 seconds
- Small R waves in leads I and aVL and small Q waves in leads II, III, and aVF
- Tall R waves in II, III, and aVF and deep S waves in I and aVL
- Exclusion of other causes of right axis deviation: chronic obstructive pulmonary disease, right ventricular enlargement, lateral myocardial infarction

BIFASCICULAR AND TRIFASCICULAR BLOCKS

Bifascicular block refers to the combination of RBBB with either left anterior superior or left posterior inferior fascicular block. Trifascicular block refers to the combination of RBBB with either left anterior or left posterior inferior fascicular block and incomplete AV block. AV block may occur at the level of the AV node or more distally (bundle of His, main left bundle, or in the remaining fascicle) (9). The level of the AV block cannot be determined with the surface ECG—only a prolonged PR interval will be noted. Figure 1.14 demonstrates an RBBB and a left posterior, inferior fascicular block.

Bifascicular and trifascicular block may be seen with the following:

- Coronary artery disease
- Cardiomyopathy
- Valvular heart disease, especially aortic
- Lenhgre's or Lev's disease—sclerodegenerative processes involving the cardiac conduction system
- Cardiac surgery—repair of a ventricular septal defect or valve replacement
- Myocarditis

Although indicative of advanced conduction system disease, chronic bifascicular or trifascicular block alone is not an indication for permanent artificial cardiac pacing because long-term follow-up studies have not revealed a high incidence of complete heart block (9). Bifascicular or trifascicular block with clinical symptoms (syncope, dyspnea on exertion, etc.) as a result of documented bradyarrhythmias or complete heart block is an indication for artificial pacing. Symptoms may be relieved, but the risk of sudden death will not be affected significantly.

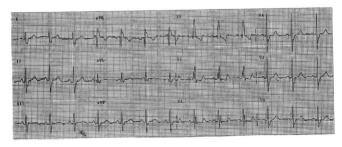

Fig. 1.14.   Bifascicular block.

ELECTROCARDIOGRAM IN ACUTE MYOCARDIAL INFARCTION

A single ECG is not the gold standard for the diagnosis of acute myocardial infarction (AMI). The initial ECG may be normal in 10% and nondiagnostic in as many as 50% of cases of AMI. The ECG diagnosis of AMI may be obscured or mimicked by a number of conditions (10,11).

ST Segment Elevation Myocardial Infarction

The ECG criteria for ST segment elevation myocardial infarction (STEMI), previously called transmural or Q wave infarction, are ST segment elevation of 1 mm or more (0.1 mV) in two or more anatomically contiguous ECG leads. ST segment amplitude is measured at 0.04 seconds (1 mm) after the J point. The J point is the position of the juncture between the end of the QRS complex and the beginning of the ST segment. The isoelectric point or baseline for this measurement is traditionally the PR segment. It has been suggested that a baseline drawn from the start of the P wave to the end of the T wave is more useful and valid (12). This measurement is critical in that such patients often will qualify for and benefit from reperfusion therapy (see Chapter 9).

ST segment elevation (especially in anterior precordial leads) is not diagnostic of AMI because it also may be seen with the following (10,11):

- LVH with strain
- LBBB
- Paced cardiac rhythm
- Pericarditis
- "Early repolarization"
- Hyperkalemia
- Use of certain drugs (digoxin, tricyclic antidepressants)
- Cerebral vascular accident
- Ventricular aneurysm
- Hypothermia (Osborne waves)

The presence of a LBBB may conceal changes of an AMI because of the repolarization changes that accompany LBBB. ECG criteria that have been found to be helpful in diagnosing AMI in patients with LBBB include the following: (a) ST segment elevation of 1 mm or more that is concordant with (in the same direction as) the QRS complex; (b) ST segment depression of 1 mm or more in lead V1, V2, or V3; and (c) ST segment elevation of 5 mm or more that was discordant with (in the opposite direction from) the QRS complex (9,13).

Non–ST Segment Elevation Myocardial Infarction

The ECG changes associated with non–ST segment elevation myocardial infarction (NSTEMI), previously called nontransmural or subendocardial AMI, are variable. The ECG changes most commonly noted include the following (10,11):

- ST segment depression—downsloping or "square wave" type of at least 1.0 mm (Fig. 1.15)
- T wave inversion
- ST segment depression and T wave inversion

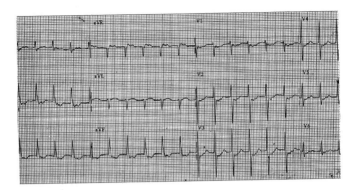

Fig. 1.15.   Anterior non–ST-segment elevation myocardial infarction.

Characteristically, abnormal Q waves do not develop during the course of NSTEMI. The ST-T wave changes may persist for a variable period but usually longer than 24 hours. The nonspecific character of these ECG changes often necessitates the use of ancillary studies (CK-MB mass, troponins, or radionuclide imaging) to confirm the diagnosis of myocardial necrosis. Patients with unstable angina may also transiently exhibit similar ST and T wave abnormalities. Patients suffering NSTEMI may experience complications similar to those noted during STEMI and have a long-term prognosis not significantly different from patients with STEMI (14).

ST-T wave changes that simulate those of NSTEMI may be noted in the following (15):

- LVH with strain
- The bundle branch blocks
- Cardiomyopathies
- WPW syndrome
- Central nervous system (CNS) disease
- Late pericarditis
- Electrolyte disturbances (especially hypokalemia)
- Association with the use of certain drugs

Infarct Localization

The ECG is able to localize the infarct artery and the site of infarction/injury with considerable accuracy based on which leads abnormal Q waves (more than 0.03 seconds) or ST-T wave changes are noted.

Abnormal Q waves or ST-T wave changes in contiguous leads:

- II, III, aVF: inferior wall infarction (Fig. 1.16)
- V1–V3: anteroseptal infarction (Fig. 1.17)
- I, aVL, V4–V6: lateral wall infarction (Fig. 1.18)
- V1 or V2 to V6: anterolateral infarction

Posterior Wall and Right Ventricular Infarction

A large R wave and ST segment depression in leads V1 and V2 are indicative of infarction of the true posterior wall of the left ventricle

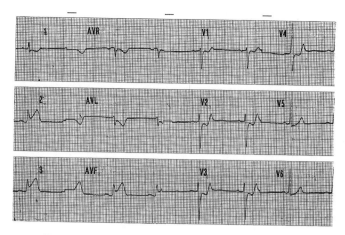

Fig. 1.16. Inferior ST-segment elevation myocardial infarction.

(Fig. 1.19) (16). The large R wave and ST segment depressions noted in the anterior precordial leads are the surface ECG manifestations of posterior infarction/injury and may be viewed as "reciprocal" changes—if ECG leads were placed dorsally, characteristic Q waves and ST segment elevation would be noted. Isolated posterior wall infarction is infrequent. This infarction pattern most commonly is seen in association with inferior wall infarction because these portions of myocardium share a common blood supply (right coronary artery in 90% of individuals). Infarction of the inferior and/or posterior wall of the left ventricle often is complicated by infarction of the right ventricle. In patients with an inferior infarction, a right precordial ECG should be obtained. ST elevation of 1 mm or more

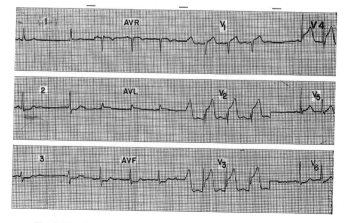

Fig. 1.17. Anteroseptal ST-segment elevation myocardial infarction.

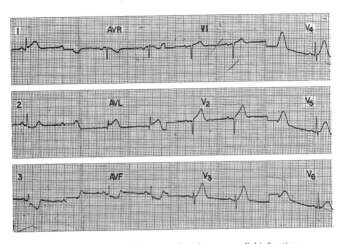

Fig. 1.18. Lateral ST-segment elevation myocardial infarction.

in lead V3R or V4R suggests right ventricular infarction (Fig. 1.20A and 1.20B) (17).

ELECTROLYTES AND THE ELECTROCARDIOGRAM

Cardiac electrical activity results from the movement of various ions across the sarcolemma membrane. Changes in electrolyte concentrations therefore may alter depolarization and/or repolarization and produce ECG abnormalities (3).

Hyperkalemia

1. Serum potassium, 5.5 to 6.6 mEq/L
   - Tall, peaked, narrow T waves in precordial leads

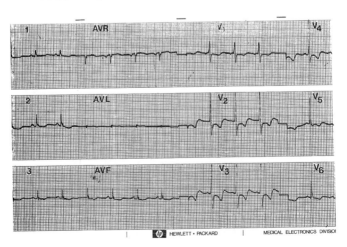

Fig. 1.19. Posterior wall infarction.

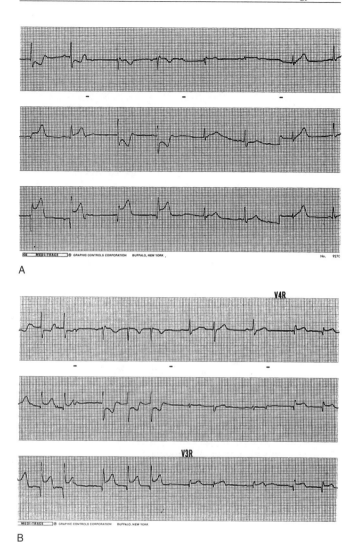

Fig. 1.20. **A:** Inferior ST-segment elevation myocardial infarction (STEMI)—standard 12-lead electrocardiogram. **B:** Inferior STEMI—right precordial ECG recording in the same patient.

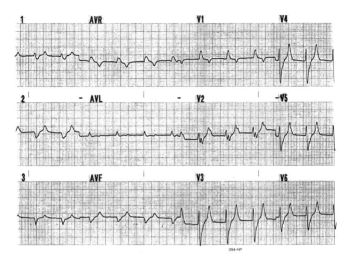

Fig. 1.21. Hyperkalemia.

- Deep S wave in leads I and V6
- QRS complex usually normal

2. Serum potassium, 7.0 to 8.0 mEq/L (Fig. 1.21)
   - QRS widening
   - Slurring of both initial and terminal portions of the QRS
   - ST segment elevation
   - Low, wide P waves
   - First- and second-degree AV block
   - Sinoatrial arrest
   - Bradycardia

3. Serum potassium, more than 8.0 mEq/L
   - Marked widening of QRS complex
   - Distinct ST-T wave may not be noted
   - High risk of ventricular fibrillation or a systole

Hypokalemia

1. Serum potassium, 3.0 to 3.5 mEq/L
   - ECG may be normal.
   - If ECG changes are present, they are most prominent in the anterior precordial leads V2 and V3 and consist of T wave flattening and the appearance of U waves.
   - QT interval and QRS duration are normal.

2. Serum potassium, 2.7 to 3.0 mEq/L
   - U waves become taller, and T waves become smaller but do not invert.
   - The ratio of the amplitude of the U wave to the amplitude of T wave frequently exceeds 1.0 in V2 or V3.

3. Serum potassium, less than 2.6 mEq/L (Fig. 1.22)
   - Almost always accompanied by ECG changes

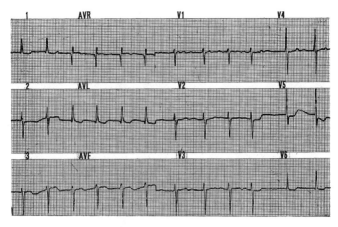

Fig. 1.22.   Hypokalemia.

- ST segment depression associated with tall U waves and low amplitude T waves
- QT interval normal, but accurate measurement may be difficult because of the close proximity of the U wave. The U wave is usually smallest in lead aVL, and this lead should be used to determine the QT interval.
- QRS duration rarely affected in adults

Hypercalcemia
- Slight increase in QRS duration
- ST segment short or absent
- Corrected QT interval shortened
- PR interval may be prolonged
- T wave amplitude and duration usually normal
- U wave amplitude may be normal or slightly increased

Hypocalcemia
- Slight decrease in QRS duration
- ST segment lengthened and corrected QT interval prolonged
- PR interval may be shortened
- T waves may become flat or inverted in severe hypocalcemia

See Fig. 1.23.

Hyponatremia or Hypernatremia
- Effects of changes in serum sodium cannot be detected electrocardiographically.

Hypomagnesium or Hypermagnesium
- Marked magnesium deficiency usually is associated with potassium depletion, and the ECG demonstrates the characteristic changes of hypokalemia. Ventricular arrhythmias may be present.
- Hypermagnesium is uncommon clinically and usually is encountered in patients with uremia who often have other electrolyte

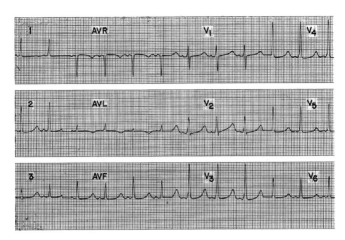

Fig. 1.23.   Hypocalcemia.

disturbances (hypocalcemia, hyperkalemia) that produce ECG changes.

- It is uncertain if changes in body magnesium alone affect the surface ECG.

ELECTROCARDIOGRAM AND NONCARDIAC DRUGS

Commonly used inotropic (digoxin) and antiarrhythmic (quinidine, procainamide) drugs produce well-defined repolarization changes that can be recognized on the surface ECG. Noncardiac drugs also can produce significant ECG changes that may be confused with organic cardiac disease. The phenothiazines and tricyclic antidepressants frequently are used in clinical practice and may produce a number of "benign" or significant ECG changes. These drugs share a number of electrophysiologic effects with the class 1 antiarrhythmic drugs (e.g., quinidine) and, thus, have a direct effect on the cardiac action potential. These drugs also possess variable anticholinergic properties and can affect the heart indirectly (3).

ELECTROCARDIOGRAM IN CENTRAL NERVOUS SYSTEM DISEASE

CNS lesions, particularly subarachnoid hemorrhage, intracerebral hemorrhage, and infarction (stroke), may produce striking ECG repolarization abnormalities (18). These alterations most commonly take the form of diffuse, deep, wide, blunted T wave inversions and QT prolongation (Fig. 1.24); U waves also may be prominent. The exact incidence of ECG changes in CNS hemorrhage or infarction is undetermined, but appears to be more common with frontal lobe lesions. These functional repolarization changes are felt to be the result of heightened cerebrocardiac autonomic stimuli.

ARTIFICIAL CARDIAC PACEMAKERS

The tip of a transvenous ventricular pacing catheter should lie in the apex of the right ventricle. Electrocardiographically, the mean

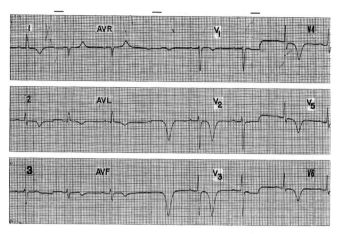

Fig. 1.24. The electrocardiogram following massive subarachnoid hemorrhage.

QRS vector of paced complexes will depend on the point of electrical stimulation of the myocardium. If the catheter tip is positioned properly, the mean QRS vector of paced complexes should be directed superiorly and posteriorly, resulting in the following:

- Large, wide QRS complexes with a dominant R wave in leads I, aVL, and commonly in V6
- Large, negative deflections (QS waves) in leads II, III, aVF, and V1–V3

The ECG pattern, thus, mimics that of a LBBB with LAD.

In Fig. 1.25, each QRS complex is preceded by a pacemaker stimulus artifact ("spike"), which is seen best in leads I and II and the

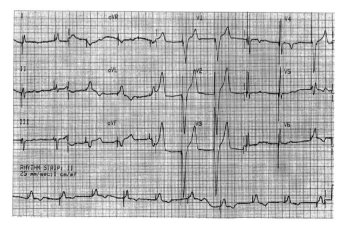

Fig. 1.25. Paced rhythm.

precordial leads. The underlying rhythm is atrial fibrillation, and the patient, in this instance, is pacemaker dependent.

WOLFF-PARKINSON-WHITE SYNDROME (PREEXCITATION)

Wolff-Parkinson-White syndrome is a form of anomalous AV conduction or preexcitation (Fig. 1.26) (19). Ventricular preexcitation is said to exist when conduction of a supraventricular impulse to the ventricular myocardium occurs via accessory pathways that bypass the AV node. Conduction via an accessory pathway in WPW permits premature activation of ventricular myocardium. Preexcitation can occur through a number of anatomic pathways. In classic WPW syndrome, a sinus impulse is conducted through the Kent's bundle, which bypasses the AV node, and initiates activation of the ipsilateral ventricle. A short PR interval and an initial slurring (delta wave) during the inscription of the QRS complex result. The bypass tract is capable of bidirectional conduction, and reentrant tachyarrhythmias (see Chapter 2) are a feature of this syndrome.

Electrocardiogram Criteria for the Diagnosis of Wolff-Parkinson-White Syndrome

- Short PR interval (less than 0.12 seconds)
- Normal P wave vector (to exclude junctional rhythm)
- Presence of a delta wave—slurring or notching of first portion of the QRS complex
- QRS duration more than 0.10 seconds

Clinical Significance of the Wolff-Parkinson-White Syndrome

- High incidence of tachyarrhythmias (usually reentrant mechanism—40% to 80% of patients)
- Frequently associated with organic heart disease (30% to 40% of

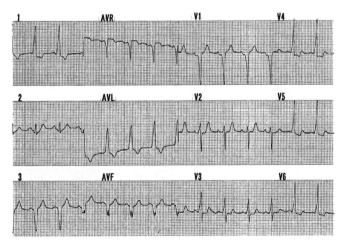

Fig. 1.26. Preexcitation (short PR and delta waves, lateral precordial leads).

cases). Disorders commonly associated with WPW syndrome include atrial septal defect, mitral valve prolapse, hypertrophic cardiomyopathy, and Ebstein's anomaly.

- ECG patterns may simulate other disease processes—myocardial infarction or ventricular hypertrophy.
- Antegrade conduction via the bypass tract and retrograde conduction through the AV node may produce regular tachyarrhythmias with wide QRS complexes, mimicking ventricular tachycardia.

REFERENCES

1. Marriott HJL: *Marriott's manual of electrocardiography: an advanced review with practice exam*, 1st ed. New York: Trinity Press, 1995.
2. Goldberger AL: *Clinical electrocardiography: a simplified approach*, 6th ed. St. Louis: Mosby, Inc., 1999.
3. Mirvis DM, Goldberger AL: Electrocardiography. In: E Braunwald, Zipes DP, Libby P, eds. *Heart disease. A textbook of cardiovascular medicine*, 6th ed. New York: WB Saunders, pp. 82–128, 2001.
4. Mehta M, Jain AC, Mehta A: Early repolarization. *Clin Cardiol* 22: 59, 1999.
5. Brady WJ: Benign early repolarization: electrocardiographic manifestations and differentiation from other ST segment elevations syndromes. *Am J Emerg Med* 16:592, 1998.
6. Ginzton LE, Laks MM: The differential diagnosis of acute pericarditis from the normal variant: new electrocardiographic criteria. *Circulation* 65:1004, 1982.
7. Chan TC, Brady WJ, Pollack M: Electrocardiographic manifestations: Acute myopericarditis. *J Emerg Med* 17:865, 1999.
8. Romhilt DW, Estes EH: Point score system for the ECG diagnosis of left ventricular hypertrophy. *Am Heart J* 75:752, 1968.
9. Sgarbossa EB, Pinski SL, Barbagelata A, et al: Electrocardiographic diagnosis of evolving acute myocardial infarction in the presence of left bundle-branch block. *N Engl J Med* 334:481, 1996.
10. Goldberger AL: *Myocardial infarction. Electrocardiographic differential diagnosis*, 3rd ed. St. Louis: CV Mosby Co., 1984.
11. Sgarbossa EB, Birnbaum Y, Parrillo JE: Electrocardiographic diagnosis of acute myocardial infarction: current concepts for the clinician. *Am Heart J* 141:507, 2001.
12. Anonymous: Acute coronary syndromes: patients with acute ischemic chest pain. In: RO Cummins, ed. *ACLS provider manual*. Dallas: American Heart Association, pp. 123–144, 2001.
13. Sgarbossa EB: Value of the ECG in suspected acute myocardial infarction with left bundle branch block. *J Electrocardiol* 33(Suppl): 87, 2000.
14. Cannon CP, McCabe CH, Stone PH, et al: The electrocardiogram predicts one-year outcome of patients with unstable angina and non-Q wave myocardial infarction: Results of the TIMI III Registry ECG Ancillary Study: Thrombolysis in Myocardial Ischemia. *J Am Coll Cardiol* 30:133, 1997.
15. Pollehn T, Brady WJ, Perron AD: Electrocardiographic ST segment depression. *Am J Emerg Med* 19:303, 2001.
16. Wung SF, Drew BJ: New electrocardiographic criteria for posterior wall acute myocardial ischemia validated by a percutaneous transluminal coronary angioplasty model of acute myocardial infarction. *Am J Cardiol* 87:970, 2001.

17. Kinch JW, Ryan TJ: Right ventricular infarction. *N Engl J Med* 330: 1211, 1994.
18. Strauss WE, Samuels MA: Electrocardiographic changes associated with neurologic events. *Chest* 106:1316, 1994.
19. Al-Khatib SM, Pritchett EL: Clinical features of Wolff-Parkinson-White syndrome. *Am Heart J* 138:403–413, 1999.

ARRHYTHMIAS

This chapter reviews the basic rules and principles of arrhythmia interpretation. Examples and descriptions of common arrhythmias are provided, and a basic approach to therapy is included for each arrhythmia.

BASIC RULES FOR RHYTHM INTERPRETATION

1. **Identify atrial activity—P wave**
   - Is there evidence of atrial depolarization (i.e., Are P waves present?)?
   - If so, do they represent normal P waves, ectopic P′ waves, the F waves of atrial flutter, or the fibrillatory waves of atrial fibrillation?
   - Do the atria depolarize in an anterograde (upright P in lead II) or in a retrograde (negative P in lead II) manner?
   - Are all P waves in a single lead of similar morphology? That is, do all P waves look the same, suggesting a single site or focus of origin?
   - What is the atrial rate? Is it regular or irregular?

2. **Identify ventricular activity—QRS complexes**
   - Does ventricular depolarization arise from a supraventricular focus [i.e., Is the QRS of normal duration (0.10 seconds or less?)]?
   - If the QRS is broad, is it the result of aberrant ventricular conduction (AVC) or an ectopic ventricular focus?
   - What is the ventricular rate? Is it regular or irregular?

3. **Evaluate atrioventricular (AV) conduction—analyze the relationship between the P wave and the QRS.**
   - Is each P wave related to a QRS? If the PR interval is less than 0.10 seconds or more than 0.40 seconds in duration, the P wave is unlikely to have "produced" the ensuing QRS complex. Consider atrioventricular dissociation (AVD).
   - Is each P wave conducted to the ventricles (1:1 AV conduction)?
   - Is the speed of AV conduction (the PR interval) normal (0.20 seconds or less)?
   - Is there any evidence of group beating (Wenckebach phenomenon)?

SUPRAVENTRICULAR ARRHYTHMIAS

Sinus Bradycardia

Description

Sinus bradycardia (Fig. 2.1) is the result of a decrease in the normal rate of discharge of the sinoatrial (SA) node. The atrial rate (P wave frequency) is less than 60/minute, but atrial depolarization is normal (i.e., the P wave vector is directed inferiorly and leftward, resulting in upright P waves in leads II, III, and aVF). The P-to-P interval is

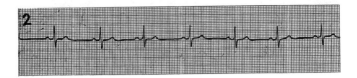

Fig. 2.1. Sinus bradycardia.

regular, and each P wave is followed by a QRS complex of normal duration (1:1 AV conduction). The PR interval is fixed or constant. In the setting of an underlying intraventricular conduction defect, QRS complexes may be of prolonged duration (longer than 0.10 seconds).

Causes

Possible causes of sinus bradycardia include the following:

Normal: increased vagal tone in the conditioned athlete.
Pathologic: intrinsic sinus node disease–sick sinus syndrome
Increased vagal tone–inferior myocardial infarction (MI), vasovagal response
Drug toxicity–beta-adrenergic blockade, calcium channel blockade, organophosphate poisoning

Therapy

Therapy is dictated by the clinical circumstances in which sinus bradycardia is noted. Acute therapy always is indicated if hemodynamic compromise/hypoperfusion is present. In the setting of acute inferior MI, acute therapy also is indicated if ventricular arrhythmias [ventricular escape beats or rhythms or premature ventricular contractions (PVCs)] are present.

ATROPINE SULFATE. Atropine is the drug of choice if sinus bradycardia is pathologic and associated with hypoperfusion. It is most effective if symptomatic bradycardia is the result of acute inferior MI, a vasovagal response, or cholinergic drug toxicity. The drug should be administered intravenously; 0.5 mg boluses administered at 3 to 5-minute intervals (to a total dose of 0.03 to 0.04 mg) are recommended (1). In the setting of acute inferior MI, a total dose of about 1 mg is usually successful in increasing the sinus rate. Atropine is of limited value in managing hemodynamically significant bradyarrhythmias associated with the sick sinus syndrome. It is unlikely to increase heart rate in the setting of drug toxicity as a result of beta-adrenergic or calcium channel blockade. Excessive use of atropine may result in sinus tachycardia and an increase in myocardial oxygen demand. This complication is of particular concern in the patient with atherosclerotic coronary artery disease.

ARTIFICIAL CARDIAC PACING. If atropine fails to produce the desired response in heart rate, temporary artificial cardiac pacing should be instituted as soon as possible. Artificial pacing initially should be attempted using the transcutaneous method. Most monitor/defibrillator devices currently available have transcutaneous pacing capability. This technique is usually successful and is well tolerated by the patient at stimulus strengths of 50 milliamperes or less.

DOPAMINE (5 TO 20 μG/KG/MINUTE) OR EPINEPHRINE (2 TO 10 μG/KG/MIN-
UTE).   These drugs may be helpful if the previously mentioned interventions are ineffective (1).

CALCIUM CHLORIDE.   Calcium chloride may be of value in the setting
of calcium channel blocker toxicity. An intravenous (IV) dose of 5
to10 mL (500 mg to 1 g) of a 10% calcium chloride solution may
reverse peripheral dilation associated with calcium blocker toxicity,
but it may not increase heart rate (2).

GLUCAGON.   Glucagon may be the drug of choice in the setting of
beta blocker toxicity (3). An IV bolus dose of 2 to 4 mg is recommended (3).

Sinus Tachycardia

Description

Sinus tachycardia (Fig. 2.2) results from an increased rate of discharge of the sinus node and is usually a physiologic response to a
demand for an increase in cardiac output. The atrial rate is typically
100 to 160/minute, and the P-to-P interval is regular. P waves are
upright in leads II, III, and aVF (normal atrial depolarization and P
wave vector). Each P wave usually is followed by a normal QRS
complex (1:1 AV conduction). However, second-degree atrioventricular block may occur, or the QRS duration may be prolonged in
patients with an intraventricular conduction defect (fixed bundle
branch block, rate-related bundle branch block, AVC). Carotid sinus
massage (CSM) or a properly performed Valsalva maneuver may
transiently slow the SA node discharge rate and be of value in diagnosis in confusing cases [e.g., sinus discharge rate of 140 to 160/minute
with 1:1 AV conduction, which can be confused with atrial flutter
with a 2:1 AV block (AVB), atrioventricular nodal reentrant tachycardia (AVNRT), or automatic atrial tachycardia]. These maneuvers will
not terminate this rhythm and may have no effect.

Causes

Causes include pain; anxiety; hypovolemia; left ventricular dysfunction; fever; pulmonary embolism; thyrotoxicosis; drug toxicity
(e.g., cocaine, amphetamines, tricyclic antidepressants, anticholinergic drugs); drug withdrawal (e.g., narcotics, alcohol); anemia; hypoxemia; hypercarbia; and autonomic insufficiency.

Therapy

Sinus tachycardia is a physiologic response of the sympathetic
nervous system to meet a demand for an increase in cardiac output.
Therefore, therapy should be directed toward correction of the physiologic stimulus. A complete history and physical examination will

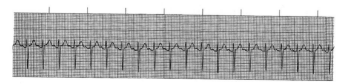

Fig. 2.2.   Sinus tachycardia.

yield the most valuable information and most often will define the cause.

Sinus Arrhythmia

Description

Sinus arrhythmia is an irregular supraventricular arrhythmia (Fig. 2.3) that occurs because of phasic alterations in vagal tone, resulting in a gradual increase and decrease in the rate of sinus node discharge. The reflex arc is initiated by normal respiration. Inspiration decreases vagal tone and produces an increase in the rate of SA discharge. Expiration results in increased vagal tone and a decrease in the rate of SA discharge. This is a normal phenomenon, especially in children and young adults. It may be accentuated in the elderly by the use of certain drugs (digoxin). Atrial depolarization is normal (upright P waves in leads II, III, and aVF) but irregular with a gradual increase and decrease in the P-to-P interval. The minimum difference between the longest and shortest P-to-P interval is usually less than 0.16 seconds. The PR interval remains constant, and each P wave is followed by a QRS complex. The resultant rhythm is irregularly irregular and must be differentiated from other causes of an irregularly irregular rhythm (see Atrial Fibrillation later in this chapter).

Causes

The cause of sinus arrhythmia is physiologic, but it may be drug induced (e.g., digoxin). Marked sinus arrhythmia may be a manifestation of the sick sinus syndrome.

Therapy

The arrhythmia is physiologic and requires no therapy. Confusion may arise when it is mistaken for another rhythm disturbance.

Premature Atrial Contractions

Description

A premature atrial contraction (PAC) is an electrical impulse that originates within the atrial myocardium but outside the SA node. It is premature (i.e., occurring before the next expected sinus discharge) and produces atrial depolarization and a P′ wave that differs in morphology from P waves of sinus node origin. A PAC usually depolarizes the SA node because the SA node is not "electrically isolated." The interval between the sinus P waves preceding and following a PAC is less than twice the normal P-P interval, resulting in a pause that is not fully compensatory. PACs originating from the same focus (unifocal PACs) have morphologically similar P′ waves

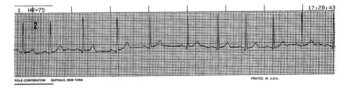

Fig. 2.3.   Sinus arrhythmia.

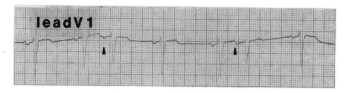

Fig. 2.4. Premature atrial contractions.

and a fixed coupling interval (the P-to-P′ interval). When PACs are multifocal, P′ waves differ in morphology and the coupling interval varies.

A PAC may be conducted normally through the AV node and ventricles. However, it may be conducted with partial AVB (PR interval more than 0.20 seconds) or be completely blocked (nonconducted PAC) at the level of the AV node if the coupling interval is short (P′ wave occurs close to T wave). Incomplete block and slow conduction at the bundle branch level may result in "aberrant" ventricular conduction (see later).

Two PACs are demonstrated in Fig. 2.4. The ectopic P′ waves are marked with arrowheads. The P′ waves occur earlier than the next expected sinus P wave. The P′R interval is longer than the PR interval of normal sinus beats (beats 1, 2, 4, and 5), indicating conduction delay. The P′ waves differ in morphology, and the ectopic coupling interval also varies. This suggests that these PACs are of multifocal origin.

Causes

Causes include increased circulating catecholamines; drug toxicity (e.g., theophylline, sympathomimetics); and pericarditis (rarely).

Therapy

Treatment of isolated PACs is rarely necessary. However, if frequent PACs precede symptomatic episodes of sustained paroxysmal supraventricular tachyarrhythmias (SVT), beta-blockers may be used, unless contraindicated, to decrease atrial automaticity.

Multifocal Atrial Tachycardia

Description

Multifocal atrial tachycardia (MFAT) is an ectopic, repetitive atrial arrhythmia that results from enhanced atrial automaticity; it frequently precedes the onset of atrial fibrillation (4). Triggered ectopic atrial electrical activity from three or more foci produces an irregular atrial rate as well as an irregular ventricular rate. The atrial rate is usually 100 to 180/minute with a varying P-to-P interval. The PR interval usually varies from beat to beat. The ventricular rate is also irregular (varying R-R interval). Ectopic P′ waves (best seen in leads II, III, and aVF) vary in morphology. MFAT can be diagnosed confidently if three consecutive P waves of different morphology at a rate of more than 100/minute are identified in a single lead. If the atrial rate is less than 100/minute, this rhythm is referred to most commonly as a "chaotic atrial rhythm" or "wandering atrial rhythm."

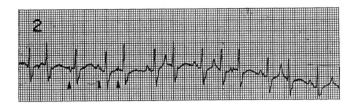

Fig. 2.5. Multifocal atrial tachycardia.

An episode of MFAT is shown in Fig. 2.5. Three consecutive ectopic P' waves are indicated by arrows. The P-to-P, PR, and R-R intervals vary in an irregularly irregular fashion.

Causes

MFAT is encountered most commonly in patients with chronic obstructive pulmonary disease (COPD) and acute respiratory failure or in patients with severe left ventricular dysfunction. Drug toxicity (sympathomimetics, theophylline) is a less common cause (4).

Therapy

Therapy initially should be directed at the underlying cause. Correction of hypoxemia and acidosis and careful use of inhaled bronchodilator therapy in the patient with COPD are essential.

Electrical cardioversion is rarely successful in producing a sustained sinus rhythm. IV verapamil, diltiazem, or beta blockers (metoprolol) are effective agents in controlling the ventricular response rate. Beta blockers should be used in patients with marginal ventricular function because of their depressant effects on myocardial contractility and in patients with respiratory failure because of bronchospasm. In patients with decreased left ventricular function, diltiazem (20-mg IV bolus) should be considered. Its effects on myocardial contractility are less pronounced than those of verapamil.

Atrial Fibrillation

Description

Atrial fibrillation is the most common of the SVTs. It is the result of multiple atrial foci discharging nearly simultaneously with multiple sites of reentry. The result is random wavelets of electrical depolarization that do not result in atrial contraction (5,6). Electrocardiographically, this chaotic electrical activity produces undulating deflections of varying sizes and shapes on the surface electrocardiogram (ECG; "f" waves best seen in V1, II, III, and aVF). There are no P waves. Although atrial electrical impulses are generated at frequencies of 400 to 700/minute, the number of impulses reaching the ventricles is limited by the refractory period of the AV node. In the absence of AV node disease or drugs that alter the refractory period or conduction velocity of the AV node, 140 to 180 impulses/minute can transverse the AV node at irregular intervals and in a random fashion. An irregularly irregular ventricular response rate (QRS complexes with varying R-R intervals) results. Atrial fibrillation with extremely low ventricular response rates (less than 70/minute), reflecting high-grade AVB, may be seen in digitalis, calcium channel

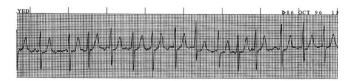

Fig. 2.6. Atrial fibrillation.

blocker, or beta blocker toxicity and in patients with sick sinus syndrome.

Figure 2.6 shows an example of atrial fibrillation in a patient who was not receiving drugs that affect AV conduction. P waves are not evident, and irregular undulations ("f" waves) can be seen between R waves. The R-R interval is irregular, and the ventricular response rate is 140/minute. Although atrial fibrillation is the most common cause of an irregularly irregular rhythm, it must be distinguished from other rhythm disturbances that may mimic it (Table 2.1).

Causes

The etiology of atrial fibrillation is thought to be associated with atrial myocardial tissue injury/damage and elevated atrial pressure. The risk of developing atrial fibrillation has been related to left atrial dimension, left ventricular wall thickness, and left ventricular fractional shortening determined by echocardiography (7). Similarly, successful conversion to and maintenance of sinus rhythm appears dependent on left atrial size and duration of atrial fibrillation (8).

Population-based data indicate that atrial fibrillation most often is associated with or caused by coronary heart disease, congestive heart failure, hypertensive cardiovascular disease, and rheumatic heart disease (9). In as many as 30% of patients, atrial fibrillation develops in the absence of clinically identifiable cardiovascular disease. In the absence of underlying clinical heart disease, atrial fibrillation has been termed "lone atrial fibrillation" and differs in its long-term complications and management (9).

Other causes include mitral and aortic valve disease of nonrheumatic origin, hypertrophic cardiomyopathy, hyperthyroidism, and idiopathic dilated cardiomyopathy. A paroxysmal form commonly is seen with alcohol abuse ("holiday heart syndrome").

Table 2.1.   Irregularly irregular rhythm: differential diagnosis

Atrial fibrillation
Atrial flutter with variable AV block
Multifocal atrial tachycardia or chaotic atrial rhythm
Sinus tachycardia with variable AV or SA block
Automatic atrial tachycardia with variable AV block
Marked sinus arrhythmia

AV, atrioventricular; SA, sinoatrial.

Therapy (Atrial Fibrillation with a Rapid Ventricular Response) (10)

PATIENT WITH HEMODYNAMIC INSTABILITY. In the hemodynamically unstable patient (e.g., systolic blood pressure of less than 90 mm Hg, cool clammy skin, altered mentation, ischemic chest pain, pulmonary edema), urgent synchronized electrical cardioversion is indicated (1,10). However, if atrial fibrillation is chronic, immediate cardioversion is unlikely to result in a sustained sinus rhythm. If the patient is conscious, sedation should be given before cardioversion. In the synchronized mode, sequential shocks of 100, 200, 300, and 360 W/second should be administered as necessary. Biphasic waveform atrial defibrillation at low energies is more effective than monophasic waveform defibrillation (11). If the patient is taking digoxin, atrial fibrillation with a rapid irregular ventricular response is not an arrhythmia associated with digitalis toxicity; it is a manifestation of subtherapeutic digoxin concentration. Cardioversion can be performed safely in patients with subtoxic serum digoxin concentrations (12).

Electrical cardioversion is usually unnecessary in the patient with clinical evidence of hypoperfusion and atrial fibrillation with a ventricular response rate of less than 120/minute. If the ventricular response rate is irregular and between 80 to 120/minute, other causes of hypoperfusion should be considered (e.g., MI and ventricular dysfunction, hypovolemia, pulmonary embolism). If the response rate is less than 80/minute and irregular or regular, digitalis toxicity should be considered if the patient is taking digoxin. Electrical cardioversion in the setting of digitalis toxicity is associated with a high complication rate.

If electrical cardioversion is unlikely to restore sinus rhythm (e.g., atrial fibrillation is chronic in duration), urgent ventricular rate control is indicated. This can be accomplished with IV diltiazem, beta blockers (metoprolol) in the absence of contraindications, or IV amiodarone (recommended in patients with decreased ejection fraction or overt congestive heart failure). Digoxin has no role in the urgent management of the ventricular response rate because of its delayed onset of action.

HEMODYNAMICALLY STABLE PATIENT.

Cardioversion. Electrical cardioversion alone is most likely to be successful (i.e., conversion to and maintenance of sinus rhythm) in patients with recent onset atrial fibrillation (less than 48 hours duration) not associated with other acute illnesses (e.g., hyperthyroidism, infection, pulmonary embolism, acute respiratory failure). In the stable patient, initial rate control with beta blockers or calcium channel blockers is recommended prior to atrial defibrillation attempts. Anticoagulation prior to electrical cardioversion is not required. Alternatively, chemical cardioversion can be attempted with an expected high degree of success using IV ibutilide or amiodarone or oral propafenone, flecainide, or dofetilide.

Left atrial thrombus formation can occur in patients with acute atrial fibrillation of more than 2 days' duration. Pharmacologic or electrical cardioversion of prolonged atrial fibrillation is associated with a small risk of systemic embolization. Randomized studies of antithrombotic therapy are lacking for patients undergoing cardioversion of atrial fibrillation, and the risk of thromboembolism is between 1% and 5% in case-control series (13). Transesophageal echocardiography (TEE) has been proposed as a method to detect the presence of left atrial thrombi to guide cardioversion (electrical or chemical) and anticoagulation therapy in atrial fibrillation of unknown duration. However, a TEE-guided strategy for elective cardioversion of atrial fibrillation (heparin before cardioversion followed by warfarin for 4 weeks after cardioversion) has been reported to result in comparable outcomes for thromboembolism and death when compared with conventional anticoagulation for 3 weeks before and 4 weeks after cardioversion. The frequency of stroke was 0.8% in the TEE group and 0.5% in the conventional group at 8 weeks of follow up (14). Using either strategy, ventricular rate control can be accomplished using digoxin, a calcium channel blocker, or a beta blocker followed by the addition of oral dofetilide, amiodarone, flecainide, or propafenone for cardioversion. If cardioversion is successful, amiodarone, dofetilide, flecainide, propafenone, and sotalol may be used to maintain sinus rhythm.

Rate Control.   In the stable patient with chronic atrial fibrillation and atrial enlargement, chemical or electrical cardioversion is unlikely to be successful. In such patients, control of the ventricular response rate should be the goal of therapy, and many treatment options are available. Digoxin is the drug of choice for chronic rate control in the setting of left ventricular dysfunction. It can be combined with beta blockers, calcium channel blockers, or amiodarone, if necessary, in selected patients. A beta blocker combined with digoxin may be efficacious for chronic therapy in patients without a contraindication to beta blocker therapy and who might benefit from other beta blocker effects (e.g., those with essential hypertension or patients who have had a MI). For patients unresponsive to pharmacologic therapy or who are unable to tolerate therapeutic doses of the previously mentioned agents, rate control is possible with AV nodal ablation therapy and implantation of a permanent transvenous pacemaker.

Anticoagulation.   Anticoagulation with warfarin is recommended for most patients with chronic atrial fibrillation, especially those with increased age (older than age 60 years), left ventricular dysfunction (ejection fraction less than 35%), hypertension, diabetes, and prior stroke or transient ischemic attacks (TIAs) (10). Chronic anticoagulation is not without risks, and its benefits and risks should be individualized for each patient. Warfarin therapy to maintain an International Normalized Ratio (INR) of 2 to 3 should be offered to all patients with chronic atrial fibrillation and the previously mentioned risk factors for thromboembolism who do not have contraindications to anticoagulation. Lone atrial fibrillation in patients younger than age 60 years is associated with a very low risk of stroke, and aspirin therapy (325 mg/day) is recommended. For patients who are not candidates for warfarin therapy, aspirin therapy (325 mg/day) may be effective in reducing the risk of stroke or systemic embolism. General considerations also include the following:

1. Long-term oral anticoagulation should be strongly considered for all patients older than age 65 with a target INR of between 2 and 3. Patients younger than age 65 with risk factors of previous TIA or stroke, hypertension, diabetes, heart failure, clinical coronary heart disease, mitral stenosis, prosthetic heart valves (INR 3 to 4), or hyperthyroidism also should be strongly considered for this therapy. Patients unwilling or unable to take warfarin should receive aspirin (325 mg/day).

2. Patients between 65 and 75 years of age without the previously mentioned risk factors should weigh the risks and benefits of warfarin versus aspirin therapy, given the low risk of stroke and the superior protection against stroke afforded by warfarin. Other factors, such as the inconvenience of frequent follow-up for INR monitoring, should enter into decision making.

3. Patients older than age 75 years, especially women, should be considered for chronic anticoagulation with warfarin (approximate INR of 2). Age-related increased risk of bleeding should be considered.

4. Patients who have been in atrial fibrillation for more than 2 days should receive oral anticoagulation to maintain an INR of 2 to 3 for 3 weeks prior to elective cardioversion and for 4 weeks after sinus rhythm has been restored.

Atrial Flutter

Atrial flutter is a disorder of atrial impulse formation, is less commonly encountered than atrial fibrillation, and most frequently is an unstable rhythm (i.e., spontaneous conversion to sinus rhythm or atrial fibrillation often occurs). Atrial flutter may be the result of localized atrial reentry or may be of focal, ectopic origin as a result of enhanced automaticity (15).

Atrial depolarization occurs at a regular rate, most commonly 280 to 320/minute, and usually is initiated by a reentry or an ectopic focus in the lower part of the right atrium. The resulting ECG deflection, representing atrial depolarization, most often is directed superiorly and leftward, in contrast to the normal inferior and leftward orientation. During atrial flutter, atrial depolarization produces flutter or "f" waves, which are recognized most easily as regular negative deflections in leads II, III, and aVF. The absence of an isoelectric period between R waves may result in the typical "sawtooth" pattern in leads 2 and 3 and aVF.

The ventricular rate (frequency and regularity of QRS complexes) during atrial flutter is primarily dependent on the refractory period of the AV node. Atrial flutter almost always is associated with a physiologic AVB. A physiologic 2:1 AVB occurs most often and results in QRS complexes that occur at a regular rate of 140 to 160/minute. At this AV response rate, atrial flutter often is misdiagnosed as sinus tachycardia because the typical sawtooth pattern in the inferior leads (II, III, aVF) is present infrequently. The sawtooth pattern is recognized more often in the inferior leads at higher degrees of AVB (Fig. 2.7B). The AV conduction ratio during atrial flutter may be altered by AV node disease, autonomic nervous system variability, or drugs that affect AV node conduction velocity or refractory period

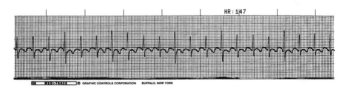

Fig. 2.7.   Atrial flutter.

(digoxin, beta blockers, etc.). AVB may be "fixed" (regular R-R interval) or variable (varying R-R interval, which is divisible by the inherent atrial rate, such as 3:1 or 4:1). Atrial flutter may be conducted infrequently in 1:1, resulting in a rapid ventricular response.

The diagnosis of atrial flutter diagnostic ECG findings can be facilitated by physiologic maneuvers that increase the degree of AVB (e.g., properly performed CSM) or the IV administration of adenosine, which has an extremely short half-life and effectively serves as a "pharmacologic vagal maneuver." These interventions will increase the degree of AVB and facilitate recognition of "f" waves, but will not terminate atrial flutter.

Figure 2.7 shows an example of atrial flutter recorded in standard lead II. The R-R intervals are regular at a rate of 150/minute (2:1 AVB).

Causes

Etiologies are similar to those of atrial fibrillation.

Therapy

The management of atrial flutter is similar to that of atrial fibrillation and is dictated by the overall hemodynamic response to the rhythm disturbance. In the hemodynamically compromised patient (systolic blood pressure of less than 90 mm Hg, cool clammy skin, altered mentation, and/or chest pain) with atrial flutter and a rapid ventricular response rate, urgent synchronized electrical cardioversion is indicated. A conscious patient should be sedated (see Atrial Fibrillation Management). In the synchronized mode, the first shock should be delivered at an energy dose of 50 J. Conversion of atrial flutter usually can be accomplished at low energy levels. Countershock most often is followed by one of three outcomes.

1. **Sinus rhythm.** The patient should be monitored closely. If frequent PACs are noted, therapy with an oral beta blocker can be initiated to decrease atrial automaticity, as well as prolong AV conduction time if atrial flutter recurs or atrial fibrillation develops. The addition of a rate control agent such as digoxin or a calcium channel blocker can be helpful as well. Long-term therapy with beta blockers, calcium channel blockers, or low-dose amiodarone can be used to prevent recurrences, but rarely is needed.

2. **Atrial fibrillation.** Atrial flutter is an unstable cardiac rhythm and often spontaneously "converts" to atrial fibrillation; countershock of atrial flutter may be followed by atrial fibrillation. Electrical cardioversion of atrial fibrillation should be attempted as outlined earlier.

3. **Persistent atrial flutter.** Countershock energy dose should be increased at increments of 50 J over the first energy dose until atrial flutter is terminated.

In the hemodynamically stable patient, several options are available.

1. Electrical cardioversion (see earlier). Electrical cardioversion is the treatment of choice for atrial flutter. Because atrial flutter is most often an unstable or transitional rhythm that does produce organized atrial contraction, the risk of systemic embolism with cardioversion is low but not zero. Anticoagulation should be considered

in selected patients, especially if atrial enlargement is present, because flutter can recur and alternate with atrial fibrillation.

2. Control of ventricular response rate. See section on rate control of atrial fibrillation.

REENTRANT SUPRAVENTRICULAR TACHYARRHYTHMIAS

Overview

The concept of functional or anatomic dissociation of conduction tissue into two pathways with different conduction velocities and refractory periods is postulated to explain reentry. With dissociation into two pathways, a premature impulse encounters refractoriness (unidirectional block) in one pathway and is conducted slowly in the other. During this period of delayed conduction, the blocked pathway recovers responsiveness. If the two pathways are connected, the impulse can reenter the previously blocked pathway and can be conducted to the chamber of origin in a retrograde fashion. During retrograde conduction, the pathway previously used for antegrade conduction regains responsiveness. Once initiated, impulse conduction over the pathways becomes self-perpetuating. Longitudinal dissociation of conducting tissue into two pathways, one with unidirectional block and the other with prolonged conduction time, is necessary for reentry to occur. In humans, reentry has been demonstrated in the SA and AV nodes, atrium, and the His-Purkinje system (16).

Atrioventricular Nodal Reentrant Tachycardia

The pathways used for reentry lie within the AV node. An episode of SVT is initiated by a closely coupled PAC. The P′ wave produced by the premature atrial depolarization is morphologically different from the sinus P wave, and the P′R interval of the PAC is usually longer than the PR interval of sinus beats. This is because atrial depolarization has occurred prematurely, and the AV node has not completely repolarized following the preceding sinus beat. If "longitudinal dissociation" has occurred, a regular tachyarrhythmia will result. The ventricular rate is regular and usually between 160 to 260/minute. Each impulse is conducted back to the atria, but the sequence of atrial depolarization is abnormal, proceeding superiorly and leftward. Abnormal atrial depolarization may be recognized by "inverted" P waves in the inferior ECG lead. In approximately 30% of patients with SVT and AV nodal reentry, an inverted retrograde P wave will be seen to closely follow each QRS complex. If P waves are seen, they are regular and occur at a rate equal to the ventricular rate (there is no AVB), and the RP interval is usually less than one-half the RR interval. However, in most cases (more than 60%), atrial depolarization occurs during inscription of the QRS complex, and a retrograde P wave is not seen (17).

Figure 2.8 (lead 2) demonstrates an episode of SVT as a result of

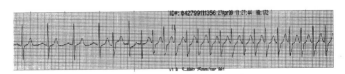

Fig. 2.8.   Atrioventricular node reentrant tachycardia.

AV node reentry. The underlying sinus rhythm (first four complexes from left to right) is interrupted by a PAC (fifth QRS complex), which induces a rapid, regular tachyarrhythmia (ventricular rate 160/minute) as a result of AV nodal reentry. As is typical, retrograde P waves are not seen during the tachyarrhythmia.

Reentry Using a Concealed Bypass Tract

The concealed bypass tract (CBT) is similar to that of SVT with AV node reentry; however, an extra nodal conduction pathway is used for retrograde conduction to the atria. This extra nodal pathway can conduct impulses only in a retrograde direction. Patients with Wolff-Parkinson-White (WPW) syndrome also have an extra nodal conduction pathway (bypass tract), but it can conduct impulses in both a retrograde or antegrade direction. Antegrade conduction via the extra nodal pathway during normal sinus rhythm in WPW produces the characteristic "delta wave." Patients with an extra nodal conduction pathway capable of only retrograde conduction are said to have a CBT because a delta wave is not inscribed during sinus rhythm.

An episode of SVT is initiated in the same manner as described previously for SVT with AV node reentry. The ventricular rate is regular but slightly faster than in SVT with AV node reentry. The sequence of atrial depolarization is again abnormal or inverted P waves (leads II, III, and aVF) following each QRS complex, which will be seen in almost all patients. The RP interval is usually less than one-half of the RR interval. During the SVT, a negative P wave usually is seen in lead I in patients with a CBT but not in patients with SVT and AV node reentry.

Sinoatrial Node Reentry

A PAC usually depolarizes the SA node, resulting in a characteristic noncompensatory pause. However, an early PAC can encounter block in one portion of the sinus node, enter sinus nodal tissue in another portion, and traverse the nodal tissue slowly enough so that the emerging impulses are able to excite the atria. Thus, the SA node, in a manner similar to the AV node, can provide pathways for reentry. SVT is initiated by a PAC, but subsequent P waves are normal (upright in leads II, III, and aVF) and morphologically similar to sinus beats because the SA node serves as the site of origin. The atrial rate is regular (160 to 260/minute). AVB (fixed or variable) may occur because the AV node is not a part of the reentrant loop. A 1:1 AV conduction ratio also can occur. The RP interval is usually greater than one-half the RR interval. Carotid sinus massage or a Valsalva maneuver may terminate the rhythm disturbance. SVT with SA node reentry is uncommon and frequently is misdiagnosed because it may mimic sinus tachycardia with AVB and SVT as a result of an automatic atrial ectopic focus.

AUTOMATIC ATRIAL TACHYCARDIA

An episode of SVT also may result from the rapid firing of an automatic ectopic focus within the atria. This rhythm disturbance traditionally has been called "nonparoxysmal atrial tachycardia." Although it is initiated by a PAC, the coupling interval typically is not short. The ectopic P' wave electrical vector is usually normal (directed inferiorly and leftward); hence, upright P waves will be noted

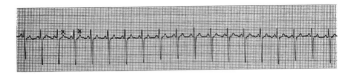

Fig. 2.9.   Automatic atrial tachycardia.

in leads II, III, and aVF. P wave morphology will be slightly different from that of sinus beats. The RP interval is usually greater than one-half the RR interval. AVB may occur; it does not occur in SVT with AV node reentry or SVT with a CBT. The ventricular rate may be regular or irregular, depending on whether the degree of AVB is variable or fixed. 1:1 AV conduction can occur. Because this rhythm does not involve a reentry "loop," vagal maneuvers that alter AV conduction (CSM, Valsalva maneuver) will not terminate the arrhythmias but may increase the degree of AVB.

An automatic atrial tachycardia is shown in Fig. 2.9 (lead III). P′ waves are shown with an "x." These P′ waves deform the T wave of the preceding QRS complex, are upright in lead III (normal atrial depolarization vector), and are regular at a rate of 280/minute. The ventricular rate is also regular at 140/minute (2:1 AVB).

VALUE OF THE ELECTROCARDIOGRAM IN DEFINING SUPRAVENTRICULAR TACHYCARDIA MECHANISM

Careful inspection of the 12-1ead ECG during an episode of SVT may be of value in suggesting the underlying electrophysiologic mechanism (Table 2.2) (17).

THERAPY

Short runs of these tachyarrhythmias are usually well tolerated and require no specific therapy other than possible PAC suppression to prevent further recurrence. Prolonged episodes may require medical therapy and/or electrical cardioversion. Because these tachyarrhythmias typically result from "reentry" within the AV node, one must interrupt the critical relation of conduction and refractoriness in the pathways of the AV node.

If the patient is hemodynamically stable, proceed with medical management as outlined in the following section. If the patient is clinically unstable, proceed with sedation and synchronized cardioversion using 100 W/second.

Treatment of Supraventricular Tachycardia of Reentrant Origin

1. **Carotid sinus massage.** Massage either the right or left carotid independently for 10 to 15 seconds while observing a monitor. The arrhythmia either will convert to normal sinus rhythm or will remain unchanged.

2. **Valsalva maneuver.** This frequently is helpful, especially when combined with CSM. Continue CSM after the Valsalva maneuver is released.

3. **Adenosine.** Adenosine is an endogenous nucleoside that inhibits AV nodal conduction (18,19). It has a very brief half-life of 10 to 30 seconds and few side effects, which are transient (most commonly

Table 2.2. Summary of electrocardiogram findings in supraventricular tachycardia

	AVNRT	SVT-CBT	Sinoatrial node reentry or automatic atrial focus
Frequency as cause of SVT	70%	20%	10%
P waves in II, III, aVF	30%	Always	Always
P wave morphology in II, III, aVF	Inverted	Inverted	Upright
P wave in I	Upright	Inverted	Upright
R-P interval	$<^1/_2$ R-R interval	$<^1/_2$ R-R interval	$>^1/_2$ R-R interval
AV block	Never	Never	Common
Rate-related bundle branch block	Uncommon	Common	Uncommon
Effect of carotid sinus massage	No change or terminates rhythm	No change or terminates rhythm	May increase AV block, but does not terminate rhythm

AV, atrioventricular; AVNRT, atrioventricular node reentrant tachycardia; SVT-CBT, supraventricular tachycardia-concealed bypass tract; SVT, supraventricular tachycardia.

flushing). It is the drug of choice for terminating a SVT that involves the AV node as a part of the reentrant loop. The dose is 6 mg via rapid IV bolus. Two subsequent 12-mg doses can be given minutes later if the first dose is ineffective. The successful conversion rate is more than 90%. The drug must be given as a bolus (followed by a flush injection of normal saline into the IV tubing) because of its rapid plasma breakdown. Adenosine also can be useful in the diagnosis and treatment of wide complex tachycardias. Adenosine can terminate SVT with aberrant conduction, yet not cause adverse effects in patients with ventricular tachycardia (VT) because of its short half-life.

4. **Calcium channel blockers:** Diltiazem is preferred. The recommended dose is 0.25 mg/kg or 20 mg IV for the typical adult patient. Conversion usually occurs within 3 to 7 minutes.

5. **Beta blockers.** Propranolol, metoprolol, and esmolol are available for IV use. As with other drugs, these should be titrated carefully to effect with close monitoring and blood pressure determinations. Contraindications include left ventricular dysfunction, asthma, high-degree AVB, and sick sinus syndrome.

6. **Digoxin.** IV doses are generally of little value in acute therapy as a result of slow onset of action.

7. **Atrial pacemaker.** This method frequently will capture the

atria and lead to normal sinus rhythm. Set the atrial pacer to a rate faster than the SVT and then abruptly terminate pacing, looking for resumption of normal sinus rhythm. This method is especially helpful in open-heart surgery patients who may have atrial epicardial wires in place postoperatively.

8. **AV node ablation.** Catheter-based techniques in the electrophysiology laboratory allow for the precise analysis and localization of the mechanism of tachycardia. AV nodal reentry mechanisms can be treated by ablating one of the pathways and thereby interrupting the reentry circuit. Some supraventricular rhythms that are difficult to define on the 12-lead ECG can be definitively diagnosed and treated, such as atrial flutter and CBTs.

ATRIOVENTRICULAR CONDUCTION DEFECTS

A disturbance in impulse conduction from atria to ventricles may occur at the level of the SA node, internodal pathways, AV node, His bundle, bundle branches, or Purkinje network. Although the terms *AVB* and *AV dissociation* often are used interchangeably, they are separate entities with markedly differing mechanisms.

AVB may be the result of an organic lesion along the conduction pathway, an increase in inherent refractoriness of the conduction pathway, or marked shortening of the supraventricular cycle with encroachment on the normal refractory period. The first two causes are pathologic; the last is physiologic (as exemplified by atrial flutter). AVB may be classified as partial or complete, permanent or temporary, or according to the site of the block (AV nodal or infranodal) (20).

First-Degree Atrioventricular Block

Description

Each supraventricular impulse is conducted to the ventricles but more slowly than normal. Electrocardiographically, first-degree AVB (1° AVB) is reflected by a prolonged PR interval (more than 0.20 seconds) that is constant from beat to beat. In Fig. 2.10, the PR interval is 0.32 seconds. The AV node is usually the site of block, but delay may occur at the level of the intranodal pathways, His bundle, or bundle branches. (One bundle branch may be completely blocked with delay occurring in the opposite bundle branch.) The intensity of the first heart sound tends to decrease as the PR interval becomes longer.

Causes

Causes include increased parasympathetic tone, drugs that prolong AV conduction (e.g., digoxin, propranolol, verapamil), and conduction system disease (e.g., fibrosis, inflammation associated with myocarditis).

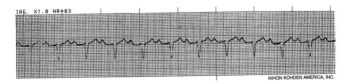

Fig. 2.10.   1° atrioventricular block.

Therapy

First-degree AVB alone does not produce symptoms and requires no therapy. Digoxin may cause 1° AVB, but this ECG finding is usually not considered a sign of digoxin toxicity unless the PR interval exceeds 0.24 seconds.

Second-Degree Atrioventricular Block

Some supraventricular impulses are conducted to the ventricles, whereas others are blocked. There are two types of second-degree AVB 2° AVB, and this distinction is prognostically and therapeutically important.

Second-Degree Atrioventricular Block, Mobitz Type I (Wenckebach)

DESCRIPTION. Type I 2° AVB is characterized by progressive prolongation of the PR interval, indicating a progressive decrease in conduction velocity ("decremental conduction") before a P wave is blocked completely. This form of block almost always occurs at the level of the AV node, but the phenomenon of decremental conduction and "Wenckebach periodicity" has been reported in other conducting tissue. Usually, only a single impulse is blocked, and the cycle is repeated. Longer pauses may be interrupted by escape beats (junctional, ventricular). Repetition of such cycles results in "group beating" (e.g., three sinus beats are conducted with progressively increasing PR intervals, and the fourth sinus beat is completely blocked, and a QRS complex is not inscribed). Such a "group" would be referred to as 4:3 conduction. The conduction ratio is usually constant, but it may vary (e.g., 4:3 to 3:2).

In addition to gradual prolongation of the PR interval, typical Wenckebach periodicity is characterized by a decreasing RR interval prior to the blocked sinus impulse. This is because the increment of PR prolongation becomes progressively less with each conducted beat (i.e., while the absolute length of the PR interval increases with each beat, the amount of increase is less with each beat after the second beat of the cycle). The PP interval is usually constant.

In Fig. 2.11, 4:3 (four P waves, three QRS complexes) Wenckebach periodicity is demonstrated. The atrial rate is regular (constant PP interval). The PR interval increases from beat to beat. The fourth sinus impulse of the cycle is not conducted to the ventricles, and a junctional escape beat follows the nonconducted P wave. During the Wenckebach cycle, the R-R interval can be seen to decrease before the dropped beat because the increment in the PR interval is decreasing. The increment from 0.28 seconds to 0.40 seconds is 0.12 seconds, whereas the next increment is only 0.06 seconds; the R-R, thus, decreases by 0.06 seconds.

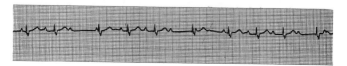

Fig. 2.11. Typical Wenckebach (Mobitz type I atrioventricular block).

Atypical Wenckebach

DESCRIPTION.   Rhythms that manifest all the features outlined previously represent the typical Wenckebach phenomenon. If many, but not all, of these features are found, then atypical Wenckebach is said to be present and is the result of inconsistent change in the degree of conduction delay from beat to beat. In typical Wenckebach conduction, each impulse is delayed progressively but with a progressive decrease in the increment of that delay. In atypical Wenckebach, the increment may fail to decrease (PR interval does not change between two consecutive beats), the increment may increase, or a PR interval may be less than the one preceding it. In atypical Wenckebach, conduction delay will tend to increase through the cycle as a whole, but will not demonstrate progression from beat to beat. The frequency of atypical Wenckebach conduction increases as the conduction ratio increases. At a conduction ratio greater than 6:5, Wenckebach conduction is almost always atypical.

Figure 2.12 demonstrates a Mobitz type I AVB with a 9:8 conduction ratio. PR and RR intervals are included in the ladder diagram. The first four QRS complexes from the right represent the start of the sequence. QRS complexes one through five from the left represent the end of the cycle. The PR interval does not progressively increase from beat to beat, but over the sequence increases from 0.18 seconds to 0.38 seconds.

CAUSES.   Causes for 2° AVB, Mobitz type I, are the same as for 1°AVB. In addition, this arrhythmia frequently occurs during acute inferior MI as a result of AV nodal ischemia, resulting in increased vagal tone at this level of conduction. (In approximately 90% of hearts, the right coronary artery supplies the inferior wall, as well as the AV node.) This rhythm is a sign of digoxin toxicity in patients taking the medication.

THERAPY.   In the hemodynamically stable patient, acute therapy is not indicated. Intensive care unit observation with ECG monitoring is suggested for patients with acute infarction, suspected drug toxicity, or suspected acute myocarditis. In the setting of acute inferior infarction, this arrhythmia is usually transient and well tolerated.

In the hemodynamically unstable patient, acute intervention is required. Signs and symptoms of hypoperfusion as a result of this rhythm disturbance are usually not encountered until the ventricular rate falls below 60/minute. In such cases, management is the same as that for symptomatic sinus bradycardia (see earlier).

If hypoperfusion persists after an effective ventricular rate increase (more than 70/minute) with atropine or pacing in the setting of acute inferior MI, associated right ventricular infarction should be suspected and diagnosed and appropriate interventions should be started (see Chapter 9).

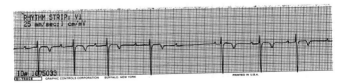

Fig. 2.12.   Atypical Wenckebach.

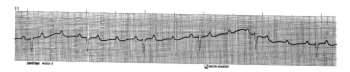

Fig. 2.13.   2° atrioventricular block, Mobitz type II.

Second-Degree Atrioventricular Block, Mobitz Type II

DESCRIPTION.   Block usually occurs below the level of the AV node (infranodal and within the His Purkinje system). The PR interval is usually normal, but may be slightly prolonged. PR intervals do not change measurably from beat to beat, although the PR interval following a blocked impulse may be somewhat shorter. The QRS complexes may be wide (QRS duration, more than 0.10 seconds) because fascicular or bundle branch block (or both) is often present because the infranodal block commonly occurs within the bundle branches. On occasion, QRS complexes of normal duration may be encountered (Fig. 2.13). The conduction ratio may be fixed or variable.

Figure 2.13 demonstrates Mobitz type II second-degree block (lead II). The sinus rate is 90/minute, and the ventricular rate is 30/minute (3:1 AVB).

When AVB occurs with a conduction ratio of 2:1, the distinction between type I or type II 2 AVB may be difficult because there is no progressive prolongation of the PR interval in 2:1 type I block. Type I should be suspected if the QRS duration of conducted beats is normal, and the presence of more typical Wenckebach periodicity is noted at other times; 2:1 AVB and wide QRS complexes most often result from infranodal type II 2 AVB if the PR interval is normal.

CAUSES.   This arrhythmia most commonly is encountered in chronic degenerative diseases (e.g., Lev's disease). It may be seen in acute myocarditis, following cardiac surgery, and in acute anterior MI as a result of distal conduction system ischemia/necrosis.

THERAPY.   This arrhythmia is usually not a transient phenomenon; it tends to be persistent or recurrent and may progress to complete heart block. It has a more serious prognosis because it is associated with extensive structural damage to the ventricular conduction system. Artificial demand ventricular pacing will be required in most instances. Atropine administration in the acute management is unlikely to be successful, but can be attempted as described in Mobitz type I AVB.

Third-Degree Atrioventricular Block, Complete Heart Block

Description

Third-degree AVB (3° AVB) indicates complete absence of AV conduction. There are two types that represent a progression in severity from types I and II 2° AVB.

Third-Degree Atrioventricular Block at Atrioventricular Nodal Level

When conduction of supraventricular impulses is blocked completely at the AV node, a "junctional" or AV nodal escape pacemaker initiates ventricular depolarization. This is a stable pacemaker with an inherent firing rate of 40 to 60 minutes. Because the escape pacemaker is located above the His bundle, the sequence of ventricular depolarization is normal, resulting in a normal QRS (QRS duration of less than 0.10 seconds). This type of 3° AVB is not uncommon following acute inferior MI as a result of an increase in vagal tone at the level of the AV node. It is usually transient, but it may last up to a week.

Infranodal 3 Degree Atrioventricular Block

The ventricles are depolarized by an intrinsic pacemaker located in the bundle branch-Purkinje system. Because the pacemaker lies below the site of the block and the bifurcation of the His bundle, ventricular depolarization does not occur via the normal conducting system and QRS complexes will have a wide configuration (Fig. 2.14). A ventricular escape pacemaker has an inherent firing rate of 30 to 40/minute and is relatively unstable [i.e., episodes of ventricular asystole may occur (Fig. 2.4)].

Infranodal 3° AVB is indicative of extensive conduction system disease and is often a complication of acute anterior MI. In both types of 3° AVB, atrial and ventricular depolarization are independent, the PR intervals vary in a random fashion, and the atrial rate is faster than the ventricular rate. The ventricular rate is regular. The atrial rate is usually regular, but may show sinus arrhythmia (ventriculophasic sinus arrhythmia: P-P intervals that bracket a QRS are shorter than those that do not). Critical differentiating features are QRS morphology and escape pacemaker rate.

Therapy

1. *Third-degree AVB at AV node level.* Same as for 2° AVB, Mobitz type I.
2. *Infranodal 3° AVB.* An artificial demand pacemaker almost always will be required. Acutely, IV atropine can be given, but it is unlikely to be of value in the hemodynamically compromised patient.

Atrioventricular Dissociation

Description

Atrioventricular dissociation is never a primary diagnosis; it is always secondary to some other rhythm disturbance. In AVD, the atria and ventricles are depolarized by separate pacemakers. The atria are activated by the sinus node. The ventricles are depolarized by a lower-level pacemaker at the level of the AV node or within the ventricular conduction system. The ventricular rate is either equal to the atrial rate (isorhythmic AVD) or greater than the atrial rate.

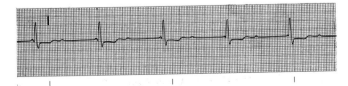

Fig. 2.14.   Infranodal 3° atrioventricular block.

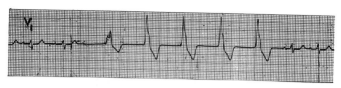

Fig. 2.15. Passive atrioventricular dissociation.

In AVB, the atrial rate is faster than the ventricular rate. The lower pacemaker depolarizes the ventricles because it encounters a nonrefractory myocardium. AVD may be passive or active.

Passive Atrioventricular Dissociation

When the sinus node fails to depolarize within approximately 1 second, a junctional or ventricular escape beat or rhythm may emerge. If a sinus impulse should reach the AV junction between escape beats when the AV node is not refractory, the sinus beat will be conducted to the ventricles. Therefore, AVB is not present.

Figure 2.15 demonstrates the passive type of AV dissociation. The first two sinus beats are conducted normally to the ventricles. A long pause follows the second QRS as a result of sinus arrest. The pause is interrupted by a fusion beat and then an accelerated idioventricular rhythm (AIVR). Sinus rhythm resumes at the end of the strip.

Active Atrioventricular Dissociation

The discharge rate of the lower pacemaker exceeds or usurps that of the sinus node in the absence of bradycardia. Hence, it is the result of an accelerated junctional or idioventricular rhythm or VT.

Therapy

In the asymptomatic patient, therapy is often unnecessary. Therapy should be directed at the underlying cause of the primary rhythm. Atropine may be effective in increasing the sinus rate in passive AVD. Suppressing an AIVR in the presence of a slow sinus rhythm may be deleterious.

VENTRICULAR ARRHYTHMIAS

Ventricular Extrasystole (Premature Ventricular Contraction)

Description

A premature ventricular contraction is a premature impulse of ventricular origin occurring before the next expected sinus beat. It may arise from a ventricular focus with enhanced automaticity or may represent a form of reentry within the His-Purkinje system. Both mechanisms may be operative under different circumstances. PVCs may be unifocal (identical or nearly identical QRS morphology with a fixed coupling interval) (Fig. 2.16) or multifocal (varying QRS morphology and coupling intervals).

Because a PVC originates in the ventricle, ventricular depolarization and repolarization are abnormal, resulting in a wide QRS complex (more than 0.12 seconds) and an ST segment and T wave directed opposite the QRS complex. The SA node is anatomically and "electrically" separated from the ventricles, and a PVC usually does

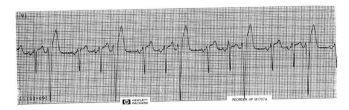

Fig. 2.16.   Unifocal premature ventricular contractions.

not depolarize the SA node as a result of refractoriness to retrograde conduction in the AV node. Therefore, the rhythm of the SA node is not disturbed, and there is usually a fully compensatory pause. On occasion, the SA node may be depolarized, and a noncompensatory pause will result. In the presence of a slow sinus rhythm, a PVC may occur between two sinus beats, resulting in an "interpolated" PVC. (The PP interval remains unchanged because there is no pause.) The sinus impulse following an interpolated PVC usually has a prolonged PR interval because the AV node is still refractory from incomplete penetration (concealed conduction) by the PVC.

The second, fifth, eighth, eleventh, and fourteenth QRS complexes in Fig. 2.16 are PVCs of unifocal origin (same morphology and coupling interval) followed by a fully compensatory pause (RR interval of sinus beats bracketing a PVC is twice that of the basic sinus rate). This is an example of ventricular trigeminy.

Causes

Causes include acute and chronic myocardial ischemia; cardiomyopathy; electrolyte disturbances (hypokalemia, hypomagnesia); and drug toxicity (sympathomimetics, digoxin).

Therapy

No therapy is indicated in the asymptomatic patient.

Ventricular Escape Beats (Idioventricular Rhythm)

Description

A ventricular escape beat is an impulse originating from a pacemaker within the His-Purkinje network. It occurs after the next expected supraventricular impulse has failed to occur or be conducted to the ventricles. Such a pacemaker has an intrinsic rate of 30 to 40/minute, and the interval preceding the escape beat is usually greater than 1.5 seconds. If more than one escape beat occurs in succession, a ventricular escape (or idioventricular) rhythm and atrioventricular dissociation are present. If the rate is greater than 40/minute but less than 100/minute, an AIVR is said to be present (Fig. 2.17). Escape

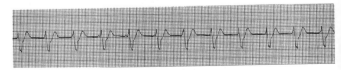

Fig. 2.17.   Accelerated idioventricular rhythm.

beats and rhythms have wide QRS complexes, abnormal ST segments, and secondary T waves changes as seen in PVCs.

Figure 2.17 (lead 2) demonstrates AIVR at a ventricular escape rate of 80/minute. The ventricular escape rate is just slightly more rapid than the sinus rate. Dissociated P waves can be seen preceding the fourth, fifth, and sixth QRS complexes.

Therapy

Ventricular escape beats and AIVRs are not uncommon following acute MI. Suppressant drugs such as lidocaine should not be used in the event that they may represent the only reliable pacemaker. IV atropine sulfate given in 0.5-mg increments every 3 to 5 minutes (total dose 0.03 to 0.04 mg/kg) may accelerate the SA node or allow the atria to "capture" the ventricles. Artificial pacing may be required if the dominant rhythm is too slow for adequate perfusion.

Ventricular Parasystole

Description

Ventricular parasystole refers to the presence of concurrent impulse formation by two pacemakers, one in the SA node and the other in the ventricle (21). Independent pacemakers also may be noted during AVD, but differences exist between AVD and parasystole. The ventricular parasystolic pacemaker has three important properties not shared by a lower pacemaker in AVD.

1. **Entrance block.** An electrical impulse cannot enter the parasystolic focus and depolarize it; hence, the parasystolic pacemaker fires at a fixed rate and is not reset by ventricular depolarization.

2. **Intermittent exit block.** Although impulses are generated repetitively by the parasystolic pacemaker, impulse conduction to the surrounding myocardium does not always occur.

3. **Constant rate of discharge.** The constant rate of discharge is evidenced by the fact that the interval between parasystolic beats (interectopic interval) remains constant or is a multiple of a basic interval. Each impulse may not produce a QRS complex because of existing block or refractoriness of the myocardium from a preceding depolarization.

Parasystolic beats are ventricular ectopic beats with constant QRS morphology, but the coupling interval is usually variable. "Fusion beats" may be seen if the sinus beat reaches the ventricle at approximately the same time that the parasystolic focus discharges.

In the example of ventricular parasystole (Fig. 2.18), the interectopic interval is nearly constant (varies by less than 2%). The first

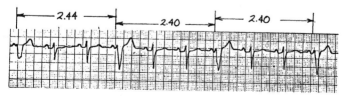

Fig. 2.18. Ventricular parasystole.

ectopic beat immediately follows the P wave, and there is no fusion. The subsequent three ectopic beats demonstrate fusion, and with progressively more influence from the conducted beat the QRS complex narrows and the T wave amplitude declines because the ectopic beat is occurring progressively later after the P wave.

Therapy

Ventricular parasystole frequently occurs in the presence of severe underlying heart disease. Parasystole can lead to VT or fibrillation, particularly in the setting of myocardial ischemia or infarction. In the absence of ischemia, the rhythm can be stable for many years.

Ventricular Tachycardia

Description

Ventricular tachycardia is a ventricular arrhythmia that may result from either an abnormality of impulse generation (automatic arrhythmia focus or triggered activity) or impulse propagation (reentry within the His-Purkinje system) (22). PVCs usually presage its occurrence (see Chapter 15). An episode of VT is constituted by at least three successive ventricular ectopic beats at a rate in excess of 100/minute (usual rate, 140 to 220/minute). Because the sequence of ventricular depolarization and repolarization is abnormal, QRS complexes during VT are wide and distinct ST segments and T waves may not be evident. The basic sinus rhythm may remain intact, leading to antegrade atrial depolarization with AV dissociation. On occasion, the sinus node may "capture" the ventricle (capture beat) or cause fusion beats if the AV node and ventricular myocardium are not refractory. VT is usually a regular rhythm, except when a capture beat occurs, or multifocal in origin (polymorphic VT). Conduction from the ventricle to the atria may occur, resulting in retrograde atrial depolarization. Capture and fusion beats will not occur during ventriculoatrial conduction.

Figure 2.19 is a 12-lead ECG demonstrating a brief episode of VT. During the recording of the limb leads, atrial fibrillation with a ventricular response rate of 85/minutes is seen. The third QRS complex seen in the augmented limb leads is a PVC that initiates a sequence

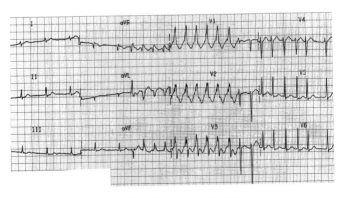

Fig. 2.19.   Ventricular tachycardia.

of nine wide QRS complexes at a regular rate 180/minute. The QRS morphology varies from lead to lead. This episode of VT is terminated by a fusion beat and a resumption of atrial fibrillation, with a ventricular response rate of 140/minute.

Causes

Causes are similar to those of PVCs.

Therapy

If the patient is hemodynamically stable, lidocaine or amiodarone may be administered. If the patient has clinical signs of hypoperfusion or is in cardiopulmonary arrest, countershock (200 J) should be administered immediately and cardiopulmonary resuscitation should be initiated (1).

Ventricular Ectopy Versus Aberrant Ventricular Conduction

Premature, morphologically bizarre QRS complexes may result from discharge of a ventricular ectopic focus (PVC) or from abnormal or "aberrant" ventricular conduction of a supraventricular impulse. AVC occurs when a premature impulse encounters partially refractory ventricular conduction tissue, usually the right bundle branch. The right bundle branch has a longer refractory period than the left bundle branch. The more premature the supraventricular impulse, the more likely that AVC will occur. Because of the disparity in refractory periods of the bundle branches, AVC usually takes the form of a right bundle branch block pattern. Left bundle branch aberration also may occur, but it is infrequent (23).

The length of the refractory period of the bundle branches is determined by the preceding RR interval; the refractory period is longer with slow heart rates (long RR interval) and shorter with fast rates (short RR interval). A long RR interval preceding a PAC will facilitate AVC.

Close inspection of the ECG may allow differentiation of a PVC from AVC of a supraventricular impulse, usually a PAC (23). The following ECG features are suggestive of a PAC with AVC (Fig. 2.20):

- An rSR′ pattern in lead V1.
- A premature P′ wave preceding the bizarre QRS complex. The P wave morphology may be different from that of sinus P waves, and the PR interval of the PAC is usually longer than that of the normally conducted sinus beats. The premature P wave may be "hidden" in the preceding T wave.
- A noncompensatory pause follows the bizarre QRS complex.
- A QRS duration of less than 0.12 seconds.
- In atrial fibrillation or in MFAT, aberrantly conducted beats resembling PVCs may be seen when short RR intervals follow long RR

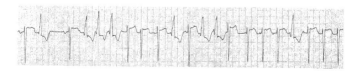

Fig. 2.20. Premature atrial contractions with aberrant ventricular conduction.

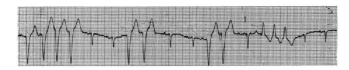

Fig. 2.21. Ventricular ectopy.

intervals ("long-short cycle sequence"). These beats often are called Ashman beats in recognition of their characterization by Gouaux and Ashman in 1947.

In Fig. 2.20 (lead V1), wide QRS complexes are seen to interrupt sinus rhythm. These eight QRS complexes are triphasic (rSR' or right bundle branch block morphology), and the QRS duration is less than 0.12 seconds. Premature P waves can be recognized on the downslope of the preceding T wave, and the PR intervals of the PACs are greater than those of normally conducted sinus beats. The wide QRS complexes are therefore the result of aberrant conduction of PACs.

The following ECG features are suggestive of a PVC (Fig. 2.21):

- A monophasic or biphasic QRS complex in lead V1.
- If the QRS complex is notched ("rabbit ear" pattern), the amplitude of the R wave is greater than that of the R' wave in V1. If R' wave amplitude is greater than that of the R wave, a PVC may not be confidently distinguished from a PAC with AVC.
- A QS wave in V6.
- A P wave does not precede the bizarre QRS complex.
- QRS duration of more than 0.12 seconds.
- Bizarre QRS complex followed by a fully compensatory pause.

Multiple PVCs of different morphology (multifocal PVCs) are shown in Fig. 2.21 (lead V1). These complexes have QRS durations of more than 0.12 seconds, and the QRS complexes have a monophasic or biphasic morphology.

A number of ECG criteria have been reported to aid in the differentiation of sustained VT from a sustained SVT with AVC. These are summarized in Table 2.3 (24,25).

Table 2.3. Ventricular tachycardia versus Supraventricular tachycardia with aberrancy

Electrocardiogram finding	SVT-AVC	Ventricular tachycardia
QRS morphology in V1	Triphasic (rSR')	Monophasic or biphasic
R/S ratio in V6	>1	<1
Frontal plane QRS axis	Normal or rightward	leftward ($<-30°$)
Ventricular rate	>170/min	<170 min
QRS duration	≤0.14 sec	≥0.14 sec
Fusion beats	Never	May be seen
AV dissociation	Never	May be seen

AV, atrioventricular; SVT-AVC, supraventricular tachycardia with aberrant ventricular conduction.

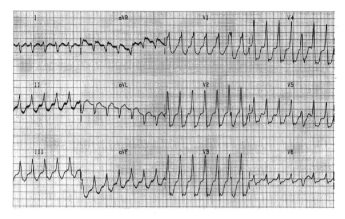

Fig. 2.22. Ventricular tachycardia (12-lead electrocardiogram).

An algorithmic approach also has been proposed to differentiate regular, wide QRS complex tachyarrhythmias. These algorithms have been demonstrated to have a sensitivity and specificity as great as >95% in delineating the origin of the rhythm disturbance (26,27). However, the Brugada algorithm performs poorly in the setting of preexisting conduction defects (28) The algorithm proposed by Griffith is similar to use and relies on the high prevalence of VT in the population with wide QRS complex tachycardias (29). Careful inspection of the 12-lead ECG with the previously mentioned differences in mind most often will lead to a correct diagnosis. In more difficult cases, the physical examination may be helpful. The presence of AV dissociation during VT may produce "cannon a" waves in the jugular venous pulse pattern and a first heart sound of varying intensity. The presence or absence of hypotension is of no differential diagnostic value (30). Figure 2.22 is an example of VT. The fifth QRS complex in the lateral precordial leads represents a fusion beat that is highly specific for VT.

Therapy

In the hemodynamically unstable patient, cardioversion is the treatment of choice, regardless of the origin of the wide QRS complex tachycardia. In the stable patient, without classic ECG findings for VT or SVT with aberrant conduction, IV adenosine (6-mg IV push) can be administered. In SVT with AVC, there is a high likelihood (approximately 90%) that the rhythm will convert to sinus. If adenosine fails to terminate the arrhythmia, amiodarone or lidocaine can be administered or cardioversion can be performed. In rare instances, adenosine may convert VT (31).

Torsade de Pointes

Description

The term *torsade de pointes* ("twisting of the points") was chosen by Dessertenne in 1966 to describe a new ventricular arrhythmia with unusual characteristics. As initially described, the limb leads

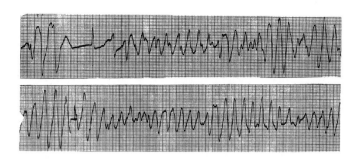

Fig. 2.23.   Torsade de pointes.

show cycles of alternating QRS polarity such that the peaks of the QRS complexes appear to be twisting around the isoelectric line of the recording. In each cycle, the amplitude of consecutive ventricular complexes increases and decreases in a sinusoidal fashion. However, these sinusoidal cycles make up only a portion of the arrhythmia. At other times, the rhythm is that of typical VT (uniform morphology and polarity of wide ventricular complexes in the monitor lead) (Fig. 2.23, lead 2 continuous strip). This rhythm also is characterized by frequent spontaneous conversion and recurrence. If spontaneous conversion occurs, it usually does so within 30 seconds of onset of the arrhythmia. Electrical cardioversion may be required to terminate the arrhythmia. Current opinion is that torsade de pointes should be diagnosed only if the previously mentioned morphologically distinct ECG pattern is associated with a prolonged correct QT interval between occurrences. In most instances, the corrected QT interval will be more than 0.60 seconds. In the absence of QT prolongation, a diagnosis of polymorphous or atypical VT is suggested. This distinction is extremely important for acute and chronic management of this unusual ventricular arrhythmia.

The majority of data indicate that torsade de pointes is a reentrant ventricular tachyarrhythmia resulting from increased temporal dispersion of myocardial recovery times (repolarization rates). The arrhythmia usually is precipitated by a ventricular premature beat occurring in late diastole and usually falling on the summit of a prolonged T wave.

Causes

Causes include (a) congenital QT prolongation syndromes; (b) drug-induced acquired QT prolongation [class IA antiarrhythmics (quinidine, procainamide), phenothiazines, tricyclic antidepressants]; (c) complete heart block; (d) hypokalemia; (e) hypomagnesemia; (f) intrinsic heart disease (ischemic heart disease, myocarditis); and (g) central nervous system disease.

Therapy

A correct diagnosis is critical in acute and chronic management. Use of class IA antiarrhythmics for this rhythm disturbance may adversely affect outcome. Treatment aims are to remove or correct the predisposing cause when possible (e.g., stop drugs, correct electrolyte disturbances) and to suppress the arrhythmia until either the

QT interval decreases or a diagnosis of congenital QT prolongation is confirmed.

Cardioversion should be used for prolonged episodes. However, because this arrhythmia tends to recur, the therapeutic objective should be to prevent recurrence (32).

IV magnesium sulfate (effective dose approximately 2 g) has been shown to be of value in preventing recurrence, even in patients with normal serum magnesium levels. Its mechanism of effect has not been established conclusively. Because this drug has not produced adverse effects and can be administered rapidly in the acute setting, magnesium may be the drug of first choice for management of this arrhythmia.

An **isoproterenol infusion** (210 μ/minute) can be used for acute control. Isoproterenol reduces the dispersion of myocardial recovery by a direct effect and indirectly by increasing the sinus node discharge rate. The QT interval decreases with increasing heart rate. However, this drug increases myocardial oxygen demand and decreases peripheral vascular resistance. It should be used with caution, especially in patients with intrinsic heart disease.

Temporary overdrive pacing has been particularly successful in preventing recurrence. If AV conduction is intact, atrial pacing is the preferred technique. Most agree that overdrive pacing is the definitive method for preventing recurrence.

The class IA antiarrhythmics should not be used because they will further increase the QT interval. Lidocaine produces inconsistent results.

In patients with acquired QT prolongation, overdrive pacing can be discontinued when the predisposing cause has been corrected and the QT interval has returned to normal. Prophylactic drug therapy is not needed.

In patients subsequently diagnosed as having congenital QT prolongation, long-term treatment with oral propranolol has been shown to be effective in symptomatic patients. Complete electrophysiologic studies with possible implantation of an automatic defibrillator should be considered.

Ventricular Fibrillation

Description

This is a chaotic ventricular rhythm (Fig. 2.24) felt to result from multiple reentrant foci within the ventricle. Organized electrical activity is not present, and because the ventricle does not depolarize as a unit, no ventricular contraction occurs.

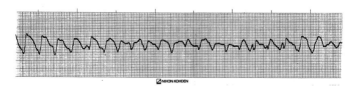

Fig. 2.24. Ventricular fibrillation.

Therapy

Therapy involves immediate defibrillation beginning with 200 J and initiation of cardiopulmonary resuscitation.

REFERENCES

1. Guidelines 2000 for cardiopulmonary resuscitation and emergency cardiovascular care. *Circulation* 102(Suppl):I-1, 2000.
2. Pearigen PD: Calcium channel blocker poisoning. In: LM Haddad, Shannon MW, Winchester JF, ed. *Clinical management of poisoning and drug overdose.* Philadelphia: WB Saunders Co., pp. 1020–1031, 1998.
3. Wolf LR: β-adrenergic blocker toxicity. In: LM Haddad, Shannon MW, Winchester JF, ed. *Clinical management of poisoning and drug overdose.* Philadelphia: WB Saunders Co., pp. 1031–1040, 1998.
4. McCord J, Borzak S: Multifocal atrial tachycardia. *Chest* 113:203, 1998.
5. Allessie MA, Boyden PA, Camm AJ, et al: Pathophysiology and prevention of atrial fibrillation. *Circulation* 2013:769, 2001.
6. Nattel S: New ideas about atrial fibrillation 50 years on. *Nature* 415: 219, 2002.
7. Vaziri SM, Larson MG, Benjamin EJ, et al: Echocardiographic predictors of nonrheumatic atrial fibrillation. The Framingham Heart Study. *Circulation* 89:724–730, 1994.
8. Golzari H, Cebul RD, Bahler RC: Atrial fibrillation: restoration and maintenance of sinus rhythm and indications for anticoagulation therapy. *Ann Intern Med* 125:311–323, 1996.
9. Chugh SS, Blackshear JL, Shen W, et al: Epidemiology and natural history of atrial fibrillation: clinical implications. *J Am Coll Cardiol* 37:371, 2001.
10. Fuster V, Ryden LE, Asinger RW, et al: ACC/AHA/ESC guidelines for the management of patients with atrial fibrillation: a report of the American College of Cardiology, American Heart Association Task Force on Practice Guidelines and the European Society of Cardiology Committee for Practice Guidelines and Policy Conferences. *J Am Coll Cardiol* 38:1266i, 2001.
11. Mittal S, Ayati S, Stein KM, et al: Transthoracic cardioversion of atrial fibrillation. Comparison of rectilinear biphasic versus damped sine wave monophasic shocks. *Circulation* 101:1282, 2000.
12. Mann DL, Maisel AS, Atwood JE, et al: Absence of cardioversion induced ventricular arrhythmias in patients with therapeutic digoxin levels. *J Am Coll Cardiol* 5:883, 1985.
13. Naccarelli GV, Dell'Orfano JT, Wolbrette DL, et al: Cost-effective management of acute atrial fibrillation: role of rate control, spontaneous conversion, medical and direct current cardioversion, transesophageal echocardiography, and antiembolic therapy. *Am J Cardiol* 84:36D, 2000.
14. Klein EA: Assessment of cardioversion using transesophageal echocardiography (TEE) multicenter study (ACUTE I): clinical outcomes at eight weeks. *J Am Coll Cardiol* 36:324, 2000.
15. Waldo AL: Pathogenesis of atrial flutter. *J Cardiovasc Electrophysiol* 9(Suppl):S18, 1998.
16. Chauhan VS, Krahn AD, Klein GJ, et al: Supraventricular tachycardia. *Med Clin N Am* 85:193, 2001.
17. Akhtar M, Jazayeri MR, Sra J, et al: Atrioventricular nodal reentry.

Clinical, electrophysiological, and therapeutic consideration. *Circulation* 88:282–295, 1993.

18. Shen W, Kurachi Y: Mechanisms of adenosine-mediated actions on cellular and clinical cardiac electrophysiology. *Mayo Clin Proc* 70: 274–291, 1995.

19. Gamm AJ, Garratt CJ: Adenosine and supraventricular tachycardia. *N Engl J Med* 325:1621–1629, 1991.

20. Olgin JE, Zipes DP: Specific arrhythmias: diagnosis and treatment. In: E Braunwald, Zipes DP, Libby P, eds. *Heart disease. a textbook of cardiovascular disease*, 6th ed. Philadelphia: WB Saunders, pp. 815–889, 2001.

21. Castellanos A, Moleiro F, Saoudi NC, et al: Parasystole. In: DP Zipes, Jalife J, eds. *Cardiac electrophysiology. From cell to bedside*. Philadelphia: WB Saunders, p. 619, 1990.

22. Saliba WI, Natale A: Ventricular tachycardia syndromes. *Med Clin N Am* 85;267, 2001.

23. Marriott HJL, Conover MHB: Differential diagnosis in the broad QRS tachycardia. In: Marriot HJL, Conover MHB, eds. *Advanced concepts in arrhythmias*. St. Louis: Mosby Co., p. 218–246, 1983.

24. Wellens HJJ, Bar FWHM, Lie KI: The value of the electrocardiogram in the differential diagnosis of a tachycardia with a widened QRS complex. *Am J Med* 64:27, 1978.

25. Akhtar M, Shenasa M, Jazayeri M, et al: Wide QRS complex tachycardia. Reappraisal of a common clinical problem. *Ann Intern Med* 109: 905, 1988.

26. Brugata P, Brugata J, Mont L, et al: A new approach to the differential diagnosis of a regular tachycardia with a wide QRS complex. *Circulation* 83:1649–1659, 1991.

27. Griffith MJ, Garratt CJ, Mounsey P, et al: Ventricular tachycardia as default diagnosis in broad complex tachycardia. *Lancet* 343:386, 1994.

28. Alberca T, Almendral J, Sanz P, et al: Evaluation of the specificity of morphological electrocardiographic criteria for the differential diagnosis of wide QRS complex tachycardia in patients with intraventricular conduction defects. *Circulation* 96:3527, 1997.

29. Lau EW, Ng GA: Comparison of two diagnostic algorithms for regular broad complex tachycardia by decision theory analysis. *PACE* 24: 1118, 2001.

30. Garratt CJ, Griffith MJ, Young G, et al: Value of physical signs in the diagnosis of ventricular tachycardia. *Circulation* 90:3103–3107, 1994.

31. Lerman BB, Stein KM, Markowitz SM: Adenosine-sensitive ventricular tachycardia: a conceptual approach. *J Cardiovasc Electrophysiol* 7:559, 1996.

32. Tan HL, Hou CJY, Lauer MR, et al: Electrophysiologic mechanisms of the long QT interval syndromes and torsade de pointes. *Ann Intern Med* 122:701–714, 1995.

EXERCISE STRESS TESTING

Exercise stress testing (EST) is a sensitive and informative examination of the cardiovascular response to exercise. EST is particularly useful in the detection and quantitation of ischemic heart disease (IHD) in those patients at increased risk for its occurrence. For the purposes of this discussion, IHD is used to represent impairment of coronary perfusion usually the result of, but not limited to, atherosclerotic coronary artery disease (CAD).

The electrocardiogram (ECG) is the most common parameter used to evaluate the ischemic response during exercise. This may be combined with cardiac imaging (echocardiography, nuclear perfusion scintigraphy, etc.) to increase the sensitivity and specificity of the test (see Chapters 4 and 5) (1–4). Additionally, exercise testing combined with cardiac imaging can be used to evaluate physiologic responses in certain valvular abnormalities (e.g., mitral stenosis).

EXERCISE PHYSIOLOGY—BASIC PRINCIPLES (5)

1. The heart extracts 70% of the oxygen carried by each unit of blood perfusing the myocardium and myocardial metabolism is nearly entirely aerobic. Therefore, an increase in myocardial oxygen demand during exercise must be matched by an increase in coronary blood flow (supply) or ischemia will result.

2. Major factors affecting myocardial oxygen demand the following:
- Heart rate (HR)
- Contractility (inotropic state)
- Wall tension (directly proportional to ventricular pressure $\times$ radius)

3. There is a good correlation between the "double product" [blood pressure (BP) $\times$ HR] and measured myocardial oxygen consumption during dynamic exercise. Angina occurs at a remarkably constant double product in a given patient with IHD and is often independent of duration, intensity, or type of exercise performed. In practice, EST is designed to produce an increase in HR of known magnitude, defined as a percentage of the maximal predicted HR of a normal population of matched age and sex (Table 3.1).

4. In the presence of IHD, coronary blood flow cannot increase adequately to meet the demands of the myocardium for oxygen, resulting in ischemia and manifested by (a) pain (angina), (b) ECG ST segment changes, (c) ventricular dysfunction, (d) arrhythmias, or (e) a combination of these.

5. Types of exercise include the following:
- Static: isometric sustained muscular contraction against a fixed resistance (e.g., hand grip)
- Dynamic: rhythmic contractions of extensor and flexor muscle groups (e.g., a bicycle or treadmill exercise)
- Combination of static and dynamic exercise

Table 3.1. Expected heart rate response to graded exercise

Age	Mild	Moderate	Moderately severe	Near maximal	Maximal
20–29	115	135	155	175	195
30–39	110	130	150	170	190
40–49	106	126	146	166	186
50–59	102	122	142	162	182
>60	98	118	138	158	178

6. There are several reasons why dynamic exercise is preferred in EST:
- Isometric exercise can produce exaggerated BP response, which may be detrimental to patients with high BP or CAD.
- HR response is variable in isometric exercise, although it will increase reliably during dynamic exercise.
- Angina pectoris is less reliably provoked during isometric exercise.
- Isometric exercise frequently provokes ventricular arrhythmias.
- ECG changes during isometric exercise may be subtle and obscured by muscle tremor artifact.

7. Alternatives to conventional EST in patients who cannot exercise include pharmacologic agents (dobutamine, adenosine, or dipyridamole) administered in conjunction with cardiac imaging (echo, nuclear scanning) to determine the physiologic consequences of ischemia (wall motion abnormalities, areas of reversible hypoperfusion) (see Chapters 4 and 5) (1,2,5,6).

INDICATIONS FOR EXERCISE STRESS TESTING (5)
- Differential diagnosis of chest pain (i.e., evaluation of patients with symptoms suggestive of IHD)
- Assessment of the level of exercise at which ischemic manifestations occur in a patient with known IHD
- Evaluation of therapy for arrhythmias and angina
- Evaluation of functional disability secondary to organic heart disease (e.g., valvular heart disease)
- Evaluation of the asymptomatic patient older than age 40 who has multiple risk factors for IHD

CONTRAINDICATIONS TO EXERCISE STRESS TESTING
- Recent acute myocardial infarction (AMI) (4 to 6 weeks), except for submaximal (65% of predicted maximum HR) or symptom-limited EST prior to hospital discharge
- Angina at rest
- Rapid ventricular or atrial arrhythmias
- Advanced atrioventricular (AV) block (unless chronic)
- Uncompensated congestive heart failure
- Acute noncardiac illnesses
- Severe aortic stenosis
- BP greater than 170/100 before the onset of exercise

SAFETY OF EXERCISE STRESS TESTING

Serious complications (AMI, cardiac arrest, arrhythmias requiring treatment, stroke, or death) of EST are extremely uncommon (0.8 complications per 10,000 maximal tests) (7). Therefore, EST is a safe procedure when done under proper supervision and with the necessary safeguards and equipment (8). These include the following:

1. Physician's knowledge of the patient's history and physical findings prior to the EST
2. Physician, a qualified physician's assistant, or a nurse present for the entire test
3. Continuous monitoring of HR and rhythm and frequent BP determinations during the procedure and for 6 to 10 minutes thereafter
4. Emergency equipment readily available, including a defibrillator, airway management equipment, and emergency drugs
5. Termination of the EST at the appropriate time (see later in this chapter)

TERMINATING THE EXERCISE STRESS TESTING

1. Achievement of predicted HR (Table 3.1)
2. Patient unable to continue because of symptoms of excessive fatigue, claudication, and/or dyspnea
3. Premature ventricular contractions increasing in frequency and/or ventricular tachycardia
4. Onset of advanced AV block
5. Occurrence of severe angina
6. Diagnostic ST segment changes clearly obtained on ECG
7. Systolic BP greater than 220 and diastolic BP greater than 120 during exercise, or during exercise BP drops to a level below baseline (may indicate left ventricular [LV] dysfunction)
8. Failure of the ECG monitoring system

Following the termination of the EST, the patient should be observed for 6 to 10 minutes with continuous ECG monitoring. Obtain BP frequently, and look for ECG ST segment changes and arrhythmias, which commonly occur postexercise. The ECG should return to baseline before releasing the patient.

EXERCISE STRESS TESTING PROCEDURE

1. Protocols are used that utilize dynamic exercise on a treadmill up to a predicted maximal HR for age. There are many multistage protocols that use increments in treadmill elevation and speed; each protocol has its advantages, depending on the patient being tested (5). Small increments in workloads of short duration (Ellestad protocol) may be better tolerated than larger workloads of longer duration (Bruce protocol), especially in older patients in poor physical condition. To obtain the maximal amount of information from the EST, a protocol can be altered somewhat to meet the clinical situation. The Bruce and the Ellestad protocols are shown in Table 3.2.

2. If a single lead is to be used for ECG monitoring in EST, lead V5 usually provides the largest R wave and, therefore, the greatest likelihood for detecting ECG changes. Sensitivity is enhanced by

Table 3.2.   Exercise stress test protocols

Bruce protocol		
3	1.75	10%
3	2.5	12%
3	3.4	14%
3	4.2	16%
3	5.0	18%
Ellestad protocol		
3	1.6	10%
3	2.2	10%
2	2.6	10%
2	3.0	10%
2	3.6	10%

15% by using a 12-lead ECG system, which also detects ST segment changes from the anterior and inferior walls (Fig. 3.1).

ECGs routinely are done supine and standing prior to the EST, at each step in the EST protocol, immediately postexercise, and at 2-minute intervals thereafter for 6 to 10 minutes.

INTERPRETATION

1. ST segment changes are the most reliable electrocardiographic indicators of myocardial ischemia (5). Six major types of ST segments may occur in response to exercise (Fig. 3.2).

2. A horizontal or downsloping ST segment that is depressed at least 1 mm below the isoelectric at the J point and that persists for 80 msec thereafter is interpreted as a positive test (Fig. 3.2, patterns C and D). The incidence of false positives is reduced significantly when a 2-mm ST segment depression requirement is used for a positive test. Three consecutive beats without baseline variation are required for reliable measurement of ST segments. Two examples of a positive EST are shown in Figs. 3.1 and 3.3. Most modern treadmill equipment has filtering software to assist in correcting for artifact.

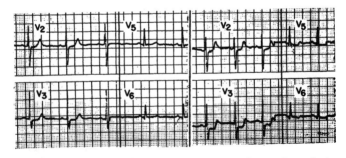

Fig. 3.1.   Control and immediate postexercise electrocardiograms in a patient with ischemic heart disease. Note the 2-mm horizontal ST segment depression in lead V3. This diagnostic change would not have been detected if only lead V5 had been monitored.

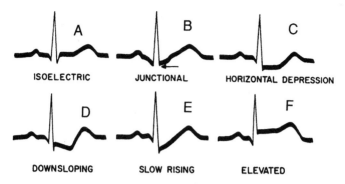

Fig. 3.2. ST segment response to exercise.

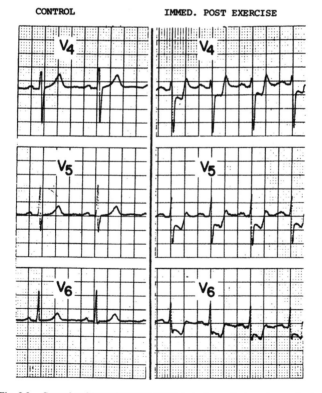

Fig. 3.3. Control and immediate postexercise electrocardiograms in a patient with ischemic heart disease. Note the 3-mm downsloping ST segment depression in leads V5 and V6.

3. The depth of the ST segment depression correlates roughly with the extent of CAD (i.e., patients with a 3-mm or greater ST segment depression 80 msec after the J point have a high incidence of triple-vessel disease). In addition, ST segment changes that occur in the first 3 minutes of exercise and/or persist past 8 minutes during recovery correlate with an 85% prevalence of two- and three-vessel disease (7).

4. Other patterns of ST segment depression include the following (Fig. 3.2):

Pattern B: Depression of the J point with a rapid rise in the ST segment is a normal occurrence with exercise and correlates poorly with IHD.

Pattern E: Depression of the J point with a slow-rising ST segment and 2.0-mm ST depression at 80 msec from the J point has been shown to correlate well with IHD, but there is a high incidence of false positives (32%). Therefore, this pattern is not widely used for the diagnosis of IHD.

Pattern F: ST segment elevation occurs rarely in EST and probably represents a severe degree of myocardial ischemia or an LV aneurysm. No quantitative criteria are established for EST interpretation.

5. Interpretation of the EST also must include the following:

- An evaluation of the workload performed
- The HR and BP response
- The presence or absence of arrhythmias
- The presence or absence of symptoms

6. ST segments changes can be difficult to interpret for the following reasons:

- The resting ECG demonstrates a left bundle branch block (LBBB), left ventricular hypertrophy (LVH) with repolarization abnormalities, Wolff-Parkinson-White syndrome, changes of digitalis, or significant ST segment depression.
- The patient does not achieve his or her 85% maximum HR, and the ST segments do not change. However, if a patient develops ST segment depression or angina at a submaximal pulse rate, this may indicate significant ischemia.

PHYSIOLOGY OF ST SEGMENT DEPRESSION

The electrophysiologic basis for ST changes during EST is an intracellular potassium loss resulting from an imbalance between myocardial oxygen supply and demand. The subendocardial layer of the left ventricle is most vulnerable because it is subjected to a high wall tension, which adversely affects tissue perfusion. Subendocardial loss of potassium ion results in an ST segment shift toward the affected subendocardial area, which is manifested on the surface ECG as ST depression.

OTHER CAUSES OF ST SEGMENT DEPRESSION

1. Supply/demand imbalance as a result of anemia, aortic stenosis, coronary spasm, severe hypertension, LVH, and/or hypertrophic cardiomyopathy

2. LBBB induces secondary repolarization changes unrelated to supply/demand imbalance
3. Drugs: digitalis (this drug usually is discontinued 10 days prior to the EST if atrial fibrillation is not present) and antihypertensives
4. Miscellaneous: cardiomyopathies, mitral valve prolapse, syndrome X (chest pain with angiographically normal coronary arteries), and autonomic dysfunction
5. Hypokalemia, recent glucose or food ingestion, and vasoregulatory asthenia

DIAGNOSTIC ACCURACY OF EXERCISE STRESS TESTING IN DETECTION OF ISCHEMIC HEART DISEASE

The predictive value of any test will vary with the prevalence of the disease in the population being tested. Thus, the greater number of patients with IHD in the population being tested, the greater the predictive value. Therefore, populations tested with few risk factors for IHD will have a larger number of false-positive responses and a decreased predictive value. Females of any age have a high incidence of false-positive tests as compared to males of the same age group (5).

Using the criterion of 1 mm of ST segment depression (patterns C and D) as an indicator of IHD, conventional EST has a sensitivity of about 68% (the proportion of people who truly have CAD who are identified by EST), a specificity of about 77% (the proportion of people who are truly free of CAD who are so identified by EST), and a predictive value of 70% to 80% (the likelihood of IHD if EST is positive) (9).

Results also are influenced by the severity of CAD present (e.g., only 9% of patients with triple vessel disease had false negative tests, whereas 63% of patients with single vessel disease had a false-negative EST).

COMMON MISCONCEPTIONS ABOUT EXERCISE STRESS TESTING

1. EST is the definitive tool to verify the existence of IHD. Overall sensitivity is 64%; therefore, 36% of patients with CAD will have a false-negative test.

2. There is little benefit from the EST in subjects with known IHD, especially those considered stable post-myocardial infarction (MI). The treadmill may be used to determine those patients at high risk for future coronary events (i.e., a patient with a positive EST 2 months post-MI is twice as likely to have a future coronary event as a patient with a negative EST post-MI). In addition, EST is useful to establish efficacy of drugs (antianginal agents/antiarrhythmics) and to establish an exercise prescription in cardiac rehabilitation programs.

3. ST segment depression is the only manifestation of IHD. Many other aspects of EST may correlate with the presence and severity of IHD. Look for the following:

- Submaximal pulse response (chronotropic incompetence correlates with LV dysfunction)
- Fall in BP
- Exercise-induced chest pain
- Ventricular ectopy
- Magnitude and configuration of ST segment depression

- Time of onset of ST segment depression (i.e., earlier onset correlates with more severe disease)
- Length of time ST segment abnormalities persist in recovery phase; longer lasting abnormalities correlate with more severe disease

REFERENCES

1. Chou TM, Amidon TM: Evaluating coronary artery disease noninvasively—which test for whom? *West J Med* 161:173, 1994.
2. Mayo Clinic Cardiovascular Working Group on Stress Testing: Cardiovascular stress testing: a description of the various types of stress tests and indications for their use. *Mayo Clin Proc* 71:43, 1996.
3. Jain A, Murray DR: Detection of myocardial ischemia. *Curr Prob Cardiol* 20:773, 1995.
4. Botvinick EH: Stress imaging. Current clinical options for the diagnosis, localization, and evaluation of coronary artery disease. *Med Clin N Amer* 79:1025, 1995.
5. Fletcher GF, Balady G, Froelicher VF, et al: Exercise standards. A statement for healthcare professionals from the American Heart Association. *Circulation* 91:580, 1995.
6. Stratmann HG, Kennedy HL: Evaluation of coronary artery disease in the patient unable to exercise: alternatives to exercise stress testing. *Am Heart J* 117:1344, 1989.
7. Gibbons L, Blair SN, Kohl HW, et al: The safety of maximal exercise testing. *Circulation* 80:846, 1989.
8. Pina IL, Balady GJ, Hanson P, et al: Guidelines for clinical exercise testing laboratories. A statement for healthcare professionals from the Committee on Exercise and Cardiac Rehabilitation, American Heart Association. *Circulation* 91:912, 1995.
9. Gianrossi R, Detrano R, Mulvihill D, et al: Exercise-induced ST depression in the diagnosis of coronary artery disease. A meta-analysis. *Circulation* 80:87, 1989.

ECHOCARDIOGRAPHY

The ability to see a real-time motion picture of a beating heart and to observe the direction of blood flow through normal and abnormal valves by merely placing a hand-held transducer painlessly on the chest wall of a conscious patient is taken for granted by today's physicians, but it could not have been imagined by even the most visionary thinkers at the midpoint of the last century. It is the purpose of this chapter to present an overview of the history of this truly amazing technology, working definitions of the various terms and procedures that are considered to be in the purview of echocardiography, and examples of its clinical usefulness. At the same time, some of its potential limitations will be emphasized in an attempt to mitigate overreliance on reported findings that are at odds with considered clinical judgment. The performance and interpretation of echocardiographic procedures require considerable skill and experience, as well as a clear understanding of the clinical problem being assessed in the individual patient.

HISTORIC EVOLUTION OF ECHOCARDIOGRAPHY

In the early 1950s, Edler and Hertz in Lund, Sweden experimented with World War II sonar technology to record the movement of cardiac wall and valve motion and instigated a revolution that has had a major impact on cardiac diagnosis and therapy. Their discovery led to the development and widespread dissemination in the 1960s of M-mode (M for motion) imaging that plots depth against time through a narrow "ice pick" path. M-mode imaging is still in current usage to measure chamber and wall thickness dimensions and to establish the timing of events such as valve or cardiac wall motion because it provides high-resolution one-dimensional images of these structures. The images display vertical dimension (depth) on the y axis and time on the x axis. The rate of depth sampling is greater than 1,000/second, compared to 30/second imaging frequency of two-dimensional (2-D) echocardiograms (ECGs), and therefore is suited ideally to tracking rapidly moving structures such as the opening and closing motions of cardiac valves or contraction and relaxation of ventricular walls. The relationship between M-mode and 2-D images of the mitral and aortic valves is depicted in Fig. 4.1.

The first experimental 2-D ECGs were fabricated manually from thin vertical slices manually cut from paper printouts of M-mode echocardiographic recordings. These strips then were pasted together with strips from adjacent regions, in spatial and temporal sequence using the electrocardiographic signals for timing within the cardiac cycle. These cumbersomely animated 2-D "cartoons" provided evidence that functional anatomic images of the beating hearts could provide a considerable diagnostic advantage to ultrasound imaging. In the early 1970s, linear array transducers consisting of comblike strips of crystals created real-time depictions of the beating heart that appeared to be taken through venetian blinds, but

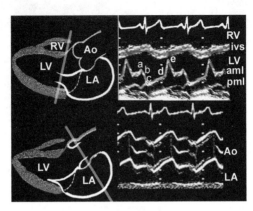

Fig. 4.1. Two-dimensional and M-mode echocardiography of the mitral and aortic valves. Two-dimensional depictions are shown on the left, with the direction of the M-mode ultrasound beam indicated by the white line traversing the valve under study. M-mode recordings are shown on the right, with the mitral valve motion in the upper panel and the aortic valve below. The anterior mitral valve leaflet (*aml*) inscribes the letter "M," whereas the posterior mitral leaflet (*pml*) reciprocates, inscribing a "W." The initial diastolic opening excursion (*d-e*) of the aml approaches the interventricular septum (*IVS*), followed by partial closure (*e-f*), then reopening with atrial systole (*a*), and finally closure (*a-b-c*). The aortic valve M-mode resembles boxes on a string enclosed between parallel undulating lines representing the front and back walls of the aortic root. The "string" represents the aortic valve leaflets pressed together in diastole, and the "boxes" represent the opened aortic valve leaflets pressed against the aortic walls.

sufficient distortion of cardiac structures to limit their usefulness to the imaging of surface arteries and veins.

Next, spinning-head transducers containing sending and receiving crystals generated fanlike sweeps that were assembled by computers into sector scans that reproduced, in real time, the handmade cartoons described previously. These spinning transducers soon were replaced by multicrystal phased-array transducers that sweep electronically in a windshield-wiper fashion to record a 900 fan-shaped image sector of the heart 30 times per second. The evolution of computers required to process and refine images, and the ability to conveniently store and replay the images on videotape, established echocardiography as the premiere noninvasive imaging modality during the 1980s.

Further refinements and applications made possible by miniaturization and enhanced computer processing resulted in the development of simultaneous echo and color-coded Doppler velocity transthoracic echo (TTE), multiplane transesophageal echocardiography (TEE) imaging, hand-held point of care echocardiographic recorders, intravascular ultrasound, intracardiac echo, and real-time three-dimensional (3-D) imaging. Much of this technology is beyond the scope of this chapter, but is worthy of mention because of the ongoing and seemingly endless evolution of Edler and Hertz's discovery a half century ago.

CONTEMPORARY ECHOCARDIOGRAPHY

The term echocardiography now encompasses an array of related procedures that use ultrasound to provide moving 2-D and 3-D images of the cardiac chambers and valves, dimensions of these structures, and flow-velocity profiles. All of these modalities are integrated in time and space, so that it is possible to depict diseased valves, abnormal chamber dimensions, altered wall motion, and abnormal flow-velocity patterns simultaneously in real time. These noninvasive procedures do not use harmful ionizing radiation or potentially nephrotoxic contrast media and, therefore, are invaluable in the initial assessment of patients with suspected cardiac valve disease as well as in serial examinations in long-term follow-up.

Ultrasound waves are propagated in a liquid medium (blood or pleural or pericardial fluid) or through tissues with high water content (e.g., muscle and liver) and reflect off interfaces between dissimilar structures (blood versus valves, blood versus myocardium, etc.). To create an image, an ultrasound wave must be reflected back to the receiver, so that its distance from the receiver can be computed from the time delay between emitted and received ultrasound. Objects with reflecting surfaces at approximately right angles relative to the ultrasound beam vector produce clear images and measurable Doppler waves, whereas surfaces that are nearly parallel will not return the signals to the receiver and will drop out. An analogy can be made with bouncing a tennis ball off a wall as opposed to skipping a rock over a pond; the ball will return, whereas the rock will disappear from sight.

Ultrasound waves cannot penetrate dense media such as bone, heavily calcified valves, or prosthetic materials. Gas-filled organs like the lung and gut scatter the waves. In addition, structures within 1 to 2 cm of the transducer are poorly defined ("near field effect"). Objects at a distance greater than 15 cm from the transducer are also poorly seen. Another limitation of echo is the paucity of suitable "windows" through which the cardiac structures can be imaged. The lung, sternum, and rib cage cover most of the heart from an anterior approach, but a small window exists to the left of the sternum between the ribs, as shown in Fig. 4.2. Diagnostic images usually can be obtained from apical, subcostal, or suprasternal windows and through one or more of the 2nd, 3rd, or 4th intercostal space windows without intervening lung.

TRANSESOPHAGEAL ECHOCARDIOGRAPHY

On occasion, the images from transthoracic windows are not diagnostic because of emphysema, severe obesity, or chest wall deformities that prevent the ultrasound waves from reaching the structures of interest. Additionally, acoustic shadowing may occur when the ultrasound beam cannot penetrate a prosthetic heart valve or a heavily calcified pericardium. Under these circumstances, TEE can be used whereby a small transducer is attached to a flexible probe, which is inserted through the patient's mouth and down the esophagus. Because the esophagus lies just behind and contiguous with the left atrium, superb images of the heart can be obtained in most patients without interference from the lungs, bones, or prosthetic valves. Additionally, the esophagus is positioned closely near the aorta, allowing superb views of the thoracic aorta that can define aortic dissection. These transducers can be steered or directed from

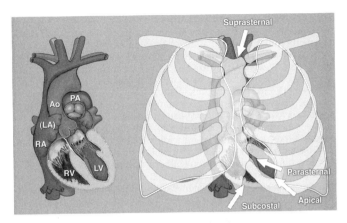

Fig. 4.2. Transthoracic echocardiographic windows. A frontal view of the thorax (**right**) reveals that most of the heart is covered by ribs and air-filled lungs that block ultrasonic access. The inferomedial aspect of the left lung is reflected away from the heart permitting parasternal access windows between the ribs, as well as an apical port. Other windows are seen in the subcostal (transhepatic) and suprasternal areas. The uncovered heart is shown on the left to reveal the central position of the aortic valve and its contiguity with the mitral and tricuspid valves. The ascending aorta is surrounded on all sides by blood-filled chambers: on the left and anteriorly by the right ventricular outflow tract (removed in this picture), dorsally by the left atrium, and on the right by the right atrium. In viewing echocardiograms from many different windows, the aortic valve serves as a "North Star" to help orient the viewer to a fixed reference point.

0 degrees to 180 degrees by the operator and allow a greater level of flexibility and image-specific orientation.

DOPPLER ULTRASONOGRAPHY

The Doppler shift, the change in pitch that affects sound emanating from a structure approaching or receding from the point where sound is received, can be used to depict direction and velocity of flowing blood elements. The modified Bernoulli equation permits estimation of the pressure change that occurs when blood flows between high- and low-pressure chambers or sites (e.g., across a stenotic or regurgitant valve or a septal defect). The pressure gradient, or $P_1 - P_2$, can be calculated by $P_1 - P_2 = 4 \times \text{velocity}^2$, a modification of the Bernoulli principle.

Three Doppler techniques are used currently:

1. **Pulsed wave (PW)**
2. **Color flow (CF)**
3. **Continuous wave (CW)**

Each depicts flow and velocity relative to the transducer, but all are unable to define flow parameters accurately because the angle of incidence between the path of the target element and the emitted/received sound waves is greater than 20 degrees. When the flow-velocity vector approaches 900, the reflecting targets (the blood cells) are neither moving toward nor away from the transducer; thus, flow escapes detection.

Pulsed wave Doppler samples from a specific point in a cardiovascular chamber (the sample volume) as though the sensors were positioned in a selected spot to detect the direction and velocity of flow relative to that site. The transducer alternately sends and receives ultrasound pulses, so that by appropriate positioning of the sample volume within the 2-D image, regurgitant flow from a valve or shunts can be detected. PW Doppler is limited by its inherent sampling rate (the Nyquist limit) in its ability to quantitate high-velocity flow; when high-velocity flow is encountered, "aliasing" of the signal occurs and the Doppler signal wraps around the zero line.

Color flow Doppler is based on PW Doppler sampling from hundreds of sampling pixels that are assigned a color code that permits detection of the direction of blood flow at each specific site. The color assigned to flow toward the transducer is red, and the color assigned to flow away from the transducer is blue. As the velocity increases, there is a shift in color from red to orange to yellow in approaching flow and from dark blue to turquoise on receding flow as the Nyquist limit is approached. High-velocity flow causes "wrap-around" color aliasing, so that approaching flow will appear turquoise or blue, and receding flow shades will be orange or red. Turbulent flow leads to colorful mosaic patterns containing the entire spectrum of color-coding. For these reasons, still images from CF Doppler studies can be difficult to interpret, but observation of motion and timing of these colorful patterns provides additional diagnostic information.

Continuous wave Doppler transducers continuously emit and receive ultrasound, so CW is not limited in high-velocity tracking, but it cannot localize the depth from which the signals emanate (Fig. 4.5). All velocity signals along the path of the beam are superimposed, with the highest velocity dominating the signal. With sequential use of PW and CW Doppler techniques, the site of high-velocity signals can be localized by PW, and the magnitude can be determined by CW interrogation.

USE OF DOPPLER METHODS TO ASSESS HEMODYNAMIC PARAMETERS

Noninvasive estimation of intracardiac pressures is made possible by combining Doppler recordings of velocity and measurements of blood pressure and/or estimates of jugular venous pressure. These estimates of intracardiac pressure are dependent on the ability to measure accurately high-velocity anterograde or regurgitant flow across valves, which is not always possible. Almost all hearts, normal or abnormal, will manifest regurgitant flow across the tricuspid valve. These estimates can be extremely useful in the management of patients. The following examples will illustrate the estimation of pressures (Figs. 4.3 and 4.4).

The pulmonary artery systolic pressure is equivalent to right ventricular systolic pressure in the absence of pulmonic stenosis. These estimates obviously require the presence of a tricuspid regurgitant jet. Doppler jets can be detected in many normal hearts and in most hearts with elevated right ventricular systolic pressures, making it possible to estimate right ventricular and pulmonary artery pressure

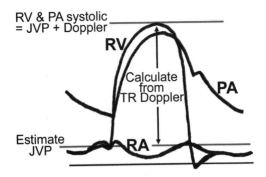

Fig. 4.3. Noninvasive estimation of right ventricular and pulmonary artery systolic pressures. After estimating the jugular venous pressure (*JVP*), this value is added to the systolic pressure difference between the right ventricle (*RV*) and right atrium (*RA*) calculated from the tricuspid regurgitant (*TR*) Doppler signal and the Bernoulli equation: Pressure difference = 4 (velocity)^2. If the JVP is thought to be normal (e.g., 5 mm Hg) and the TR Doppler velocity is 2 M/second, the RV and PA systolic pressures would be approximated as $5 + 4(4)^2 = 21$ mm Hg. The right atrial pressure can be assumed to be high (more than 10 mm Hg) if the echocardiogram demonstrates right atrial or inferior vena caval enlargement.

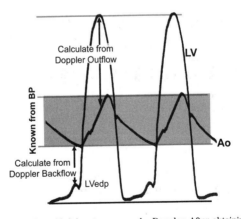

Fig. 4.4. Estimation of left heart pressures by Doppler. After obtaining the blood pressure of 130/80 in a hypothetic patient with mixed aortic valve disease, the left ventricular systolic and diastolic pressures can be estimated. For example, if the outflow velocity is 5 M/second, the systolic pressure gradient between the left ventricle (*LV*) and aorta (*Ao*) would be $4 \times (5)^2 = 100$ mm Hg, and the LV systolic pressure is $130 + 100 = 230$ mm Hg. If the backflow velocity from the regurgitant jet at the end of diastole is 3 M/second, the LV end-diastolic pressure (*LVedp*) would be $80 - 4 (3)^2 = 44$ mm Hg.

in the majority of studies. Doppler values also can be used in combination with blood pressures (measured at the time of the Doppler study with a sphygmomanometer) to estimate hemodynamic parameters in the left heart, as shown in Fig. 4.4.

VENTRICULAR FUNCTIONAL ASSESSMENT BY ECHOCARDIOGRAPHY

Systolic and diastolic ventricular function may be assessed by echocardiography. Although accurate determinations of ventricular ejection fraction can be made by planimetry and conversion to end-diastolic and end-systolic volume by Simpson's rule (similar to the estimation of the volume of an egg from the sum of slices), these determinations are rarely, if ever, performed in most echocardiographic laboratories. In truth, most determinations of ejection fraction are "guesstimates" by the reader, and depending on experience, may vary from reader to reader. Global or regional wall motion abnormalities at rest and/or with stress (exercise, dobutamine, adenosine, etc.) usually are apparent to the experienced observer.

Diastolic functional analysis of ventricular function is complex and constantly evolving technology. Observation of the ventricular wall motion and rate of filling during relaxation can indicate problems with ventricular compliance, especially in hypertrophy, cardiomyopathy, or pericardial disease. Diastolic inflow Doppler signals in ventricles with impaired relaxation may reveal reversal of the usual ratio between passive and active filling, in which a normal ventricle receives more blood at higher velocity during passive filling than with active, atrial systolic filling (with reversal of the E/a ratio). The terminology applied to Doppler flow peaks matches the M-mode terminology (see Fig. 4.1), with the e-wave coincident with the initial opening of the mitral valve and the a-wave matching the reopening attendant with atrial systole. More recently, **tissue Doppler** analysis has been used to detect diastolic filling abnormalities.

ECHOCARDIOGRAPHY IN VALVE DISEASE AND CARDIOMYOPATHY

Virtually every form of heart disease either can be diagnosed definitively or can be strongly suspected by a skillfully performed and interpreted ECG in a suitably "echogenic" subject. The vignettes in Figs. 4.5–4.11 highlight the value of the combined use of echocardiographic modalities in the study of patients with heart disease.

ECHOCARDIOGRAPHY IN ISCHEMIC HEART DISEASE

Echocardiography may be useful in the evaluation of acute myocardial infarction and its complications. Ischemic manifestations of acute coronary thrombosis may include wall motion abnormalities (hypokinesis, akinesis, or dyskinesis); acquired ventricular septal defect; mitral regurgitation as a result of papillary muscle dysfunction or rupture; and left ventricular thrombi. In chronic ischemic cardiomyopathies, myocardial thinning or scarring commonly may be seen in the area of a previous infarction. Left ventricular ejection fraction can be determined accurately and can be very useful in determining the future prognosis of the patient. The presence of segmental wall motion abnormalities in a patient with a dilated cardiomyopathy favors ischemia as an etiology in the differential diagnosis.

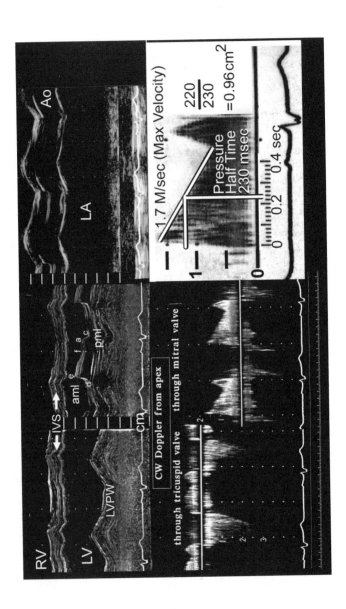

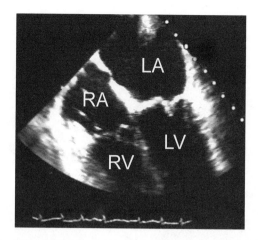

Fig. 4.6. Left atrial thrombus detected by transesophageal echocardiography. A patient with moderate mitral stenosis and atrial fibrillation was to undergo elective countershock, but a transesophageal echocardiogram (TEE) revealed a large mural thrombus (*top center*) on the dorsal aspect of the left atrium. It is recommended that TEE should be performed routinely to detect thrombus prior to cardioversion, especially if there is left atrial enlargement, left ventricular dysfunction, or mitral stenosis.

Fig. 4.5. Echocardiography in a patient with mitral stenosis. M-mode depictions are shown in the upper panels, and **continuous wave (CW)** Doppler recordings are shown in the lower panels. **Mitral valve area** is calculated in the lower right panel. The M-mode recording through the left ventricle demonstrates a normal end-diastolic dimension of 4.6 cm, "paradoxical" systolic interventricular septal (*IVS*) motion, moving toward the right ventricle suggesting right ventricular volume and/or pressure overload. The anterior mitral leaflet (*aml*) is held open by a persistent pressure gradient, demonstrated by the reduced closing slope (*e-f*), and the posterior leaflet (*pml*) is pulled anteriorly by commissural fusion with the anterior leaflet. The left atrium is enlarged (5.5 cm). The Doppler tricuspid regurgitant velocity is 2.7 M/second, representing a 30 mm Hg systolic pressure difference. The maximum diastolic mitral valve velocity is 1.7 M/second, which equates to 11.6 mm Hg. The mitral valve area is calculated by the **pressure half-time** method in which the time (in msec) required to fall to half the maximum gradient is divided into 220, an empirically derived constant. A valve area of 0.96 is less than one-fourth the normal valve area, suggesting moderately severe stenosis.

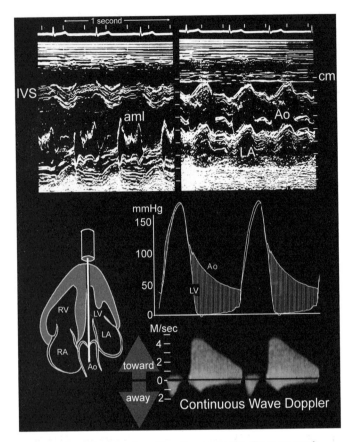

Fig. 4.7. Bicuspid aortic valve with aortic regurgitation. The upper panels show M-mode images of the mitral valve (**left**) and aortic valve (**right**). The anterior mitral leaflet (*aml*) has high frequency vibratory motion caused by the aortic regurgitant stream cascading along the ventricular aspect of the valve leaflet. The ventricular dimensions are increased: end diastolic 6.5 cm and end systolic 4.7 cm, with increased excursions of the septum and posterior walls indicative of a well-tolerated "volume overload" state. The closure line of the aortic leaflets is eccentric (i.e., closer to the posterior aortic wall), suggesting a bicuspid aortic valve (confirmed by angiography). The continuous wave Doppler velocity signal in the lower panel indicates a small systolic pressure gradient (1.7 M/second, 12 mm Hg) from high-volume outflow, whereas the diastolic signal shows a rapid decline compatible with a rapid fall in aortic pressure and/ or a rapid rise in ventricular filling pressure. Left ventricular (*LV*) and aortic (*Ao*) pressures confirm the rapid dissipation of the pressure difference between the Ao and LV in diastole.

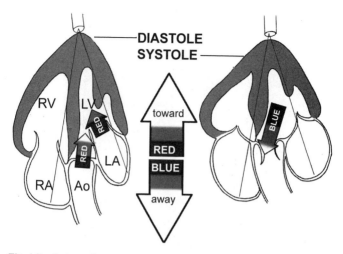

Fig. 4.8. Cartoons demonstrating color flow Doppler in aortic regurgitation. The color spectra of flow toward and away from the transducer at the left ventricular apex, with red indicating mitral inflow and aortic backflow and blue indicating aortic outflow. Because the high velocities (see Fig. 4.7) exceed the Nyquist limit for pulsed wave Doppler on which color flow Doppler is based, some aliasing is indicated.

EXERCISE STRESS ECHOCARDIOGRAPHY

Combining an imaging modality such as echocardiography with an exercise stress test has many advantages. A wall motion defect is the final common pathway for the physiologic response to a significantly ischemic region of myocardium. The echocardiographic equipment is a portable system that can be used easily in the office or in the hospital. It provides immediate information without using ionizing radiation. Intravenous lines are not necessary, unlike with other nuclear scanning techniques. Additionally, stress echo is comparable with nuclear imaging in cost effectiveness. Many of the indications of stress echo are similar to those of stress thallium, isonitrile (technetium-99m sestamibi), and radionuclide angiography. These include the following:

- Patients with abnormal resting ECGs (left ventricular hypertrophy, left branch bundle block digitalis effect, ST segment depression)
- Patients with a high likelihood of false-positive ECG results (middle-aged women)
- Patients for whom a therapeutic procedure is planned (such as angioplasty or bypass surgery), so that the physiologic significance of the lesion can be assessed and followed

The disadvantages of stress echo include difficulty in obtaining a good image (because of body habitus or technician inexperience), the need to image during or as close to peak exercise as possible, and difficulty in interpreting new wall motion defects in the presence of resting hypokinesis or akinesis. However, the use of digitized, on-line cine loop technology has greatly facilitated the interpretation

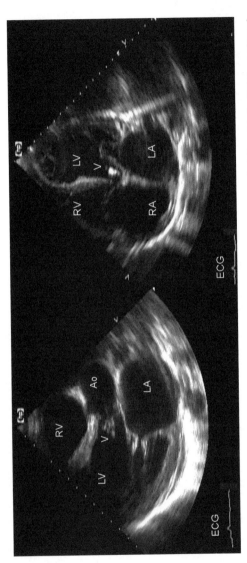

Fig. 4.9. Aortic valve endocarditis. An aortic valve vegetation (*V*) is seen prolapsing into the left ventricular (*LV*) in parasternal long axis (**left**) and apical views taken in diastole. The radial array of dots indicates 1-cm depth. In motion sequences, the vegetation could be seen to traverse the aortic valve to enter the aortic root and then fling back into the outflow tract with diastole.

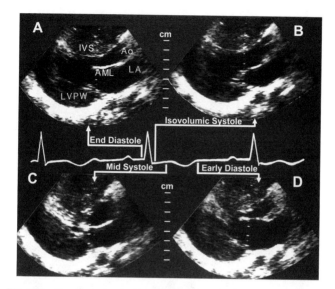

Fig. 4.10. Two-dimensional echocardiography in hypertrophic cardiomyopathy. Four sequential frames from a left parasternal long axis view of a patient with hypertrophic cardiomyopathy. The thick interventricular septum (*IVS*) and left ventricular posterior walls (*LVPW*) obliterate the small left ventricular cavity and impinge on the mitral apparatus by midsystole.

of stress echo images. Whereas the specificity of stress echo is high, the sensitivity may not be as high as thallium or isonitrile techniques. Certain groups of investigators, however, have achieved excellent results when comparing it to nuclear imaging. Intravenous injection of sonicated albumin can enhance the visualization of the endocardium in patients who are difficult to image with standard ultrasound. For patients unable to perform exercise, pharmacologic stress with dobutamine can be used in conjunction with echocardiography to assess the presence and severity of ischemic heart disease. Dipyridamole and adenosine also have been used but less so than dobutamine. Exercise echo remains the best modality for predicting the extent of coronary artery disease, followed by dobutamine stress ultrasound imaging and, lastly, dipyridamole.

DOBUTAMINE ECHO FOR ASSESSMENT OF MYOCARDIAL VIABILITY

Dobutamine echocardiography also can be used in the assessment of myocardial viability before anticipated coronary revascularization. Both acute and chronic ischemia can impair contractility of viable myocardium. Revascularization of viable but ischemic myocardium can improve significantly the morbidity and mortality of patients with coronary disease and left ventricular dysfunction. A biphasic response to dobutamine stimulation with improvement in wall motion and increased systolic thickening at low doses (5 to 7.5 µg/kg/min) with worsening at higher doses (more than 7.5 µg/kg/

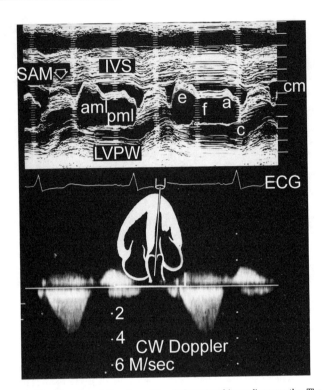

Fig. 4.11. M-mode and Doppler outflow in hypertrophic cardiomyopathy. The interventricular septum (*IVS*) is 4-cm thick, whereas the left ventricular posterior wall (*LVPW*) is 1.6 cm, indicating asymmetric hypertrophy. Systolic anterior motion (*SAM*) of the multilayers of the mitral apparatus is seen in systole. In diastole, the anterior mitral leaflet (*aml*) affects the IVS and the e-f slope is reduced by the slow emptying of the left atrium into the noncompliant LV (similar to mitral stenosis in Fig. 4.5). The continuous wave Doppler signal has a late peak velocity at 4 M/second, indicating a dynamic pressure gradient of 64 mm Hg.

min) suggests dysfunctional but viable myocardium. Continued improvement in wall motion can be seen in myopathic ventricles of nonischemic etiology and has poor predictive value. Nonviable, scarred myocardium would not show improvement in wall motion with either low- or high-dose dobutamine. Myocardial contrast echocardiography involves injecting sonicated albumin into a coronary artery during cardiac catheterization and observing by transthoracic echo the distribution of the agent into the myocardium. Collateral flow to ischemic myocardium indicates viability.

ECHOCARDIOGRAPHY IN CARDIOVASCULAR EMERGENCIES

As noted earlier in this chapter, echocardiography is heavily dependent on the technical expertise in obtaining diagnostic images and in their interpretation. This expertise is especially important in

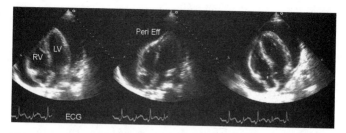

Fig. 4.12. Acute pericardial tamponade with electrical alternans. Three sequential systolic frames from an apical window in a patient with pericardial tamponade demonstrate the pendular swinging of the heart is at half the frequency of the heart rate, so that alternate systoles find the heart pointing left and then right, registering alternating QRS complexes on the electrocardiogram.

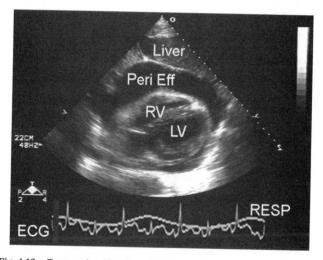

Fig. 4.13. Tamponade with right ventricular diastolic collapse. This is the same patient shown in Fig. 4.10, demonstrating a subcostal view in diastole with the right ventricular collapse. The phase of respiration is shown on the undulating line; this frame was exposed during expiration. The right ventricle's ability to fill is disadvantaged during expiration because the left ventricle is receiving venous return from the lungs at higher pressure. During inspiration (*not shown*), the right ventricle fills at the expense of the left because the pulmonary veins are intrathoracic and subjected to negative inspiratory pressure, whereas the right heart fills from extrathoracic veins.

cardiovascular emergencies in which the patient may be unable to cooperate and time is of the essence. Some noteworthy scenarios would include the following:

- **Pericardial tamponade** (Figs. 4.12 and 4.13)
- **Aortic dissection**
- **Ventricular septal rupture (in myocardial infarction)**
- **Acute valvar regurgitation**
- **Prosthetic valve malfunction**
- **Myxoma of the left atrium**

When used appropriately, echocardiography can play a vital role in the diagnosis and management of patients with suspected cardiovascular emergencies because of its unique ability to define the functional anatomy of the heart at the bedside noninvasively and in real time. Rapid detection of potentially salvageable life-threatening emergencies such as pericardial tamponade (see Fig. 4.9) and aortic dissection can lead to early intervention. Similarly, detection of a wall motion abnormality in a patient with a suspected acute coronary syndrome but equivocal electrocardiographic changes can lead to the earlier application of percutaneous coronary intervention and myocardial salvage.

CONCLUDING REMARKS

This chapter is going to press on the fiftieth anniversary of the discovery of echocardiography. The early promise of this invaluable technique has been exceeded beyond any expectations, and its future is bright. The number of lives it has saved by timely diagnosis is incalculable.

The invaluable assistance of David Criley, Blaufuss Multimedia, LLC, in the preparation of the illustrations is gratefully acknowledged.

SELECTED READINGS

Edler I, Hertz CH: Use of ultrasonic reflectoscope for continuous recording of movement of heart walls. *Kungl Fysiogr Sallsk I Lund Forhandl* 24:40, 1954.

Feigenbaum H: *Echocardiography*, 4th ed. Philadelphia: Lea & Febiger, 1994.

Hatle L, Angelsen B: *Doppler ultrasound in cardiology: physical principles and clinical applications*, 2nd ed. Philadelphia: Lea & Febiger, 1985.

Nishimura RA, Abel MD, Hatle LK, et al: Assessment of diastolic function of the heart: background and current applications of Doppler echocardiography. Part II. Clinical studies. *Mayo Clin Proc* 64:181, 1989.

Nishimura RA, Housmans PR, Hatle LK, et al: Assessment of diastolic function of the heart: background and current applications of Doppler echocardiography. Part I. Physiologic and pathophysiologic features. *Mayo Clin Proc* 64:71, 1989.

Nishimura RA, Miller FA, Callahan MI, et al: Doppler echocardiography: theory, instrumentation, technique, and application. *Mayo Clin Proc* 60:321, 1985.

Oh JK, Seward JB, Tajik AJ: *The echo manual*. Philadelphia: Lippincott-Raven Publishers, 1998.

Popp RL: Echocardiography (Part 1). *N Engl J Med* 323:101, 1990; (Part 2) *N Engl J Med* 323:165, 1990.

NUCLEAR CARDIOLOGY

In the last 25 years, nuclear cardiology has developed rapid, accurate, noninvasive means for evaluating regional myocardial perfusion and quantitating cardiovascular performance. The technical advances that have made this possible include the availability of appropriate radiopharmaceutical agents, high-performance gamma-scintillation cameras, and low-cost computer equipment that allows rapid data acquisition and analysis. The noninvasive nature of these techniques has resulted in widespread applicability and acceptance.

Cardiac imaging procedures can be separated into four broad categories:

1. Gamma imaging
2. Positron emission tomography (PET)
3. Computed tomography (CT)
4. Magnetic resonance imaging (MRI)

GAMMA IMAGING

Myocardial perfusion imaging assesses myocardial blood flow by using radiopharmaceutical agents, which are injected into the bloodstream and accumulate in the myocytes (1). **Thallium-201** and **technetium-99 (Tc99m) sestamibi or tetrofosmin** are radioisotopes delivered to all organs of the body in relative proportion to the blood flow each organ receives. The heart accumulates thallium-201 in areas of viable myocardium in proportion to blood flow to those regions. The greater the perfusion of blood to a region of the myocardium, the greater the uptake of thallium-201 to that region. Regions with decreased blood flow are represented by decreased or absent thallium uptake and are seen as "cold spots." Imaging can be performed either in planar or tomographic format; the latter procedure is referred to as **single photon emission computed tomography (SPECT).**

The most widely used clinical application for myocardial perfusion imaging is stress testing with either thallium-201 or Tc99m radiopharmaceutical (discussed later in this chapter) (2). During this procedure, the patient undergoes stress testing with an intravenous line in place. Approximately 1 minute before stopping exercise, the radiopharmaceutical agent is injected intravenously, and soon thereafter the patient is taken to the nuclear medicine department where the gamma-scintillation camera is used to image the myocardium (stress phase). In areas of decreased myocardial blood flow, diminished uptake of pharmaceutical agent can be seen (2). If repeat images are obtained 3 or 4 hours later at rest (redistribution phase), changes from the stress images will reflect changes in regional myocardial blood flow occurring with exercise. Thus, "cold spots" that are seen with maximal exercise and disappear with rest indicate regions of the myocardium that have decreased blood flow with exercise but adequate blood flow at rest. Areas of reversible hypoperfusion, corresponding to reversible ischemia, indicate areas of significant obstructions to coronary artery blood flow. A "fixed defect" is an area of hypoperfusion that is seen on both rest and stress imaging and implies that there is myocardial scarring. Homogeneous uptake of the radioisotope on both rest and stress imaging suggests normal myocardial perfusion.

The standard treadmill stress test has specificity of 70% to 80%, depending on the population under study. A nuclear stress test has a specificity of more than 90% (depending on the experience and quality control of the laboratory). Soft-tissue attenuation can be seen in patients who are obese or who have large breasts or elevated diaphragms. This can lead to a significant incidence of false-positive results. A normal nuclear stress test makes the diagnosis of significant coronary artery disease (CAD) very unlikely. However, balanced coronary stenosis (such as significant left main, as well as right coronary stenosis) can appear as homogeneous hypoperfusion and may be missed by nuclear scintigraphy. The sensitivity of the nuclear stress testing is more than 85%. In contrast, the sensitivity of standard electrocardiogram (ECG) treadmill testing is 60% to 70% (3–5).

Nuclear "cold spot" imaging is useful in a number of situations, including the following:

1. Diagnosis of CAD, particularly in patients with a conflicting database (e.g., suspected false-positive stress ECG; false-negative stress ECG with a convincing history for angina; preexisting ST-segment and T-wave ECG abnormalities such as left bundle branch block, digitalis therapy, left ventricular hypertrophy, etc.)

2. Evaluation of patency of coronary artery bypass grafts, particularly in patients with chest pain after bypass surgery

3. Determination of the physiologic significance of coronary artery stenosis discovered by coronary angiography

4. Detection of additionally jeopardized myocardium after a myocardial infarction suggesting multivessel CAD

5. Diagnosis, sizing, and localization of acute myocardial infarction, with an accuracy approaching 100%, if a resting nuclear study is done within 6 hours of the onset of symptoms. "Cold spot" defect resolution strongly suggests coronary artery spasm. Small infarcts, subendocardial infarcts, and scans performed later than 24 hours after the onset of symptoms all can result in negative scans.

6. Patients with dilated cardiomyopathy may have characteristic nuclear scans. Patients with ischemic disease as an etiology for their dilated cardiomyopathy typically demonstrate multiple large perfusion defects. In contrast, patients with idiopathic dilated cardiomyopathy generally have homogeneous uptake of perfusion radioisotopes in the myocardium.

7. Patients with sarcoidosis and myocardial involvement may have nuclear scans with multiple patchy left ventricular (LV) perfusion defects.

8. Assessment of viable myocardium is helpful in ischemic cardiomyopathy with depressed LV function, as well as in fixed perfusion defects. In the former, determination of viable myocardium is helpful when deciding whether a patient would be a suitable candidate for myocardial revascularization versus cardiac transplantation. In the

latter, imaging can assist in deciding if revascularization is indicated for myocardium that may be viable or have significant periinfarction ischemia. Although PET scanning (discussed later) is more accurate, thallium can be used when PET scanning is unavailable (6). Several protocols can be used. In one method, the patient is injected with thallium-201 at peak exercise and scanned at 4 to 6 hours. If a fixed defect is seen, then rescanning at 24 hours may show redistribution suggesting viability and potential benefit from revascularization. Another method of assessing viability is by injecting thallium at peak exercise with scanning 3 to 4 hours later, followed by reinjection of thallium the next day and rescanning at 24 hours. Early and delayed rest thallium imaging (performed at 3 and 24 hours) without exercise is yet another way to assess myocardial viability and may be the most accurate of the techniques using thallium.

Tc99mm agents (Tc99mm complexed with 2-methoxy isobutyl isonitrile or tetrofosmin) accumulate in myocardium in proportion to blood flow (1). This combination also is known as Cardiolyte (produced by DuPont), RP-30, Tc99m-MIBI, Tc99m-isonitrile, and Tc99m-hexamibi. Tc-99m agents are accumulated rapidly in proportion to regional blood flow by passive diffusion and bind to mitochondrial membranes. The agent remains in myocardium several hours but is cleared from the blood rapidly, allowing for excellent contrast. Logistically, the patient exercises, and the agent is administered intravenously 1 minute before the end of exertion. The patient usually waits 30 to 60 minutes before being brought to the nuclear medicine department (or the nuclear camera) for image acquisition. If a defect is seen in the myocardium (indicative of regional hypoperfusion as a result of coronary narrowing), then the patient must return the following day for a reinjection and repeat image acquisition. If on repeat scan the defect remains, then this indicates myocardial scar or old infraction. However, if on repeat injection, the defect is no longer present, then this indicates that the patient has ischemia and probably a high-grade stenosis in the coronary artery supplying that segment of myocardium.

Dual isotope imaging using thallium-201 at rest and technetium agents with exercise allows same day imaging and obviates the need for the patient to return on the second day (7). The advantages that Tc-99m agents have over thallium include the following:

1. Because Tc-99m agents have no redistribution and slow washout, image acquisition can be done up to 4 hours after the injection. In contrast, thallium imaging must be done within minutes of injection, so that redistribution does not begin, and potential perfusion defects do not fill in.

2. The photon energy of Tc-99m agents is higher (140 keV) than that of thallium (80 keV), allowing better contrast and potentially fewer false-positive results because of artifact or soft-tissue attenuation.

3. If administered while the patient is under the nuclear camera, Tc-99m agents can be used for first-pass ventriculography of the right and left ventricle (see later in this chapter). This allows for the determination of wall motion and biventricular function, as well as regional perfusion with the same agent. Thallium does not provide adequate counts for radionuclide angiography.

4. Tc-99m agents can be prepared easily, whereas thallium must be generated in a linear accelerator and then delivered to the institution.

5. Tc-99m agents can be used to assess the efficacy of thrombolysis in the setting of acute myocardial infarction (8).

Tc99mm teboroxime is another isonitrile perfusion agent that has high myocardial extraction and washout. Two injections must be made, as in the Tc-99m sestamibi examination. However, because of the rapid washout, the patient must be imaged within 2 minutes of exercise and image acquisition must be completed within 10 minutes. Although Tc-99m teboroxime may have an advantage in pharmacologic vasodilator imaging studies where the patient is usually near the scintillation camera, it may be impractical when patients cannot be transported or imaged quickly. Because it is a technetium compound, first-pass wall motion and ejection fraction can be performed. As a result of the rapid washout, reinjection and imaging can be done within 2 hours of the initial injection, allowing for a more expeditious examination (9,10).

Some patients are unable to perform adequate exercise because of severe claudication, orthopedic disability, poor exercise tolerance, or chronotropic incompetence. The use of intravenous vasodilator substances in conjunction with nuclear perfusion imaging (thallium or Tc-99m isotopes) can assist in the evaluation of patients who cannot exercise (11,12). Dipyridamole is a phosphodiesterase inhibitor that dilates the resistance coronary vessels and produces a relative hypoperfusion in myocardium served by stenotic coronary arteries. Adenosine is a purine molecule that is naturally produced intracellularly in the body and used in various metabolic pathways. When administered intravenously, it is a potent coronary vasodilator and can be used with perfusion agents to detect relative areas of hypoperfusion. These agents are contraindicated in patients with asthma or bronchospastic lung disease. Adenosine is contraindicated in patients with significant conduction system disease. Vasodilator perfusion imaging has been demonstrated to be useful in evaluating cardiac patients anticipating noncardiac surgery, as well as in predicting postmyocardial infarction complications (13,14).

Dobutamine administered intravenously with or without atropine also can be used to increase the heart rate and simulate exercise, especially in patients who cannot tolerate dipyridamole or adenosine. Generally, an infusion is started at a rate of 10 μg/kg/minute for 3 minutes and then increased by 10 μg/kg/minute increments every 3 minutes to a maximum of 40 μg/kg/minute. If the heart rate is not 85% predicted maximum for age, then atropine, 0.2 mg, is given incrementally to a maximum of 1 mg (15).

RADIONUCLIDE ANGIOGRAPHY

Another class of cardiac imaging procedures is radionuclide angiography, sometimes called radionuclide ventriculography, multigated acquisition (MUGA), or intravenous ventriculography. This technique allows visualization of the atria and ventricles using radioactive intravascular indicators to create pictures of the great vessels and chambers of the heart (16).

There are two types of radionuclide ventriculography: the first-pass method and the gated-equilibrium method. In the first-pass method, a bolus of a technetium compound (e.g., technetium sodium pertechnetate) is injected intravenously, and sequential cardiac images are obtained at a rapid rate during the initial passage of the radiotracer through the great vessels and chambers of the heart. The tracer first passes through the superior vena cava and the right-sided chambers of the heart. Because the tracer moves through the lungs rapidly, good separation of the right and left heart chambers can be achieved. Background activity is minimized because most of the radiopharmaceutical is in the heart itself during imaging. The first-pass study can be done rapidly.

Using the gated-equilibrium method of blood pool imaging, red blood cells are labeled with technetium, which allows continuous imaging of the heart chambers. Gating means obtaining a repetitive image of the heart at a predetermined time after the QRS complex. Each cardiac cycle is divided into a series of segments by the computer, and tracer counts from corresponding segments of the cardiac cycle from multiple heart beats are added together to create one summed picture of the cardiac chambers at one set time in the cardiac cycle. This allows for an averaged picture of the cardiac chambers from systole to diastole.

Both methods allow the calculation of end-systolic and end-diastolic counts. Therefore, calculation of ventricular ejection fractions can be performed using the end-diastolic counts minus end-systolic counts (stroke count) divided by end-diastolic counts. The ejection fractions so calculated are highly correlated with values obtained by standard contrast ventriculography at cardiac catheterizations.

Regional wall motion abnormalities can be detected by displaying the end-diastolic and end-systolic images in a static format. In addition, sequential frames of the cardiac cycle can be displayed on a video monitor to create a "movie" of ventricular function over an entire cardiac cycle. This helps in the precise localization of regional wall motion abnormalities.

Ventricular volumes can be determined using data from gated radionuclide ventriculograms. Geometric formulas usually used with routine contrast ventriculograms have been utilized to approximate ventricular volumes. Another technique for volume determination compares the isotope activity in a known volume of the patient's blood drawn at the time of the radionuclide ventriculogram. This allows conversion of isotope counts in the ventricle to volume in the ventricle.

A priori, the right ventricular (RV) stroke volume and LV stroke volume should be equal. In the presence of aortic regurgitation (AR) or mitral regurgitation (MR), however, LV stroke volume will be greater than RV stroke volume, and the difference will represent the regurgitation fraction.

LV aneurysms can be detected using radionuclide ventriculography. LV aneurysms result in systolic images protruding beyond diastolic images and the regional difference representing aneurysmal dilatation.

RV ejection fractions can be calculated from both first-pass and gated studies. Radionuclide ventriculograms revealing dilation of the right ventricle and a reduced RV ejection fraction are seen in RV infarcts.

In normal hearts, exercise results in an increase in the LV ejection fraction. However, CAD results in a decline or no change in ejection fraction with exercise. Radionuclide ventriculography detects this decrease in ejection fraction, as well as regional wall motion abnormalities with exercise. The sensitivity of exercise radionuclide ventriculography for detecting coronary disease is better than that using exercise electrocardiography alone and is similar to exercise thallium-201 scans. The specificity of the technique is similar to that of the stress ECG. Advantages of radionuclide ventriculography include a lower cost for Tc99mm than for thallium-201 and the ability of radionuclide ventriculography to assess ventricular function—information thallium scans cannot provide. Disadvantages include the requirement for computer acquisition and processing of the study information. Tc99mm radioisotopes, however, can provide both perfusion and wall motion information and essentially has replaced radionuclide ventriculography in the assessment of patients with suspected CAD in many centers.

Radionuclide ventriculography provides useful information about chronic valvular heart disease, particularly regarding aortic and mitral regurgitation. These data may be useful in the timing of valve replacement surgery. Compensated regurgitant lesions (AR, MR) result in an increased stroke volume. There is an increased end-diastolic volume with a normal end-systolic volume. With time, chronic valvular regurgitant lesions result in progressive dysfunction of the left ventricle, marked by a decrease in resting ejection fraction and failure to increase ejection fraction with exercise. In addition, an increase in end-systolic volume is seen. These very sensitive indicators of worsening LV function may be of value in assessing a patient's need for valve replacement.

The first-pass method can predict accurately the presence and extent of left-to-right cardiac shunts. A technetium compound is injected intravenously and followed as it passes through the right heart, the lungs, and then the left heart. A computer-derived region of interest is placed over the area of interest (e.g., lung), and the computer plots the counts that occur in that region over time. In normal patients, the pulmonary time-activity curve shows an initial peak as the tracer moves through the lungs, followed by a later smaller secondary peak resulting from "recirculation" as part of the tracer bolus reappears in the lungs after having traveled through the systemic circulation. A left-to-right intracardiac shunt results in the early and prominent reappearance of the secondary peak curve because of the early reappearance of the tracer that took a "shortcut" through the shunt back to the right heart rather than the longer route through the systemic circulation. A normal shunt study effectively excludes an intracardiac left-to-right shunt of any clinical significance. Right-to-left shunts may be detected by early appearance of tracer in the left-sided chambers, in the aorta, or over the kidneys.

Echocardiography (with transesophageal imaging, if necessary) has been more useful in the qualitative detection of intracardiac shunts. However, in larger shunts, nuclear-derived shunt ratios can be complementary in the evaluation of patients that have undergone echocardiographic examinations. It is now also possible to quantitate shunts with MRI.

INFARCT AVID IMAGING

The other type of myocardial imaging is the infarct avid imaging or **technetium pyrophosphate** scan. This discussion is largely historical, especially now that we have MRI delayed enhancement. Pyrophosphate forms complexes with deposits of calcium. Infarction results in the influx of calcium and phosphate ions. In infarcted areas, interaction of the pyrophosphate and calcium occurs in the damaged myocardial tissue and subsequently is detected as a "hot spot" when viewed with a gamma camera (1,2). Additional information about infarct avid imaging can be found in previous editions of this book.

POSITRON EMISSION TOMOGRAPHY

PET scan imaging is useful in the detection of CAD and in the assessment of myocardial viability in patients with coronary disease and LV dysfunction (17,18). Rubidium-82 and ammonia labeled with nitrogen-13 are tracers used for the evaluation of regional myocardial blood flow. Fluorodeoxyglucose (FDG) and carbon-11 acetate are used for evaluation of glucose and fatty-acid metabolism, respectively. If perfusion testing with rubidium-82 or nitrogen-13 ammonia demonstrates decreased flow and metabolic testing with FDG or carbon-11 acetate demonstrates absent metabolic activity, then that region of myocardium would be considered nonviable or necrotic (matched depression of perfusion and metabolism). However, if flow appeared reduced by the perfusion tracers but metabolic activity was preserved, then that region of myocardium would be considered ischemic and viable (mismatched depression of perfusion with preserved metabolism) (7). Limited widespread availability and cost have prevented general use of PET scanning (19).

Although PET is considered the gold standard for assessment of viability, thallium techniques are a cost-effective alternative (see earlier in this chapter). **Fluorine-18** (F-18) injection combined with **SPECT** imaging allows the use of a metabolic agent with a standard SPECT camera, which is more widely available than PET. Perfusion assessed by thallium-201 imaging combined with F-18 metabolic imaging compares favorably with thallium-201 stress-reinjection and dobutamine echo in assessing myocardial recovery after revascularization (20).

Dobutamine echocardiography is another technique that can be used in the assessment of myocardial viability. (See Chapter 4.)

COMPUTED TOMOGRAPHY

CT can be performed with electron beam and multidetector machines. Electron beam computed tomography (EBCT) has been used to quantify and localize coronary calcium. Because the atherosclerotic plaque commonly is associated with calcium, detection of coronary artery calcium may be helpful in the screening of patients at risk for CAD. This test can be performed quickly, noninvasively, and with no need for contrast injection. The absence of calcium in the coronaries has a high negative predictive value (95%) for significant lesions of greater than 50% luminal diameter stenosis. However, the specificity of an abnormal scan is not good, ranging from 45% to 66% for significant disease. Many atherosclerotic plaques have calcium, but are not flow limiting. EBCT may be useful for screening high-risk individuals to help guide risk-factor modification, as well as for the evaluation of patients at low risk for coronary disease who have atypical features for angina. Because this test does not exclude the presence of obstructive or unstable plaques, it should not be used as an alternative for angiography in the definition of coronary anatomy (21,22). CT angiography provides cross-sectional imaging of coronary arteries with intravenous injection of contrast. EBCT angiography requires patients to hold their breath for approximately 40 seconds. Furthermore, it has been shown that substantial segmental calcifications may lead to false-negative results (23). Multidetector angiography requires lowering the patient's heart rate to less than 60 beats per minute in addition to a 40-second breath hold for proper imaging (24). Future developments with faster and enhanced acquisition will help facilitate the detection and grading of stenoses of coronary arteries.

CARDIAC MAGNETIC RESONANCE IMAGING

The clinical role of MRI in cardiology has been limited, but is increasing as a result of its improved clinical efficiency and the lack of ionizing radiation or an iodinated contrast agent. An MRI machine uses magnets and electricity to cause hydrogen ions within cells to resonate and emit radiofrequency energy. This energy is detected by the machine and converted into an image. With current MRI machines, these images can be generated into 3-D projections, allowing the analyzer to "slice" an image in any plane for precise and detailed anatomic evaluation of structures. Current uses of cardiac MRI include evaluating aortic dissection in the preoperative patient, studying rare cardiac tumors, and mapping congenital anomalies to better plan corrective surgery. Recent innovations have boosted the role of cardiac MRI to include the evaluation of cardiac viability, ischemia, and cardiomyopathy (25). Coronary magnetic resonance angiography has been used to detect CAD (26–28). However, the role of CT likely will be better suited for imaging CAD, whereas MRI will be used for assessment of plaque composition (24).

REFERENCES

1. Zaret BL, Wackers FJ: Nuclear cardiology. Part 1. *N Engl J Med* 329: 775, 1993.
2. Mayo Clinic Cardiovascular Working Group on Stress Testing: Cardiovascular stress testing: a description of the various stress tests and indications for their use. *Mayo Clin Proc* 71:43, 1996.
3. Kotler TS, Diamond GA: Exercise thallium-201 scintigraphy in the diagnosis and prognosis of coronary artery disease. *Ann Intern Med* 113:684, 1990.
4. Beller GA: Diagnostic accuracy of thallium-201 myocardial perfusion imaging. *Circulation* 84 (Suppl I):I-1, 1991.
5. Ritchie JL, Bateman TM, Bonow RO, et al: Guidelines for clinical use of cardiac radionuclide imaging. A report of the American Heart Association/American College of Cardiology Task Force on Assessment of Diagnostic and Therapeutic Cardiovascular Procedures (Committee on Radionuclide Imaging)—developed in collaboration with the American Society of Nuclear Cardiology. *Circulation* 91: 1278, 1995.
6. Hendel RC, Chaudhry FA, Bonow RO: Myocardial viability. *Curr Prob Cardiol* 21:145, 1996.
7. Berman DS, Kiat H, Friedman JD, et al: Separate acquisition rest thallium-201/stress technetium-99m sestamibi dual-isotope myocardial perfusion single-photon emission computed tomography: a clinical validation study. *J Am Coll Cardiol* 22:1455, 1993.

8. Gibbons RJ: Perfusion imaging with 99mTc-sestamibi for the assessment of myocardial area at risk and the efficacy of acute treatment in myocardial infarction. *Circulation* 84(Suppl I):I-37, 1991

9. Berman DS, Kiat H, Maddahi J: The new 99m-Tc myocardial perfusion imaging agents: 99mTc-sestamibi and 99mTc-teboroxime. *Circulation* 84(Suppl I):I-7, 1991.

10. Johnson LL: Clinical experience with technetium 99m teboroxime. *Semin Nucl Med* 21(3):182,1991.

11. Coyne EP, Belvedere DA, Vande Streek PR, et al: Thallium-201 scintigraphy after intravenous infusion of adenosine compared with exercise thallium testing in the diagnosis of coronary artery disease. *J Am Coll Cardiol* 17:1289, 1991.

12. Taillefer R, Amyot R, Turpin S, et al: Comparison between dipyridamole and adenosine as pharmacologic coronary vasodilators in detection of coronary artery disease with thallium-201 imaging. *J Nucl Cardiol* 3:204, 1996.

13. Eagle KA, Brundage BH, Chaitman BR, et al: Guidelines for perioperative cardiovascular evaluation for noncardiac surgery. Report of the American College of Cardiology/American Heart Association Task Force on Practice Guidelines (Committee on Perioperative Cardiovascular Evaluation for Noncardiac Surgery). *Circulation* 93:1278, 1996.

14. Heller GV, Herman SD, Travin MI, et al: Independent prognostic value of intravenous dipyridamole with technetium-99m sestamibi tomographic imaging in predicting cardiac events and cardiac-related hospital admissions. *J Am Coll Cardiol* 26:1202, 1995.

15. Geleijnse ML, Elhendy A, Van Domburg RT, et al: Prognostic value of dobutamine-atropine stress technetium-99m sestamibi perfusion scintigraphy in patients with chest pain. *J Am Coll Cardiol* 28:447, 1996.

16. Aurigemma GP, Gaasch WH, Villegas B, et al: Noninvasive assessment of left ventricular mass, chamber volume, and contractile function. *Curr Prob Cardiol* 20:361, 1995.

17. Keck A, Hertting K, Schwartz Y, et al: Electromechanical mapping for determination of myocardial contractility and viability. A comparison with echocardiography, myocardial single-photon emission computed tomography, and positron emission tomography. *J Am Coll Cardiol* 40(6):1067–1074, 2002.

18. Rohatgi R, Epstein S, Henriquez J, et al: Utility of positron emission tomography in predicting cardiac events and survival in patients with coronary artery disease and severe left ventricular dysfunction. *Am J Cardiol* 87(9):1096–1099, A6, 2001.

19. Bonow RO, Berman DS, Gibbons RJ, et al: Cardiac positron emission tomography. A report for health professionals from the Committee on Advanced Cardiac Imaging and Technology of the Council on Clinical Cardiology, American Heart Association. *Circulation* 84(1): 447, 1991.

20. Bax JJ, Cornel JH, Visser FC, et al: Prediction of myocardial dysfunction after revascularization. Comparison of fluorine-18 fluorodeoxyglucose/thallium-201 SPECT, thallium-201 stress-reinjection SPECT, and dobutamine echocardiography. *J Am Coll Cardiol* 28:558, 1996.

21. Rumberg JA, Sheedy PF, Breen JF, et al: Electron beam computed tomography and coronary artery disease: scanning for coronary artery calcification. *Mayo Clin Proc* 71:369, 1996.

22. Wexler L, Brundage BB, Crouse JC, et al: Coronary artery calcification: pathophysiology, epidemiology, imaging methods, and clinical applications. A statement for health professions from the American Heart Association. *Circulation* 94:1175, 1996.

23. Schmermund A, Rensing BJ, Sheedy PF, et al. Intravenous electron-beam computed tomographic coronary angiography for segmental analysis of coronary artery stenoses. *J Am Coll Cardiol* 31: 1547–1554, 1998.

24. Fayad ZA, Fuster V, Nikolaou K, et al: Computed tomography and magnetic resonance imaging for noninvasive coronary angiography and plaque imaging: current and potential future concepts. *Circulation* 106(15):2026–2034, 2002.

25. Hundley WG, Morgan TM, Neagle CM, et al. Magnetic resonance imaging determination of cardiac prognosis. *Circulation* 106(18): 2328–2333, 2002.

26. Plein S, Ridgway JP, Jones TR, et al. Coronary artery disease: assessment with a comprehensive MR imaging protocol—initial results. *Radiology* 225(1):300–307, 2002.

27. Kim WY, Danias PG, Stuber M, et al: Coronary magnetic resonance angiography for the detection of coronary stenoses. *N Engl J Med* 345:1863, 2001.

28. Schwitter J, Nanz D, Kneifel S, et al: Assessment of myocardial perfusion in coronary artery disease by magnetic resonance: a comparison with positron emission tomography and coronary angiography. *Circulation* 103(18):2230–2235, 2001.

CARDIAC CATHETERIZATION

Many cardiac problems can be properly diagnosed and treated without the need for invasive procedures. In some clinical situations, cardiac catheterization may be required to manage the patient with cardiac problems. The decision to study a patient invasively is one that should be considered carefully. The clinician must take into consideration the clinical setting, the patient's age, and past medical and/or surgical history of the suspected cardiac problem. The individual performing the procedure is performing a high-level consultation—not merely a laboratory test. He or she should have a thorough knowledge of the patient and, most importantly, of what questions must be answered by the procedure in the specific patient undergoing study.

Before the patient consents to an invasive study, he or she must be informed of the risks of the procedure. Although the risks vary depending on the type of case, cardiac catheterization in a stable patient is very safe with competent personnel and carries a less than 1% probability of morbidity. The risks are amplified in patients who are elderly or infirm and in patients who are not physiologically or psychologically stable at the time of the procedure. Coronary angiography is a safe procedure, with the risks of a major adverse event [e.g., stroke, myocardial infarction (MI), major bleeding] being less than 0.5%. Overall mortality is less than 0.2% (1). Other complications include local thrombosis, embolism, cardiac perforation, significant arrhythmias, and allergy to contrast media.

The referring physician should be satisfied that the procedure can be done safely and adequately and that the laboratory has the ability to answer the clinical questions. Not all catheterization laboratories are equipped properly with a wide range of laboratory equipment, and not all catheterization personnel have adequate training and experience.

Patients with ischemic heart disease constitute the majority of cases in the average cardiac catheterization laboratory. The principal information needed in these cases is an angiographic demonstration of the nature and extent of disease in the coronary arteries, the left ventricular filling pressure, ejection fraction, size, wall motion, and valvular competence. Patients with congenital or valvular heart disease require more elaborate physiologic studies to identify the anatomic relationships, pressures, and regional blood flow in the central circulation (2,3).

During the 1980s, the cardiac catheterization laboratory was the site of significant changes as it evolved from strictly a diagnostic arena to the place of therapeutic interventions. Balloon angioplasty was the backbone of the interventional procedures in this period. Percutaneous transluminal coronary angioplasty (PTCA) changed extensively following the first procedure by Gruentzig in 1977. Initially, PTCA was limited to single-vessel lesions in patients with coronary artery disease (CAD) who were symptomatic and undergoing medical therapy. Later this evolved to a much broader spectrum of patients undergoing this nonsurgical technique, including those with multivessel CAD, patients with previous coronary artery bypass grafting (CABG) surgery and stenosis in the native or graft vessels, patients with acute myocardial infarction (AMI) who present early in their course to a properly equipped facility, patients with total occlusions, and certain high-risk surgical cases (elderly patients with renal failure, systemic disease, and some with severe left ventricular dysfunction).

In experienced hands, PTCA is a low-risk procedure with 1% or less mortality and approximately 5% morbidity, including MI, arrhythmia, infection, bleeding, and the need for emergency CABG because of dissection or acute closure (4). The success rate for experienced operators is 90% per vessel dilated. Certain advantages of PTCA make it an attractive alternative to surgery (e.g., it is less expensive, it does not necessitate general anesthesia and thoracotomy, and duration of hospitalization is shorter). The major pitfall of PTCA is restenosis, which is a complex problem that occurs in 30% to 50% of cases. Restenosis occurs to a variable degree in virtually all lesions (5). The terms *acute gain, late loss,* and *net gain* have been used to describe the relationship between lumen diameter at baseline, immediately after intervention, and during follow-up. *Acute gain* is the difference in lumen diameter before and immediately after intervention and is the result of arterial expansion or plaque removal. *Late loss* is the difference in lumen diameter after intervention and at follow-up; late loss is the result of intimal hyperplasia, elastic recoil, and vascular remodeling.

In the majority of restenosis cases, the clinical presentation of restenosis is recurrent angina and not MI or sudden death. This may be explained by the fact that restenotic lesions, which consist of intimal hyperplasia and fibrous tissue, are less prone to rupture and acutely thrombose. Angiographic analysis suggests that early recoil is associated with a high incidence of restenosis. It appears that restenosis involves not only intimal proliferative hyperplasia but also remodeling (both positive and negative remodeling). Whatever the mechanisms involved, the most powerful indicator of restenosis is a high degree of residual plaque.

Pharmacologic approaches to the prevention of restenosis involving more than 20 candidate drugs have shown very disappointing results to this point. Stenting has had an enormous impact in lowering restenosis rates, accounting for a 30% to 50% decrease (6). Stenting prevents elastic recoil and constrictive remodeling; however, stenting increases neointimal proliferation. Because present-day use of stents involves more than 80% of interventions, in-stent restenosis is a major challenge.

The use of intracoronary radiation has been shown to be very effective in reducing neointimal hyperplasia with both beta and gamma radiation and has been approved for use (7,8). The long-term effects of brachytherapy remain to be determined. Another promising approach to restenosis is the use of a drug-eluting stent (9).

DEVICES FOR CORONARY INTERVENTION

From 1979 to 1990, balloon angioplasty was the only modality for coronary intervention. Despite an explosive growth in the use of the procedure, PTCA still was plagued by a number of limitations:

- Difficulty in crossing certain lesions, such as total occlusions
- Difficulty dilating rigid lesions, such as densely calcified lesions, or dilating osteal or elastic lesions, such as vein grafts
- Difficulty in preventing dissection-induced abrupt closure of the dilated vessel
- 30% to 50% incidence of restenosis in 6 months of follow-up

Interest in alternative modes of luminal enlargement grew with increasing recognition of the limitations of standard balloon angioplasty. Devices entered clinical testing in the late 1980s, and then gained FDA approval between 1990 and 1994.

STENTS

Stents serve as endoluminal scaffolds that resist elastic recoil and "tack up" dissections. Introduction of the intracoronary stent has revolutionized transcatheter intervention.

Kuntz and Baim postulated that a larger postprocedural lumen would affect restenosis rates favorably (i.e., "bigger is better") (5). The Palmaz-Schatz stent achieved the greatest acute gain and proved to reduce the incidence of restenosis compared to PTCA. Randomized trials such as the STRESS (Stent Restenosis Study) trial (6,10) and the BENESTENT (Belgium-Netherlands Stent) trial (11) have shown a decrease in restenosis for *de novo* lesions in native coronary arteries. The SAVED trial (Stenting of Angioplasty in Vein graft Disease) has demonstrated lower restenosis in saphenous vein (SV) grafts (12). Along with treating *de novo* lesions and SV graft lesions, stents have shown to be highly effective in the treatment of actual or threatened closure. Stenting success rates of more than 90% and reduced stent thrombosis rates of 1% to 3% with optimal higher pressure deployment techniques have catapulted the stent to *the most valuable available tool* for the interventional cardiologist (13). Stenting also has been shown to be valuable in certain aortoostial lesions, restenotic lesions, long lesions, chronic occlusions, and many cases of AMI.

Drug-eluting stents are a new technology using local delivery of immunosuppressive or antiproliferative agents, thus providing a biologic and mechanical approach to inhibit restenosis. Several agents have been studied, including sirolimus, paclitaxel, actinomycin, tacrolimus, and everolimus. The RAVEL trial (238 patients, 19 institutions) was the first multicenter trial of drug-eluting stents and the largest to date. The restenosis rate for the sirolimus drug-eluting stent group at 6 months was 0%, compared to 26.6% for the control group (14). There was also a significant reduction in angiographic late loss and major cardiac events. This new technique is the most promising technique in interventional treatment of CAD.

ATHERECTOMY

Atherectomy refers to removal rather than displacement of the plaque that comprises the lesion under treatment. Various atherectomy approaches have been developed.

Directional atherectomy (DVI Simpson AtheroCath) involves extracting plaque that has been excised by advancing a blade that is pushed down into a collecting nose cone. Early suboptimal directional atherectomy led to the disappointing results of the CAVEAT

(Coronary Angioplasty Versus Excision Atherectomy Trial) (15). Optimal directional atherectomy (aggressive tissue removal plus post-dilatation) has been shown by the BOAT (Balloon versus Optimal Atherectomy Trial) (16) and the OARS (Optimal Atherectomy Restenosis Study) trial (17) to provide significantly larger luminal diameters than seen in CAVEAT without sacrificing procedural safety. The major niche for this appears to be in the osteal lesions, which are not calcified, and in bifurcation lesions. Although the alternative stenting technique is the preferred technique in most labs, directional atherectomy still is used in a small number of interventions nationwide (less than 5%).

Rotational atherectomy involves a diamond chip–coated burr that rotates at speeds of 140,000 to 180,000 rpm and is advanced over a guide-wire. This device preferentially ablates hard or calcified tissue with resulting particles of less than 5 to 10 μ being liberated into the distal coronary circulation. Because of its unique niches in the calcified, osteal, and longer lesions, the rotablator is an important tool in most modern interventional laboratories (18,19).

Rotational coronary atherectomy combined with stenting (rotas-tenting) is an extremely effective approach in some cases by combining the benefits of debulking a lesion and then providing a maximal lumen scaffold to prevent recoil. Improvements in the technique and equipment have decreased problems of spasm, bradycardia, slow flow, and the "no flow" problems significantly.

Extraction atherectomy is performed with the transluminal extraction catheter and uses suction to remove thrombi. The device is felt to have some niche in removing thrombi in degenerated vein grafts (20); however, its cumbersome technology and complication rates have diminished its appeal. It is used in less than 1% of current interventions.

Laser atherectomy photochemically ablates plaque by using high-energy laser pulses transmitted through a catheter containing multiple optical fibers. Persistent problems of dissection, perforation, and high restenosis rates of greater than 50% have markedly diminished the enthusiasm for this device, and it accounts for less than 1% of interventions nationwide (21).

OTHER NEW DEVICES IN INTERVENTIONAL CARDIOLOGY

The **cutting balloon** performs a microsurgical dilatation with extremely sharp atherotomes, which are housed on a balloon. This device has been promising for rigid lesions, ostial lesions, and to some degree for in-stent restenosis lesions (22).

Thrombus-removing devices are thrombectomy catheters effective in removing thrombus in cases of large thrombus load, such as certain acute infarction cases (23).

Distal embolization with atherosclerotic debris or thrombotic debris presents a significant complication, especially with interventions involving old degenerated vein grafts or cases of AMI with a large thrombus burden. **Distal protection devices** help protect against this phenomenon and are being evaluated in clinical trials (24).

VALVULOPLASTY

Balloon valvulotomy is another example of a therapeutic tool used in the cardiac catheterization laboratory. Pulmonary valvulotomy is now a well-established technique for the treatment of severe pulmonary stenosis in all age groups (25). A successful procedure results in a dramatic relief of the pressure gradient with excellent long-term clinical results. Balloon dilatation of the mitral valve is an acceptable alternative to surgical valvotomy, and data indicate that the results of this procedure are similar to closed surgical valvotomy (26). The largest group of patients with severe rheumatic mitral stenosis likely to benefit from this procedure lives in the developing countries. The use of aortic valvuloplasty for severe aortic stenosis has markedly diminished because the restenosis rate is high and the natural history of the disease in most patients is unchanged (27).

DEVICES FOR INTERVENTION IN CONGENITAL HEART DISEASE

Stents and balloons are able to treat a number of congenital heart lesions. Septal closure devices are being investigated for nonsurgical procedural closure of atrial septal defects. Coils are available for closure of cases with patent ductus (28,29).

Table 6.1.   Normal values and pressures

	Normal
O_2 consumption (VO_2)	110–150/mL/min/M^2
Pulmonary arteriovenous (AV) O_2 difference	3.5–4.7 vol. %
Systemic AV O_2 difference	3.5–4.7 vol. %
Systemic O_2 saturation	$\geq 94\%$
Cardiac index (CI)	2.5–4.0 L/min/M^2
Systemic vascular resistance (SVR)	8.0–15.0 units
Pulmonary vascular resistance (PVR)	0.2–1.12 units
Total pulmonary resistance (TPR)	1.0–3.0 units
Aortic valve area (AVA)	2.6–3.5 cm^2
Mitral valve area (MVA)	4.0–6.0 cm^2
Left ventricular (LV) end-diastolic volume	<90 mL/M^2
Ejection fraction	55%–70%
His bundle electrogram AH interval	60–115 msec
HV interval	35–55 msec
Normal pressures (mm Hg)	
Right atrium (RA), mean	1–8
Right ventricle (RV), systolic	15–28
End-diastolic	0–8
Pulmonary artery (PA), systolic	15–28
Diastolic	5–16
Mean	10–22
Pulmonary artery wedge (PAW), mean	4–12
Left atrium (LA), mean	4–12
Left ventricle (LV), systolic	85–150
End-diastolic	4–12
Aortic (Ao) systolic	85–150
Diastolic	60–90
Mean	70–105

PHYSIOLOGIC DATA DERIVED FROM CARDIAC CATHETERIZATION

A thorough review of the terminology and physiologic data derived from cardiac catheterization is beyond the scope of this text. However, a table of normal values is included for the reader's reference (Table 6.1).

REFERENCES

1. ACC/AHA guidelines for cardiac catheterization and cardiac catheterization laboratories. American College of Cardiology/American Heart Association Ad Hoc Task Force on Cardiac Catheterization. *Circulation* 84:2213, 1991.
2. Criley JM, French JW: Cardiac catheterization in adults with congenital heart disease. *Cardiovasc Clin* 10:173, 1979.
3. Yang SS, Bentivoglio LG, Maranhoa V, et al: *From cardiac catheterization data to hemodynamic parameters*, 3rd ed. Philadelphia: FA Davis Co, 1988.
4. Landau C, Lange RA, Hillis LD: Percutaneous transluminal coronary angioplasty. *N Engl J Med* 330:981, 1994.
5. Kuntz RE, Baim DS: Defining coronary restenosis. Newer clinical and angiographic paradigms. *Circulation* 88:1310, 1993.
6. Fishman DT, Leon MB, Baim DS, et al: A randomized comparison of coronary stent placement and balloon angioplasty in the treatment of coronary artery disease. Stent Restenosis Study Investigators. *N Engl J Med* 331:496, 1994.
7. Teirstein PS, Massullo V, Jani S, et al: Catheter-based radiotherapy to inhibit restenosis after coronary stenting. *N Engl J Med* 336(24): 1697, 1997.
8. Waksman R, White LR, Chan RC, et al: Intracoronary beta radiation therapy for patients with in-stent restenosis: the   month clinical and angiographic results. *Circulation* 100(18):1, 1999.
9. Sousa JE, Costa MA, Abizaid A, et al: Lack of neointimal proliferation after implantation of sirolimus-coated stents in human coronary arteries: a QCA and 3-D IVUS study. *Circulation* 103:192, 2001.
10. Wong SC, Zidoc JB, Chuong YC, et al: Stents improve late clinical outcomes: Results from the combined (I + II) Stent Restenosis Study. *Circulation* 92(Suppl 1):1, 1995.
11. Macaya C, Serruys PW, Ruygrok P, et al: Combined benefits of coronary stenting versus balloon angioplasty: one year follow-up of BENESTENT trial. *J Am Coll Cardiol* 27:255, 1996.
12. Douglas JS, Savage MP, Bailey ST, et al: Randomized trial of coronary stent and balloon angioplasty in the treatment of saphenous vein graft stenosis. *J Am Coll Cardiol* 27(Suppl A): A-178, 1996.
13. Pepine CJ, Holmes DR: Coronary artery stents. *J Am Coll Cardiol* 28:782, 1996.
14. Serruys RE, Bode C, Holubarsch C, et al: Angiographic findings of the multicenter Randomized Study with the Sirolimus Eluting Bx Velocity Balloon-Expandable Stent (RAVEL): Sirolimus-eluting stents inhibit restenosis irrespective of vessel size. *Circulation* 8; 106(15):1949–1956, 2002.
15. Topol EJ, Teya F, Pinkerton CA, et al: A comparison of directional atherectomy with coronary angioplasty in patients with coronary artery disease. The CAVEAT Study Group. *N Engl J Med* 329:221, 1993.
16. Baim DS, Cutlip D, Ho KK, et al: Acute results of directional coronary

atherectomy in the Balloon versus Optimal Atherectomy Trial (BOAT) pilot phase. *Coronary Artery Disease* 7:290, 1996.

17. Dussaillant GR, Mintz GS, Popma JJ, et al: Intravascular ultrasound, directional coronary atherectomy, and the Optimal Atherectomy Restenosis Study (OARS). *Coronary Artery Disease* 7:294, 1996.

18. Ellis SG, Popma JJ, Buchbinder M, et al: Relation of clinical presentation, stenosis morphology, and operator technique to the procedural results of rotational atherectomy-facilitated angioplasty. *Circulation* 89:882, 1994.

19. Worth DC, Leon MB, O'Neill W, et al: Rotational atherectomy multicenter registry: acute results, complications and six-month angiographic follow-up in 709 patients. *J Am Coll Cardiol* 24:641, 1994.

20. Safian RD, Grines CL, May MA, et al: Clinical and angiographic results of transluminal extraction coronary atherectomy in saphenous vein bypass grafts. *Circulation* 89:302, 1994.

21. Bittl JA, Kuntz R, Estella P, et al: Analysis of late lumen narrowing after excimer laser-facilitated angioplasty. *J Am Coll Cardiol* 23:1314, 1994.

22. Ajani AE, Kim HS, Castagna M, et al: Clinical utility of the cutting balloon. *J Invasive Cardiol* 13(7):554, 2001.

23. Muller R, Gerckens U, Staberock M, et al: Clinical experience with the PercuSurge Guard Wire-a new system for prevention of peripheral embolisms in catheter interventions on degenerated coronary venous bypasses. *Z Kardiol* 89(4):316, 2000.

24. Belli G, Pezzano A, DiBiase AM, et al: Adjunctive thrombus aspiration and mechanical protection from distal embolization in primary percutaneous intervention for acute myocardial infarction. *Catheter Cardiovasc Interv* 50(3): 362,2000.

25. Rao PS, Fawzi ME, Solymar L, et al: Long term results of balloon pulmonary valvuloplasty of valvular pulmonary stenosis. *Am Heart J* 115:1291, 1989.

26. Palacios IF, Block PC: Percutaneous mitral balloon valvulotomy. Update of immediate results and follow-up. *Circulation* 78(Suppl II): II-490, 1988.

27. Bashore TM, Davidson CJ: Follow-up recatheterization after balloon aortic valvuloplasty. Mansfield Scientific Aortic Valvuloplasty Registry Investigators. *J Am Coll Cardiol* 17:1188, 1991.

28. Matitiau A, Birk E, Kachko L et al. Transcatheter closure of secundum atrial septal defects with the amplatzer septal occluder: early experience. *Isr Med Assoc J* 1:32, 2001.

29. Rao PS: Summary and comparison of PDA closure devices. *Curr Interv Cardiol Rep* 3:268, 2001.

ISCHEMIC HEART DISEASE: RISK FACTORS AND PREVENTION

Cardiovascular disease claims approximately 1.5 million American lives per year, with half of these deaths resulting from coronary artery disease (CAD). The CAD mortality rate remains higher in the United States than in other industrialized nations.

CAD continues to be the world's number-one killer, but there has been a significant reduction (more than 50%) in age-adjusted mortality rates in the United States in the last 30 years. The decline has been attributed to many causes such as better emergency care, advances in hospital treatment, and improved prehospital care, but the major credit goes to the reduction in coronary risk factors. The most impressive risk-factor changes have been the decline in prevalence of smoking, more widespread treatment and control of hypertension, and a decrease in average serum cholesterol levels. The ability to identify and manage CAD risk factors will profoundly affect efforts to maintain the trend of declining CAD mortality rates.

RISK FACTORS

A risk factor is an element whose presence is associated with an increased likelihood that disease will develop at a later time. Risk factors can be categorized as modifiable or nonmodifiable. *Modifiable* risks, such as smoking, can be changed; *nonmodifiable* risks, such as age or gender, cannot. Prevention of risk factors can be primary or secondary. *Primary prevention* involves intervention before the onset of disease. *Secondary prevention* involves intervention after the onset of disease. The risk of a coronary event in any individual increases exponentially when two or more major risk factors are present.

Modifiable risks include the following:

1. Cigarette smoking
2. Hyperlipidemia
3. Hypertension
4. Diabetes mellitus
5. Inactivity
6. Obesity

Nonmodifiable risks include the following:

1. Family history
2. Gender
3. Age

Other potential causative factors include the following:

1. Mitogens
2. Growth factors

3. Cytokines
4. Homocysteine
5. Heat-shock proteins
6. *Helicobacter pylori*
7. Chlamydia
8. Cytomegalovirus
9. Hyperfibrinogenemia
10. Elevated amyloid A protein

Modifiable Risk Factors

Cigarette Smoking

Tobacco smoking—a major modifiable risk factor for a coronary event—is the leading preventable cause of disease and death in the United States (1). Of American adults, 46 million are smokers (28% males and 22% females); despite numerous antismoking campaigns one-fourth of adult Americans still smoke. Cigarette smoking is estimated to be responsible for one in every five deaths. Nearly 25% of the deaths were the result of ischemic heart disease, and 43% were the result of a cardiovascular disease (2). Research demonstrates that smoking causes transient and reversible prothrombotic increase in fibrinogen levels and platelet adhesion, increased blood carboxyhemoglobin levels, reduced high-density lipoprotein (HDL) cholesterol, enhanced catecholamines, and coronary artery vasoconstriction.

The percentage of Americans who smoke has declined 37% since 1965. Smoking cessation increases life expectancy; smokers who quit approach mortality rates of nonsmokers within 3 years of stopping (3,4). In a 10-year follow-up of patients in the Coronary Artery Surgery Study (CASS), smokers who quit had fewer hospitalizations, less angina, and less physical limitations than those who continued to smoke (5). Physicians should counsel any patient who smokes to quit, set quit dates, provide self-help material, and arrange follow-up visits to assess compliance. The U.S. Public Health Service's guideline document released in 2000 suggests a "5A" approach to helping patients stop smoking: Ask, Advise, Assess, Assist, and Arrange (6). Nicotine-replacement products such as the patch can ease patients' withdrawal symptoms. The drug bupropion hydrochloride (Zyban) and other antidepressants also can help patients quit.

HYPERLIPIDEMIA

The central role of lipids in atherogenesis is derived mostly from the low-density lipoprotein (LDL) fraction of serum cholesterol. LDL cholesterol may be modified by oxidation within cells, such as leukocytes and endothelial cells. The oxidized form of LDL is the major contributor to atheromatous lesions.

The 2001 National Cholesterol Education Program (NCEP) recommendations state that lowering LDL cholesterol is the primary goal of coronary heart disease risk reduction (7). Three main risk categories and goals of treatment are identified.

1. Coronary heart disease or coronary heart disease risk equivalents (e.g., diabetes, other arteriosclerotic disease): treatment goal is LDL less than 100 mg/dL
2. Multiple (2 +) major risk factors: treatment goal is LDL less than 130 mg/dL

3. Zero to one major risk factor: treatment goal is LDL less than 160 mg/dL (7)

The Scandinavian Simvastatin Survival Study (4S), Cholesterol and Recurrent Events (CARE) trial, and Long-Term Intervention with Pravastatin in Ischemic Disease (LIPID) trial all evaluated the effect of lowering cholesterol as secondary prevention in patients with known coronary heart disease (8–10). The WOSCOPS (West of Scotland Coronary Prevention Study) and the AFCAPS/TexCAPS (Air Force/Texas Coronary Atherosclerosis Prevention Study) studied the effect of lowering LDL cholesterol as primary prevention in patients with no evidence of coronary heart disease (11,12). More than 31,000 patients were studied in these five trials, and several key observations can be made that are consistent with each of these trials, as summarized by Waters (13):

Statins reduce coronary event rates in patients with or without coronary disease. In the 4S, trial simvastatin treatment was associated with a 42% decrease in coronary mortality compared with placebo. In the AFCAPS/TexCAPS trial of primary prevention (6,605 patients), there was a 37% reduction in the primary composite endpoint of unstable angina, fatal or nonfatal myocardial infarction (MI), or sudden cardiac death in the pravastatin treatment group as compared with the placebo recipients.

There is greater relative risk reduction the longer the therapy lasts. In the 4S trial, simvastatin was associated with a 29% reduction in coronary death at 2 years, 36% at 4 years, and 55% at 6 years.

The risk reduction is proportional to the LDL cholesterol reduction.

Statins reduce the risk of transient ischemic attacks and stroke in patients with coronary heart disease.

Statins are safe. Significantly abnormal levels of serum aminotransferases or creatine kinase occur in less than 1% of cases.

Many angiographic studies have demonstrated that lipid-lowering therapy combined with a low-fat diet can impede progression or bring about regression of atherosclerotic lesions. Lesion regression has been shown in several studies in the 1990s such as the St. Thomas Atherosclerosis Regression Study (STARS) and the Regression Growth Evaluation Statin Study (REGRESS) (14,15).

The major lipoprotein classes are chylomicrons, very-low-density lipoproteins, LDLs, intermediate-density lipoproteins, and HDLs. Each lipoprotein has an apoprotein content. Apoproteins are distinguished alphabetically and numerically as apo A-1 through apo E. Apo A-1 is associated with HDL, and apo B-100 is associated with LDL. New factors that affect CAD have been shown to be of clinical use and may change the course of treatment approach:

1. Some investigators have found that the concentration of apo A-1 and apo B-100 are better predictors of CAD than are measurements of total plasma lipids or lipoproteins. The greater the ratio of apo A-1 to apo B-100, the less the risk for development of CAD.

2. Lipoprotein-a, or Lp(a), has been established as an independent CAD risk factor. If serum levels of both LDL and Lp(a) are elevated, the risk of CAD is markedly increased.

3. LDL cholesterol is categorized further into pattern A and pattern B, the latter being small and dense LDL, and associated with a three-fold increase CAD risk. Of importance is the treatment; gemfibrozil reduces small LDL in pattern B but not in pattern A.

Elevated levels of HDL are associated with a reduction in the risk of atherosclerosis. Elevated levels of HDL can be induced with exercise, moderate alcohol use, and antihypercholesterolemic medications.

SIMPLE APPROACH TO TREATMENT OF HYPERLIPIDEMIA

1. Virtually all patients with atherosclerotic disease (provided there are no contraindications) should be undergoing treatment (usually a statin).
2. Therapy should be implemented immediately rather than waiting for diet.

SUGGESTED GOALS FOR HYPERLIPIDEMIA THERAPY

Goals for treatment with known CAD/vascular disease include the following:

*   Total cholesterol: 150
*   LDL: 60 to 80
*   Diet: less than 20 g of saturated fat

Primary prevention involves the following:

*   Total cholesterol: less than 200
*   LDL: less than 100
*   Diet: less than 25 g of saturated fat

The rationale for these goals include the following:

*   Lipid lowering reduces rate of MI by 30% over 5 years. Benefits also are noted in decreasing frequency of angina and need for revascularization.
*   Data suggest that lowering LDL to as low as 60 mg/dL should be beneficial (13,16)

DISORDERS WHERE TREATMENT NEEDS TO GO BEYOND LDL CHOLESTEROL REDUCTION

Certain disorders require additional therapy (17):

1. Familial heterozygous hypercholesterolemia
2. Familial hyperlipidemia and hypoalphalipoproteinemia
3. Hyperbetalipoproteinemia
4. Homocystinemia
5. Disorders of Lp(a)
6. Apolipoprotein-LDL subclass pattern B

Hypertension

Nearly 60 million adult Americans, roughly 30% of U.S. adults, have hypertension (Table 7.1) (18). Both systolic and diastolic pressure are risk factors, even in the elderly. Blood pressure levels and end-organ damage are used as clinical markers in the estimation of hypertension severity. End-organ damage includes the brain (strokes), eyes (retinopathy), heart (left ventricular hypertrophy), and kidney

Table 7.1. Classification of blood pressure for adults 18 years and older[a]

Category	SBP (mm Hg)	DBP (mm Hg)
Normal	<130	<85
High normal	130–139	85–89
Hypertension[b]		
Stage 1 (mild)	140–159	90–99
Stage 2 (moderate)	160–179	100–109
Stage 3 (severe)	180–209	110–119
Stage 4 (very severe)	210	120

DBP, diastolic blood pressure; SBP, systolic blood pressure. When systolic and diastolic pressures fall into different categories, the higher category should be selected to classify the individual's blood pressure status.

[a]Classification based on the average of two or more readings on two or more occasions in individuals who are not taking antihypertensive drugs and who are not acutely ill.

[b]Optimal blood pressure with respect to cardiovascular disease risk is <120 mm Hg systolic and <80 mm Hg diastolic. However, unusually low readings should be evaluated for clinical significance. New targets for hypertension RX SBP 130; 140 in elderly DBP 80.

(decreased renal function). Hypertension causes smooth-muscle cell proliferation and increased endothelial permeability. These changes promote increased cholesterol uptake and accumulation. Endothelial dysfunction caused by hypertension promotes vasoconstrictor effects (19). There is considerable evidence that reducing blood pressure decreases the development of cardiovascular disease events, including CAD, stroke, and congestive heart failure (20). Control of hypertension involves diet, exercise, and drug therapy. Many drugs are effective in treating hypertension in patients with CAD; the most notable classes are beta blockers, calcium channel blockers, the angiotensin converting enzyme (ACE) inhibitor drugs, angiotensin receptor blockers, and diuretics.

Diabetes Mellitus

The American Diabetes Association (ADA) defines diabetes as a fasting blood sugar greater than 126 mg/dL (21). This abnormality is present in approximately 10% of adult Americans. Strong epidemiologic and clinical evidence indicates that diabetes mellitus (both insulin-dependent and non–insulin-dependent diabetes mellitus) is a major risk factor for CAD. Atherosclerosis accounts for 80% of diabetic mortality (21). CAD alone is responsible for 75% of total atherosclerotic death; the remainder results from stroke and peripheral vascular disease. It is estimated that 25% of all heart attacks in the United States occur in patients with diabetes. The connection between diabetes and CAD is becoming more important because of the increasing prevalence of diabetes in high-risk populations such as Mexican Americans, African Americans, and Native Americans.

Diabetes frequently exists in the presence of other risk factors. Roughly half of people with diabetes have hypertension, and a similar number have hyperlipidemia. Obesity is common in people with diabetes. The typical lipid disorder in a person with diabetes is increased plasma triglyceride and decreased HDL cholesterol and small dense LDL particles. Resistance to insulin may play a role in the lipid disorder of diabetes.

Diabetes contributes to vascular injury by increasing glycosylated end products and plasma lipoproteins. Platelet activity is enhanced, and platelet microemboli are common in patients with diabetes.

Treatment of diabetes should emphasize maintenance of ideal body weight, appropriate diet, and a sensible exercise program. On the basis of the known adverse effects of prolonged hyperglycemia, strict glucose control may play a major role in reducing the risk of CAD. In patients with diabetes and hypertension, tissue-avid ACE inhibitors may be particularly advantageous in improving endothelial function. The benefits of ACE inhibitors are greater than would be expected from blood pressure lowering alone (22). Current NCEP and ADA guidelines advise lowering LDL cholesterol to less than 100 mg/dL in patients with diabetes.

Obesity and Physical Inactivity

About 34 million Americans are overweight, 12.4 million severely so. Obesity itself predisposes to hyperlipidemia, diabetes, and hypertension; therefore, the role of weight reduction in the treatment of these diseases makes it an obvious choice for an intervention. Moreover, increased physical activity favorably influences lipoprotein levels, blood pressure, weight, glucose tolerance, and cardiovascular and pulmonary functional capacity.

Nonmodifiable Risks

Family History

Family history of heart disease is one of the most powerful determinants of CAD. The NCEP defines a family history of premature coronary heart disease as having a definite MI or sudden death before 55 years of age in a father or other male first-degree relative or before 65 years of age in a mother or other female first-degree relative.

Age and Gender

CAD risk increases nearly linearly with age and is greater in men compared to women until approximately age 75, when the prevalence is nearly equal. At younger than age 55, the incidence of CAD

Table 7.2. Simple summary of risk interventions and recommendations

Risk intervention	Recommendations
Smoking cessation	Complete cessation using the 5A approach
Lipid control	Usually a statin; LDL<100
Blood pressure control	SBP 130; elderly 140; DBP 80
Diabetes control	Blood sugar <100mg/dL
Weight management	Diet and exercise

DBP, diastolic blood pressure; LDL, low-density lipoprotein; SBP, systolic blood pressure.

among men is three to four times that in women. After age 55, the rate of increase with age in men declines and that in women escalates. In the post-MI setting, older patients are at higher subsequent risk of death than younger patients, and the effect of age predominates over other risk factors.

Prevention

Preventive services are provided less often than experts recommend and less frequently than patients and their physicians prefer (Table 7.2).

REFERENCES

1. Bartecchi CE, MacKenzie TK, Schriere RW: The human cost of tobacco use. *N Engl J Med* 330:90, 1994.
2. Rigotti NA, Pasternak RC: Cigarette smoking and coronary heart disease. *Cardiol Clin* 14:51, 1996.
3. Rosenberg L, Palmer JR, Shapiro S: Decline in the risk of myocardial infarction among women who stop smoking. *N Engl J Med* 322:213, 1990.
4. Rosenberg L, Kaufman DW, Helmrich SP, et al: The risk of myocardial infarction after quitting smoking in men under 55 years of age. *N Engl J Med* 313:1511, 1985.
5. Cavender JB, Rogers WJ, Fisher LK, et al: Coronary artery surgery study (CASS): 10 year follow-up. *Am Coll Cardiol* 20:287, 1992.
6. *Clinical practice guidelines.* Agency for Health Care Policy and Research, U.S. Department of Health and Human Services. Rockville, MD: Agency for Health Care Policy and Research, 2000.
7. Executive summary of the Third Report of the National Cholesterol Education Program (NCEP) Expert Panel on Detection, Evaluation, and Treatment of High Blood Cholesterol in Adults (Adult Treatment Panel III). *JAMA* 285:2486, 2001.
8. The Scandinavian Simvastatin Survival Study (4S): Randomized trial of cholesterol lowering in 4444 patients with coronary heart disease. *Lancet* 344:1383, 1994.
9. Sacks FM, Pleffer MA, Moye LA, et al: For the Cholesterol and Recurrent Events Trial Investigators: the effect of pravastatin on coronary events after myocardial infarction in patients with average cholesterol levels. *N Engl J Med* 335:1001, 1996.
10. Long-Term Intervention with Pravastatin in Ischemic Disease (LIPID) Study Group: Prevention of cardiovascular events and death with pravastatin in patients with coronary heart disease and a broad range of initial cholesterol levels. *N Engl J Med* 339:1349, 1998.
11. Shepherd J, Cobbe SM, Ford I, et al: For the West of Scotland Coronary Prevention Study Group: prevention of coronary heart disease with pravastatin in men with hypercholesterolemia. *N Engl J Med* 333:1301, 1995.
12. Downs JR, Clearfield M, Weis S, et al: For the AF-CAPS/TexCAPS Research Group: primary prevention of acute coronary events with lovastatin in men and women with average cholesterol levels: results of AFCAPS/TexCAPS. *JAMA* 279:1615, 1998.
13. Waters DD: What do the statin trials tell us? *Clin Cardiol* 24(Supp111):3, 2001.
14. Watts GF, Lewis B, Brunt JNH, et al: Effects on coronary artery disease of lipid-lowering diet, or diet plus cholestyramine. The St.

Thomas' Atherosclerotic Regression Study (STARS). *Lancet* 339:563, 1992.

15. Jukema JE, Bruschke AVG, van Boven AJ, et al: The Regression Growth Evaluation Statin Study (REGRESS). *Circulation* 9:2528, 1995.

16. Vaughn CJ, Gotto AM Jr, Basson CT: The evolving role of statins in the management of atherosclerosis. *J Am Coll Cardiol* 35:1, 2000.

17. Superko HR: Beyond LDL cholesterol reduction. *Circulation* 94: 2351, 1996.

18. The Sixth Report of the Joint National Committee on Detection, Evaluation, and Treatment of High Blood Pressure. *Arch Intern Med* 157: 2413, 1997.

19. Anderson TJ, Overhiser RW, Haber H, et al: A comparative study of four anti-hypertensive agents on endothelial function in patients with coronary disease. *J Am Coll Cardiol* 35:60, 2000.

20. The Heart Outcomes Prevention Evaluation Study Investigators: Effects of the angiotensin-converting enzyme inhibitor ramipril on death from cardiovascular causes, myocardial infarction, and stroke in high-risk patients. *N Engl J Med* 342:145, 2000.

21. Report of the Expert Committee on the Diagnosis and Classification of Diabetes Mellitus. *Diabetes Care* 20:1183, 1997.

22. Huffner SM: Coronary heart disease in patients with diabetes. *N Engl J Med* 342:1040, 2000.

8

ANGINA PECTORIS

Angina pectoris (AP) is the most common manifestation of ischemic heart disease and is the initial presenting symptom in more than one-half of patients with the illness (1). The prevalence of angina is difficult to determine, but it is likely to affect more than 6 million Americans (2).

AP results from an imbalance between myocardial oxygen supply and demand and most commonly is caused by the inability of atherosclerotic coronary arteries to perfuse the heart under conditions of increased myocardial oxygen consumption (demand). Angina also occurs in patients with seemingly normal coronary arteries subjected to acute or chronic increases in myocardial work such as aortic stenosis, hypertension, or hypertrophic cardiomyopathy or decreases in supply such as anemia. An increase in coronary vasomotor tone or frank coronary artery spasm, superimposed on normal or diseased arteries, can provoke pain in the absence of increased myocardial demands and has been shown to be responsible for variant (Prinzmetal's) angina and certain cases of unstable angina. Last, there is a sizable group of patients who have angina without evidence of coronary artery disease (CAD), with or without an increase in myocardial work. This latter syndrome has been termed "syndrome X" because of its enigmatic nature.

TYPICAL ANGINA

Description of Symptoms

Character

Typical angina most often is described as a discomfort, pressure, heaviness, or squeezing sensation—not a pain. It sometimes is described as burning or sharp. Dyspnea is less common.

Location

It most often is found in the substernal area, precordium, or epigastrium with radiation to the left arm, jaw, or neck. It less commonly is felt only in radiation areas and not in the chest.

Precipitation

Typical angina often is provoked by exertion, emotion, cold weather, eating, or smoking. It is relieved by rest, removal of provoking factors, or sublingual nitrates.

Duration

The condition usually lasts a few minutes. It rarely lasts longer than 30 minutes.

Evaluation

History

The diagnosis of AP is established by obtaining a reliable description of the chest discomfort and its relationship to activity. The likelihood of underlying CAD is enhanced by a personal history of hypertension, diabetes mellitus, hyperlipidemia, or smoking or a family history of premature ischemic heart disease in first-degree relatives younger than age 55 years.

Physical Examination

Although often normal, examination may yield important confirmatory information (i.e., hypertension, peripheral arterial disease, xanthelasma, tendinous xanthomata, tobacco-stained fingers or teeth, or diagonally creased earlobes). Episodic ischemia alters left ventricular compliance. Thus, a transient S_4, S_3, and/or apical systolic murmur (as a result of papillary muscle dysfunction) may be heard during an anginal chest pain episode.

Blood Chemistry

Basic screening is important to identify potentially treatable risk factors such as hypercholesterolemia and/or hyperglycemia. Hypertriglyceridemia is less well-established as a risk factor. High low-density lipoprotein (LDL) is a risk factor, whereas elevated high-density lipoprotein is protective against coronary heart disease. A complete blood count should be obtained to check for the presence of anemia. A fasting glucose also is recommended. Thyroid function tests should be drawn if hyperthyroidism is suspected.

Electrocardiogram

The electrocardiogram (ECG) is often normal in the absence of a myocardial infarction (MI) or a cause for left ventricular hypertrophy. An ECG during angina may show transient ST depression, T wave inversion, or ventricular arrhythmias. An ambulatory ECG (Holter) may demonstrate ischemic episodes with or without the patient having symptoms ("silent ischemia").

Chest X-ray

A chest X-ray is recommended in patients with signs or symptoms of congestive heart failure, valvular heart disease, pericardial disease, aortic dissection, or aneurysm or in patients with pulmonary disease.

Exercise Stress Testing

Exercise stress testing (EST) (see Chapter 3) is invaluable in reproducing symptoms, documenting ischemic ECG changes, and assessing the level of disability. Patients with high-grade CAD may manifest inability to increase heart rate or blood pressure during exercise, develop angina, or develop marked ST changes at low stress levels that persist after exercise. Exercise-induced arrhythmias or left ventricular dysfunction provide diagnostic information with important therapeutic potential.

Exercise imaging is a valuable adjunct to standard exercise testing, especially in patients with resting ST changes, preexcitation, paced rhythm, left bundle branch block, or left ventricular hypertrophy.

Radionuclide scintigraphy (see Chapter 5) enhances the sensitivity and specificity of EST. Patients with significant coronary arterial obstructions usually will develop exercise-induced "cold spots" during thallium or sestamibi perfusion scanning or left ventricular wall motion abnormalities during nuclear scanning.

Exercise echocardiography (see Chapter 4) helps establish the diagnosis by demonstrating regional wall motion abnormalities such as hypokinesis, akinesis, dyskinesis, or failure to thicken during systole.

Electron Beam Computerized Tomography

A positive electron beam computerized tomography (EBCT) detection of calcium for the presence of atherosclerosis has a variable predictive value (55% to 84%) (3). The proper role of EBCT testing is still controversial.

Coronary Arteriography

Although not necessary for the diagnosis of CAD in most instances, cardiac catheterization and coronary angiography permit localization and quantification of obstructive lesions, evaluation of left ventricular function, and assessment of any valvular or myocardial disease. The indications for these invasive studies vary widely in different centers. Widely accepted indications include the following:

- Angina refractory to medical management
- Angina or MI in patients younger than 45 years of age
- Unstable angina (after medical stabilization)
- Persistent angina and/or low level EST abnormalities after MI
- Marked (0.2 mV) ST changes at low-level exercise or persisting several minutes after cessation of EST
- Suspected Prinzmetal's (variant) angina (coronary vasospasm)
- Preoperative evaluation of patients with valvular or congenital heart disease
- Patients with life-threatening arrhythmias associated with ischemic heart disease
- When needed for clarification of possible causes for recurrent chest pain when noninvasive testing has yielded negative or equivocal findings

Risk Stratification

The specific approach to risk stratification varies according to the individual. However, the following general types of patient characteristics apply to most cases (Tables 8.1 and 8.2) (4,5).

1. Left ventricular function (the strongest predictor of long-term survival with CAD)
2. Anatomic extent and severity of atherosclerosis in the coronary tree
3. Evidence of a recent coronary plaque rupture (substantially increases short-term risk)
4. General health and noncoronary comorbidity

General Therapeutic Considerations

General Measures

Conditions that exacerbate or provoke angina should be sought in all patients. Treatment of anemia, arrhythmia, hyperthyroidism, and hypertension may relieve angina.

Risk-Factor Reduction

Quitting smoking, controlling hypertension and diabetes, lowering cholesterol and lipids (initially by diet), and maintaining an ideal body weight are strongly advised.

Table 8.1.   Noninvasive risk stratification

High risk (>3% annual mortality rate)
1. Severe resting left ventricular dysfunction (LVEF <35%)
2. High-risk treadmill score (score: 5–11)
3. Severe exercise left ventricular dysfunction (exercise LVEF <35%)
4. Stress-induced large perfusion defect (particularly if anterior)
5. Stress-induced multiple perfusion defects of moderate size
6. Large, fixed perfusion defect with LV dilation or increased lung uptake (thallium-201)
7. Stress-induced moderate perfusion defect with LV dilation or increased lung uptake (thallium-201)
8. Echocardiographic wall motion abnormality (involving greater than two segments) developing at low dose of dobutamine (0.5–1.0 mg/kg/min) or at a low heart rate (<120 beats/min)
9. Stress echocardiographic evidence of extensive ischemia

Intermediate risk (1% to 3% annual mortality rate)
1. Mild/moderate resting left ventricular dysfunction (LVEF = 35% to 49%)
2. Intermediate-risk treadmill score (−11 < score <5)
3. Stress-induced moderate perfusion defect without LV dilation or increased lung intake (thallium-201)
4. Limited stress echocardiographic ischemia with a wall motion abnormality only at higher doses of dobutamine involving two or fewer segments

Low risk (< 1% annual mortality rate)
1. Low-risk treadmill score (score ~5)
2. Normal or small myocardial perfusion defect at rest or with stress[a]
3. Normal stress echocardiographic wall motion or no change of limited resting wall motion abnormalities during stress[a]

LVEF, left ventricular ejection fraction; LV, left ventricular.
[a]Although the published data are limited, patients with these findings will probably not be at low risk in the presence of either a high-risk treadmill score or severe resting left ventricular dysfunction (LVEF <35%).

Exercise

The role of exercise in patients with known ischemic heart disease remains controversial. It has been established that regular exercise can lower the heart rate and blood pressure at rest and, during submaximal work loads, favorably modify the blood lipid composition, consume calories, and provide psychologic benefits. In certain patients, regular exercise may lessen cigarette smoking and result in more prudent eating habits. However, the widely held concepts that exercise causes regression of coronary atherosclerosis, increases collateral formation, improves ventricular performance, and prolongs life lack rigorous scientific proof. Also, exercise causes an increase in the cardiac double product (heart rate × blood pressure), which increases myocardial oxygen demand. Exercise can threaten the supply/demand balance of the myocardium and can produce ischemic dysfunction and arrhythmias in certain patients with latent or overt CAD. Thus, a "prescription" for exercise must be written

Table 8.2. Coronary artery disease prognostic index[a]

Extent of CAD	Prognostic weight (0–100)	5-year survival rate (%)[a]
1-vessel disease, 75%	23	93
>1-vessel disease, 50% to 74%	23	93
1-vessel disease, ≥95%	32	91
2-vessel disease	37	88
2-vessel disease, both ≥95%	42	86
1-vessel disease, ≥95% proximal LAD	48	83
2-vessel disease, ≥95% LAD	48	83
2-vessel disease, ≥95% proximal LAD	56	79
3-vessel disease	56	79
3-vessel disease, ≥95% in at least 1	63	73
3-vessel disease, 75% proximal LAD	67	67
3-vessel disease, ≥95% proximal LAD	74	59

CAD, coronary artery disease; LAD, left anterior descending coronary artery.
[a]Assuming medical treatment only. (From Calif RM, Armstrong PW, Carver JR, et al: Task Force 5. Stratification of patients into high-, medium- and low-risk subgroups for purposes of risk factor management. *J Am Coll Cardiol* 27:964–1047, 1996, with permission.)

carefully with the knowledge of each individual patient taken into consideration.

General Comments on Medical Therapy

Because the overall prognosis of stable angina is relatively good (annual mortality of 1.6% to 3.3%), many patients can be managed with medical therapy (6). The goal of drug therapy is to abolish or reduce angina and ischemia and to promote a normal life. The pharmacologic approach depends on the severity of the symptoms, side effect of the drugs, and the patient's response. Several major classes of drugs with different mechanisms of action are available and account for the improvement in medical therapy over the last decade. Optimal treatment with nitrates, beta blockers, and calcium blockers will result in marked improvement or complete relief of symptoms in most patients (7).

Drug Therapy

Antiplatelet Agents

Aspirin therapy is a Class 1 indication for therapy in the absence of contraindications. Clopidogrel is used when aspirin is absolutely contraindicated. The use of acetylsalicylic acid in stable angina reduces the risk of adverse events by 33% (8).

Lipid-Lowering Agents

Lipid-lowering therapy in patients with documented or suspected CAD and LDL cholesterol of more than 130 mg/dL is indicated, with a target goal of LDL less than 100 mg/dL. Reductions in cholesterol are significantly associated with observed reductions in CAD mortality (9).

Nitrates

The mechanism of action of nitrates in relieving angina is in large part the result of a decrease in left ventricular work (by reducing venous return and preload, a determinant of myocardial oxygen demand) and to a lesser extent the result of coronary vasodilatation and improved collateral flow (10). Other factors include decreased left ventricular end-diastolic pressure, which enhances subendocardial flow, and inhibition of coronary spasm. There is also some decrease in demand by decreasing systemic arterial compliance and lowering afterload.

Nitrates are safe and effective for the treatment of stable AP. Short-acting nitrates are used for the relief of the acute attacks, whereas long-acting nitrates are used for antianginal prophylaxis. (See Chapter 18 for individual nitrate drugs.)

NITRATE TOLERANCE. It is not possible to provide continuous antianginal and antiischemic prophylaxis throughout the dosing interval with any of the nitrate preparations. With continuous application of the drug at a constant rate, tolerance can develop within 24 hours and further therapy results in complete loss of the antianginal effect (11). The magnitude of tolerance varies with the nitrate preparation and the route of administration. Tolerance may be complete with constant dosing of patches or slow-release compounds, or it may be partial with the oral drugs, which have peaks and valleys in plasma concentrations.

Providing a nitrate-free interval is the strategy for preventing tolerance. With oral isosorbide dinitrate, dosing at 7 a.m., 12 noon, and 5 p.m. appears to avoid tolerance problems. With a patch-free interval of 10 to 12 hours, patches retain their effectiveness.

CONTRAINDICATIONS. Contraindications are hypersensitivity, hypotension, and hypovolemia. A relative contraindication may be severe nitrate-induced headaches, although the severity of headaches usually decreases with continued use of the drug. Nitrates are relatively contraindicated in hypertrophic cardiomyopathy and should be used cautiously in severe aortic stenosis. Patients should be warned strongly against the coadministration of nitrates and sildenafil because of life-threatening hypotension (12).

Beta-Adrenergic Blocking Agents

Beta blockers are extremely effective in the treatment of angina. They also have been shown to improve survival rates of patients with recent MI and in patients with hypertension (13).

These agents competitively occupy β-receptor myocardial sites (β-1-receptors) and, thus, block the chronotropic and inotropic actions of catecholamines on the heart. In combination with nitrates, they often can prevent angina in a large percentage of patients with chronic stable angina (1). Noncardiac β-receptors (β-2-receptors) in arterial walls and bronchial smooth muscle also are blocked by nonselective beta blockers. Some beta blockers have the capacity to activate the β-1-receptor and are referred to as having intrinsic sympathomimetic activity. The principal mechanism of action with beta blocker therapy is β-1-receptor blockade, which results in a reduction of heart rate and myocardial contractility. Other beneficial effects include attenuating systolic blood pressure increase during exercise, lessening exercise-induced vasoconstriction, and increasing diastolic filling time. (See Chapter 18 for individual beta-blocker drugs.)

Cardioselective agents are preferred in patients with angina and coexisting peripheral vascular disease, diabetes, or asthma. Some patients do not respond to beta blocker therapy because of the severity of their underlying CAD.

It is customary to adjust the dose of beta blocker to secure a resting heart rate between 50 to 60 beats per minute and the exercise heart rate to less than 100 beats per minute. Beta blockers should not be discontinued abruptly; if necessary, they should be tapered off gradually over a 10-day period.

Beta blockers frequently are combined with nitrates, and the combination is more effective than either agent alone (14). Beta blockers also may be used in combination with calcium channel blockers.

PRECAUTIONS AND CONTRAINDICATIONS. The absolute contraindications for the use of beta blockers are severe bradycardia, preexisting high-degree atrioventricular (AV) block, sick sinus syndrome, and severe left ventricular failure (mild congestive heart failure is, in fact, an indication for beta blockers).

Many patients with chronic obstructive pulmonary disease (COPD, nonreversible airway obstruction as a result of emphysema) or well-controlled diabetes mellitus in combination with ischemic heart disease can tolerate and benefit greatly from beta blockers administered cautiously with close follow-up observation. Similarly, patients with left ventricular dysfunction (ejection fraction 30% to 50%) that worsens with exercise also can benefit from cautious use of beta blockers because the myocardial supply/demand imbalance during exercise may be decreased substantially.

Noncardioselective beta blockers, by inhibiting β-mediated arteriolar dilation, may worsen chest pain in some patients with coronary vasospasm and may be poorly tolerated by patients with severe peripheral arterial disease. Systemic side effects in those patients at risk appear to be less with cardioselective blockers.

Calcium Blocking Agents

Calcium channel blockers are a diverse group of compounds that inhibit calcium channel currents in cardiac and smooth muscle, and have been shown to be effective for relief or prevention of angina (15). The mechanism of action is by afterload reduction, decreasing myocardial contractility, inhibiting coronary vasoconstriction, decreasing coronary resistance, and increasing coronary blood flow. (See Chapter 18 for individual calcium channel blocker drugs.)

Properties peculiar to each specific calcium blocker may be helpful in selecting a particular agent and are dependent on clinical circumstances. The hemodynamic effects of verapamil and diltiazem are similar to those of nonselective beta blockers (decrease heart rate, decrease arterial pressure, decrease contractility). Nifedipine is a more potent arteriolar dilator than verapamil or diltiazem and thus may be a preferable choice in patients with hypertension or congestive heart failure. Verapamil and nifedipine have the most negative inotropic effects and are not well tolerated in patients with moderate to severe left ventricular dysfunction. The newer generation vasoselective dihydropyridines such as amlodipine and felodipine exert much less of a negative inotropic effect. Patients with recurrent, symptomatic reentrant supraventricular tachyarrhythmias are better treated with verapamil or diltiazem. For those with sick sinus syndrome, nifedipine would be the best choice.

Side effects from the vasodilatory properties of calcium channel blockers include palpitations, headache, flushing, hypotension, ankle edema, constipation, and abdominal discomfort. The negative inotropic effects may cause myocardial depression. The AV nodal delay may cause heart block.

Overt congestive heart failure is a contraindication for the use of calcium channel blockers (although amlodipine and felodipine are tolerated in patients with moderately reduced ejection fractions). Severe bradycardia and sinus and AV nodal dysfunction are contraindications for the use of rate-modulating calcium antagonists.

Percutaneous Revascularization

Percutaneous coronary intervention is an effective treatment method for many patients with disabling symptoms and those with significantly jeopardized myocardium (16). Percutaneous transluminal coronary angioplasty (PTCA) initially was used mainly in the treatment of single and select cases of double-vessel disease, but its use has been expanded to more complex cases with multivessel disease. PTCA is an attractive alternative to bypass surgery for many patients because of the decreased hospital time, major reduction in expense, minimal recovery time, and less operative insult. Relief of symptoms usually is seen in conjunction with objective improvement in exercise performance and improvement in ST changes. Restenosis continues to be a problem in approximately 30% of patients undergoing standard balloon angioplasty and often is heralded by recurrence of symptoms. The use of coronary stenting has reduced the restenosis rate by 50% compared to standard balloon angioplasty. Coronary stenting has enhanced greatly the ability to treat patients with angina and CAD and coronary graft disease.

Two randomized trials [Angioplasty Compared to Medicine (ACME) and Randomized Intervention Treatment of Angina-2 (RITA-2)] (17,18) have compared PTCA with medical management alone for chronic stable angina. The majority of patients treated had single-vessel disease, and expected death rates were low for both groups. Compared with medical treatment, the PTCA group had improved symptoms, although reintervention often was needed.

Coronary Artery Bypass Grafting

Coronary revascularization, can provide significant relief from angina to more than 80% of patients with angina refractory to drug therapy and has a low operative mortality (1% to 2%) in patients with good left ventricular function. It continues to be a very common major operative procedure performed in the United States. Because it neither reverses the disease process nor ensures permanent revascularization, the use of the procedure should be limited to those patients who cannot be managed medically (risk factor modification, nitrates, beta blockers, and calcium channel blockers); those who have failed angioplasty; or those found to have significant obstruction of the main left coronary artery or significant obstruction (more than 70%) in all major arteries. Graft closure and recurrence of symptoms continue to be a problem with this form of therapy. The first-year saphenous vein graft closure rate is 10% to 15% and subsequently is 1% to 2% per year. The use of the internal mammary artery has increased markedly because of its superior long-term patency rates (90% in 10 years) and the unusual lack of atherosclerosis in this particular conduit.

Two U.S. trials of PTCA versus CABG are the multicenter Bypass Angioplasty Revascularization Investigation (BARI) trial (19) and the single-center Emory Angioplasty Surgery Trial (EAST) (20). Both trials included patients with stable and unstable angina. Because these trials required that patients be suitable candidates for angioplasty, they involved only a minority of the spectrum of patients with multivessel disease. The result of these trials at a 5-year follow-up showed that early and late survival rates were equivalent for the PTCA and CABG groups. The biggest difference in late outcome was the need for repeat revascularization, which was five times more frequent in the PTCA group. In the BARI trial, patients with diabetes had a significantly better survival rate with CABG.

Invasive treatment for chronic stable angina is effective for the relief of symptoms but has not been shown to improve survival. Both procedures have a low mortality rate (1% to 1.5%). Both have advantages and disadvantages. Recurrent angina and repeat procedures are, and continue to be, more frequent with PTCA.

VARIANT ANGINA

Variant angina pectoris (VAP) also has been termed Prinzmetal's angina and angina inversa because of its propensity to occur at rest and to be associated with ST segment elevation, which is the ECG inverse of typical AP. After the comprehensive clinical descriptions by Prinzmetal and associates in the late 1950s (21) and early 1960s, the first major breakthrough occurred in 1963 when Oliva and colleagues demonstrated unequivocal coronary artery spasm associated with the pain and ST segment elevation of VAP (22). Subsequently, spasm has been seen in "normal" coronary arteries and those with fixed obstructions. Coronary artery spasm and VAP are probably not synonymous. Reversible spasm has been seen during unstable AP and early in the course of typical MIs; it can be provoked by ergonovine stimulation in patients with obstructive CAD and typical AP.

VAP is not a benign syndrome. MI can occur in the region affected by coronary artery spasm in about 25% of patients, and either high-grade heart block or ventricular fibrillation can occur during an episode of spasm. Although collective knowledge of the degree of overlap between the coronary spasm in VAP and that seen in "typical" CAP (AP or unstable AP) is incomplete, advancing **a diagnosis of VAP should be limited to those patients who fulfill two or more of the following criteria:**

- **Pain occurs principally at rest** (i.e., usually unprovoked). Because CAD may coexist, pain also may be provoked by exercise.
- **Pain may occur in a circadian manner** (i.e., recurrent episodes at a similar time of day, often in the early morning hours).

- **Pain is associated with ST segment elevation.** Often, subclinical (painless) episodes occur with "silent" ST segment elevations. Less commonly, *only ST segment depression* will occur (on a 12-lead, etc.) in a patient who otherwise has typical VAP.
- **Painful or "silent" episodes often are associated with arrhythmias,** usually heart block and/or ventricular tachyarrhythmias or bundle branch block (including fascicular blocks).

Evaluation

History

The history of chest pain is often so atypical of ischemic heart disease as to be misconstrued by the physician as noncardiac in origin, particularly because VAP frequently is seen in patients who have a paucity of risk factors.

Electrocardiography

A 12-lead ECG during a spontaneous attack, demonstrating transient and reversible marked ST segment elevation, can establish the diagnosis with certainty. In those patients with ST depression only, the diagnosis is less certain. Because the episodes often are short-lived and unpredictable, an ambulatory ECG (Holter) is statistically more likely to record the ECG changes; however, the limitation of conventional lead configurations may obscure the diagnostic features.

Coronary Arteriography

Coronary arteriography is indicated in severely symptomatic patients with established or suspected CAD. The goals of coronary arteriography should be to achieve the following:

- Establish the status of the coronary vessels in an asymptomatic state.
- Establish the extent of change in the coronary arteries during spontaneous or induced (ergonovine) spasm. (A multilead ECG should be used to record simultaneous electrocardiographic and rhythm changes.)
- Establish the response of spasm to sublingual nitrates.

Important Caveats in VAP

1. Because patients with VAP may develop life-threatening arrhythmias, electromechanical dissociation, or profound spasm of major vessels unresponsive to sublingual nitrates after ergonovine provocation, it is **not** advisable to use ergonovine stimulation outside a closely monitored setting.
2. It is important to visualize both major coronary arteries during spontaneous or induced spasm because the surface ECG may reflect spasm of the more dominant artery (e.g., the right coronary artery), while another major artery branch (e.g., the left anterior descending coronary artery) is also in spasm.

Therapy

Nitrates

Sublingual nitrates (nitroglycerin 0.4 mg or isosorbide dinitrate 5 mg) usually reverse spasm within 30 to 60 seconds; oral nitrates (isosorbide dinitrate 20 to 40 mg every 4 hours) or topical nitrates can reduce the frequency of attacks. Because nitrates are not always successful and abrupt withdrawal of nitrates can provoke spasm in patients with seemingly normal coronary arteries, it is important to taper—and not to abruptly stop—nitrates, regardless of their seeming ineffectiveness.

Calcium Blockers

Calcium blockers are extremely effective in preventing spasm in patients with VAP. Use of these agents generally will result in marked reduction in frequency of episodes and need for nitroglycerin.

Beta blockers generally are ineffective in VAP and have some theoretic disadvantages by blocking adrenergic coronary vasodilation. Angioplasty or coronary bypass surgery is not effective in those patients with VAP without fixed lesions. Selected cases with fixed underlying stenosis may need revascularization along with medical therapy.

SYNDROME X

As noted in the introduction to this chapter, there is a group of patients who have chest pain of seemingly ischemic origin but in whom CAD, VAP, nor other evident cause for pain can be established. About 10% of patients with UAP and approximately 20% of patients thought to have typical AP have normal coronary arteriograms. These patients, for want of a better term, have been labeled as having **syndrome X.** It is not known if the basis for the pain is a local metabolic imbalance, small-vessel disease undetected by conventional coronary angiography, or a vasoregulatory disorder.

REFERENCES

1. Elveback LR, Connolly DC, Melton LJ 3rd: Coronary heart disease in residents of Rochester, Minnesota 7. Incidence, 1950 through 1982. *Mayo Clin Proc* 61:896, 1986.
2. Elveback LR, Connolly DC: Coronary heart disease in residents of Rochester, Minnesota V. Prognosis of patients with coronary heart disease based on initial manifestations. *Mayo Clin Proc* 60:305, 1985.
3. Wexler L, Brundage B, Crouse J, et al: Coronary artery calcification: pathophysiology, epidemiology, imaging methods, and clinical implications. A statement for health professionals from the American Heart Association. Writing Group. *Circulation* 94(5):1175–1192, 1996.
4. Gibbons RJ, Chatterjee K, Daley J, et al: ACC/AHA/ACP-ASIM guidelines for the management of patients with chronic stable angina: a report of the American College of Cardiology/American Heart Association Task Force on Practice Guidelines (Committee on Management of Patients with Chronic Stable Angina). *J Am Coll Cardiol* 33(7): 2092, 1999.
5. Califf RM, Armstrong PW, Carver JR, et al: Task Force 5. Stratification of patients into high-, medium-, and low risk subgroups for purposes of risk factor management. *J Am Coll Cardiol* 27:964, 1996.
6. Maseri A: Medical therapy of chronic stable angina pectoris. *Circulation* 82:2258, 1990.
7. Ryden T, Malberg K: Calcium channel blockers of beta receptor antagonists for patients with ischemic heart disease. What is the best choice? *Eur Heart J* 17:1, 1996.

8. Antiplatelet Trialists Collaboration. Collaborative overview of randomized trials of antiplatelet therapy-1, prevention of death, MI, and stroke by prolonged antiplatelet therapy in various categories of patients. *Br Med J* 308:81, 1995.

9. Gould AL, Rossouw JE, Santanello NC, et al: Cholesterol reduction yields clinical benefit: impact of statin trials. *Circulation* 97:946, 1998.

10. Parker JO: Nitrates and angina pectoris. *Am J Cardiol* 72:3C, 1993.

11. Mangione NJ, Glasser SP: Phenomenon of nitrate tolerance. *Am Heart J* 128:137, 1994.

12. Cheitlin MD, Hutter AM Jr, Brindis RG, et al: ACC/AHA expert consensus document. Use of sildenafil (Viagra) in patients with cardiovascular disease. *J Am Coll Cardiol* 33:273, 1999.

13. McLenachan JM, Findlay IN, Wilson JT, et al: Twenty-four-hour beta-blockade in stable angina pectoris: a study of atenolol and betaxolol. *J Cardiovasc Pharmacol* 20:311, 1992.

14. Wayshort J, Meshulam N, Brumner D: Isosorbide-5-mononitrate and atenolol in the treatment of stable exertional angina. *Cardiology* 79(2):19, 1991.

15. Opie LH: Calcium channel antagonists in the treatment of coronary artery disease: fundamental pharmacologic properties relevant to clinical use. *Prog Cardiovasc Dis* 38:273, 1996.

16. Weintraub W, King SB, Douglas JS, et al: Percutaneous transluminal coronary angioplasty as a first revascularization procedure in single-, double-, and triple-vessel coronary artery disease. *J Am Coll Cardiol* 26:142, 1995.

17. Parisi AF, Folland ED, Hartigan P: A comparison of angioplasty with medical therapy in the treatment of single-vessel coronary disease. Veterans Affairs ACME Investigators. *N Engl J Med* 326:10,1992.

18. Coronary angioplasty versus medical therapy for angina: the second Randomized Intervention Treatment of Angina (RITA-2) trial. RITA-2 trial participants. *Lancet* 350:461, 1997.

19. Comparison of coronary bypass surgery with angioplasty in patients with multivessel disease. The Bypass Angioplasty Revascularization Investigation (BARI) Investigators. *N Engl J Med* 335:217, 1996.

20. King SB 3rd, Lembo NJ, Weintraub WS, et al: A randomized trial comparing coronary angioplasty with coronary bypass surgery. Emory Angioplasty versus Surgery Trial (EAST). *N Engl J Med* 331:1044, 1994.

21. Prinzmetal M, Kennamer R, Merliss R, et al: Angina pectoris. The variant form of angina pectoris. *Am J Med* 27:375, 1959.

22. Oliva PB, Potts DE, Pluss RG: Coronary arterial spasm in Prinzmetal angina: documentation by coronary arteriography. *N Engl J Med* 288:745, 1973.

PART A. ACUTE CORONARY SYNDROMES–UNSTABLE ANGINA AND NON–ST– SEGMENT ELEVATION MYOCARDIAL INFARCTION

The new phrase *acute coronary syndromes* (ACS) refers to a combination of unstable angina pectoris (UAP), non–ST segment elevation myocardial infarction (NSTEMI), and ST segment elevation myocardial infarction in patients. The value of this terminology is that it points to similarities in pathophysiology—plaque rupture or fissuring, platelet activation, and some degree of superimposed thrombus. UAP and NSTEMI often are indistinguishable at the time of presentation and will be covered together in this chapter.

UNSTABLE ANGINA

It generally is recognized that UAP results from an interplay between fixed coronary artery disease (CAD) and dynamic factors that contribute to intermittent coronary occlusion. UAP is probably not a single entity but a combination of syndromes. It is classified clinically into crescendo angina, non–Q wave myocardial infarction (MI), new-onset angina with accelerating symptoms, and post-MI angina.

Description

The **character, location,** and **radiation** of chest discomfort may be similar to that of stable angina pectoris (AP), although it is often more intense. UAP is distinguished from AP by the presence of one or more of the following criteria:

- **Precipitation:** may occur at rest or at a lower activity level compared to AP and may be less responsive to nitrates
- **Duration:** may last longer than AP, up to several hours in some cases
- **Frequency:** may occur more frequently than stable AP
- **Electrocardiogram (ECG) changes:** More common than AP, UAP often is accompanied by reversible ECG changes of ischemia or injury. Such ECG changes may herald a poor long-term outcome (death as a result of a fatal cardiac event).

Clinical Manifestations

UAP usually presents in one of the following ways:

- Abrupt onset of ischemic symptoms at rest or precipitated by effort in a patient without a history of CAD
- Intensification or change in pattern of ischemic symptoms in a patient with stable angina
- Recurrence of ischemic symptoms soon after (after 24 hours) an acute MI

NON–ST SEGMENT ELEVATION MYOCARDIAL INFARCTION

NSTEMI also has been called a non–Q wave MI or a subendocardial MI, but the more specific terminology of NSTEMI has a more precise connotation. Diagnosis of an NSTEMI is based on two of the following features:

1. A typical prolonged angina history
2. New ST abnormalities that persist (usually ST depression)
3. Elevated troponins

It is often impossible to differentiate between UAP and NSTEMI at initial presentation; the final determination comes after the results of the enzymes are available. Of interest, the pathophysiology of both entities is similar.

Pathophysiology

Like chronic stable AP, UAP often represents an imbalance between supply and demand; however, in UAP, the level of demand is not always measurably increased. In contrast, patients with UAP develop symptoms as a result of a dynamic decrease in myocardial oxygen delivery. Angiographic studies have shown that patients with stable and unstable angina do not differ from each other when traditional indices of the severity of CAD (number of significantly diseased vessels, percent stenosis, and collaterals) are examined. However, antemortem angiographic investigations and postmortem studies show that at least 70% of patients with UAP have eccentric, irregular stenosis or hazy or radiolucent defects in the culprit lesion, whereas these features are infrequent (less than 20%) in patients with stable angina (1). These studies and information from coronary angioscopy have demonstrated the culprit lesion in UAP to be the ruptured plaque. A typical vulnerable lesion consists of an eccentric plaque rich in lipids with a thin fibrous cap. Matrix metalloproteinases may degrade and rupture the plaque, exposing the lipid core with the formation of a platelet-rich thrombus. Whatever the mechanism of plaque fissure, it may result in increasing obstruction by triggering dynamic factors that contribute to intermittent coronary occlusion. These important factors include vasomotor tone, intermittent platelet aggregation, and intraluminal thrombus (2). When plaque fissure and these factors cause brief periods of coronary occlusion, the result is UAP.

Plaque disruption leads to platelet activation, adhesion, and aggregation. **Platelet aggregation** has been shown to be an important factor in experimental studies in the setting of partially occluded coronary arteries. Pretreatment of experimental animals with aspirin before acute coronary occlusion has been shown to reduce the incidence of ventricular fibrillation and to increase collateral blood flow. Clinical evidence of platelet activation during UAP includes elevated levels of products of activation such as β-thromboglobulin, platelet factor 4, thromboxane metabolites, and prostaglandins. **Platelet microemboli** in the myocardial microvasculature downstream from the culprit coronary lesion and the protective effect of aspirin in UAP against MI underscore the importance of platelet aggregation in this setting.

Plaque rupture also leads to release of tissue factor, which interacts with factor VIIa, activates the coagulation cascade, and generates thrombin and fibrin. Several angiographic studies have shown

intracoronary thrombosis in a high percentage (50% to 80%) of patients with UAP with recent symptoms. Histopathologic studies have confirmed the high prevalence of intraluminal thrombus at the site of the fissured plaque. In this regard, the effect of heparin on the development of transmural MI in randomized patients with unstable angina has been studied. Heparin significantly decreased the occurrence of acute MI, suggesting an important role of acute coronary thrombosis.

Coronary vasoconstriction superimposed on a fixed stenotic lesion may lead to total occlusion, infarction, and cardiac death. It is unclear whether vasoconstriction alone can cause sufficiently severe ischemia to cause MI or if there is superimposed localized platelet aggregation with intimal injury and thrombus formation.

Inflammation plays a significant role in the pathophysiology of UAP. Certain infections such as herpes virus and *Chlamydia pneumoniae* have been implicated as etiologic agents. Serologic markers such as elevated C-reactive protein in UAP attest to the importance of inflammation in the pathophysiology (3).

Evaluation

The evaluation of a patient with UAP should follow along the same lines as described in stable angina (see Chapter 8) with the exception that exercise stress testing (EST) should not be performed until the patient has been hospitalized and found to be clinically stable and free of pain for more than 24 hours. The presence of ECG changes of ischemia or injury during spontaneous UAP often precludes the necessity for EST. It is important to stratify patients with UAP into high-risk, intermediate-risk, or low-risk groups because this determines the subsequent therapeutic strategies. The three major determinants of this risk stratification are the likelihood of CAD, the tempo of recent clinical events (frequency, severity, duration, precipitating causes of chest pain), and the patient's likelihood of surviving a cardiac event (4) (see Tables 9a.1 and 9a.2).

Electrocardiogram

Transient ST changes with symptoms of chest discomfort are strongly suggestive of acute ischemia. Symmetric precordial T wave inversion of more than 0.3 mV is also very suspicious for underlying CAD. Nonspecific T changes or ST segment depression of less than 0.5 is not highly predictive of ischemia. The risk of death is highest when there is a left bundle branch block (LBBB), paced rhythm, or left ventricular hypertrophy (LVH).

Serum Cardiac Markers

Cardiac-specific troponin T and troponin I are sensitive and specific markers for myocardial damage. These essentially have replaced CK-MB as the principal markers in evaluating ACS. The presence of these markers serves to differentiate between UAP (symptoms and negative enzymes) and NSTEMI (positive enzymes). The level of troponin also is related directly to the level of risk in ACS.

Other Noninvasive Testing

For many patients with clear symptoms and ECG changes and/or elevated troponins, further workup involves angiography and further

Table 9a.1.   Likelihood of significant coronary artery disease in patients with symptoms suggesting unstable angina pectoris

High likelihood	Intermediate likelihood	Low likelihood
Any of the following features:	**Absence of high likelihood and features of any of the following:**	**Absence of high and intermediate features may have:**
Known history of CAD	Definite angina	Chest pain, probably not angina
Definite angina pectoris	Probable angina	One risk factor, not diabetes
Hemodynamic and ECG changes with pain	Probably not angina in diabetics or in nondiabetics with > 2 other risk factors	
Variant angina	Extracardiac vascular disease	
ST segment increase or decrease >1 mm with pain	ST depression 0.5–1.0 mm	T wave flat or inverted. 1 mm in dominant R wave leads
Marked symmetric T wave inversion in multiple precordial leads	T wave inversion. 1 mm in leads with dominant R waves	Normal ECG

CAD, coronary artery disease; ECG, electrocardiogram.

noninvasive testing is not necessary. For those who have not had a MI, have a normal ECG, and are able to exercise, a standard exercise test without imaging is warranted. For those with resting ECG abnormalities such as LBBB, LVH, resting ST-T abnormalities whose clinical picture is still in doubt, exercise imaging is appropriate.

Therapeutic Considerations

Patients with low-risk UAP may be managed as outpatients with early follow-up evaluations. Outpatient evaluation basically consists of stress testing. Hospitalization with imposition of bed rest and sedation in an ECG-monitored environment is absolutely indicated in patients with UAP classified as high or intermediate risk. Hypertension and other extra cardiac factors increasing demand or decreasing supply should be treated aggressively.

ANTIPLATELET THERAPY

Aspirin

Because platelet aggregation has been strongly implicated in the pathogenesis of UAP and MI, aspirin (a platelet inhibitor) was studied in a large Veterans Administration (VA) cooperative double-blind

**Table 9a.2. Short-term risk of death or
nonfatal myocardial infarction in patients
with symptoms suggesting unstable angina pectoris**

High risk	Intermediate risk	Low risk
At least one of the following features must be present:	**No high-risk feature, but must have any of the following:**	**No high or intermediate risk feature, but may have any of the following:**
Prolonged ongoing (>20 min) rest pain	Rest angina now resolved, but not low likelihood or CAD	Increased angina frequency, severity, or duration
Pulmonary edema	Rest angina (>20 min or exertional angina relieved with rest or nitroglycerin)	Angina provoked at a lower threshold
Angina with new or worsening mitral regurgitation murmurs	Angina with dynamic T wave changes	New onset angina within 2 weeks to 2 months
Rest angina with dynamic ST changes of 1 mm	Nocturnal angina	Normal or unchanged ECG
Angina with S3 or rales	New onset CCSC III or IV angina in past 2 weeks, but not low likelihood of CAD	
Angina with hypotension	Q waves or ST depression. 1 mm in multiple leads Age >65 years	

CAD, coronary artery disease; CCSC, Canadian Cardiovascular Society Classification; ECG, electrocardiogram.

study to test whether endpoints of death and MI were altered. The data showed a 51% lower incidence of MI and death in the aspirin group (324 mg/day) as compared to the placebo group (5). Aspirin causes irreversible acetylation of platelet cyclooxygenase, thereby preventing the formation of thromboxane A_2, an extremely potent vasoconstrictor and platelet activator. Although the VA trial used 324-mg aspirin, it generally is conceded that lower doses (1 mg/kg/day) work as well and are less inhibitory to the arterial endothelium's production of prostacyclin than higher doses.

Thienopyridines

The thienopyridine drugs ticlopidine and clopidogrel inhibit adenosine diphosphate receptors and are effective antiplatelet agents.

These drugs are indicated for patients with UAP who are unable to take aspirin.

Ticlopidine is effective for secondary prevention of stroke and MI and has been used to prevent stent closure. Ticlopidine has been shown to reduce the rate of fatal and nonfatal MI at 6 months by 46% (13.6% versus 7.3%) when compared to placebo in patients with UAP (6). Adverse effects of ticlopidine include diarrhea, abdominal pain, nausea, and vomiting. Hematologic side effects include neutropenia.

The Clopidogrel Aspirin Stent International Cooperative Study (CLASSICS) trial compared clopidogrel with ticlopidine in patients undergoing stenting. Both agents were equally effective, but clopidogrel was better tolerated. Generally, clopidogrel is the preferred thienopyridine over ticlopidine because it is safer, more potent, and faster acting and can be taken once a day (7).

Glycoprotein IIb/IIIa Receptor Antagonists

The GP IIb/IIIa receptor has an affinity for fibrinogen and is the final common pathway involved in platelet aggregation (8). The antagonist drugs occupy the receptor, prevent fibrinogen binding, and prevent platelet aggregation. Three GP IIb/IIIa receptor antagonists are currently available—abciximab, eptifibatide, and tirofiban. Abciximab is a humanized murine antibody whose long duration of action affects platelets for more than 12 to 24 hours after discontinuing the drug. Abciximab is nonspecific for the GP IIb/IIIa receptor, and it also inhibits vitronectin.

Both tirofiban and eptifibatide are small molecules with short half lives of 2 to 3 hours. These drugs are highly specific for the GP IIb/IIIa receptor. Platelet function returns to normal within hours of discontinuing the drug.

The GP IIb/IIIa receptor antagonists have been studied and analyzed in 10 large trials involving more than 32,000 patients with ACS and those undergoing percutaneous coronary intervention (PCI). A metaanalysis of these randomized placebo-controlled trials showed the incidence of death or MI at 30 days of 9% with the GP IIb/IIIa receptor antagonists versus 11.1% for the placebo group.

Although bleeding rates are increased with GP IIb/IIIa receptor blockers, it is usually mild to moderate mucocutaneous bleeding or involves the access site. Severe thrombocytopenia (less than 20,000/mL) is seen in 0.5% of patients. It should be emphasized that the subset of patients with ACS who benefits the most from GP IIb/IIIa receptor antagonists are those patients at high risk and those undergoing PCI (8).

ANTICOAGULATION

Heparin

Evidence shows that unfractionated heparin (UFH) reduces the risk of sudden cardiac death, MI, and recurrent ischemic events when combined with ASA in the setting of UAP. Unless there is a contraindication, full-dose heparin anticoagulation appears to be a logical therapy in the early coronary care unit setting followed by chronic low-dose aspirin in patients with intermediate- or high-risk UAP (9). Most of the benefit is short term, and most trials have limited heparin use to 2 to 5 days. Most predictable results occur when UFH is dosed by weight adjustment; a bolus of 60 to 80 U/

kg is given followed by an infusion of 12 to 18 U/kg/hour. Severe thrombocytopenia (less than 100,000/mL) occurs in 1% to 2%. UFH autoimmune-induced thrombocytopenia with thrombosis (HIT) occurs in less than 0.2% of cases.

Low Molecular Weight Heparin

Low–molecular-weight heparin (LMWH) has been compared to UFH in four randomized trials (10–13). Two trials showed modest benefits, whereas the other two were neutral or negative. LMWH has the advantages of subcutaneous administration, no need for activated partial thromboplastin time testing, less stimulation of platelets, and a lower incidence of HIT.

BETA BLOCKERS

Acute use of beta blockers is advised in ACS with an aim of reducing pulse rate and blood pressure. Beta blockers are effective in stabilizing patients and relieving chest discomfort. Beta blockers have been shown to reduce the progression of UAP to MI by 13% (14).

NITRATES

Nitrates reduce angina and improve clinical stability in patients with ACS. However, there are no data to show that nitrates lower mortality or reduce morbidity (15,16). Usually, nitrates are given intravenously for 24 to 48 hours. There does not appear to be a role for chronic nitrates.

CALCIUM CHANNEL BLOCKERS

Calcium blockers have been added to nitrates and beta blockers to control ongoing pain, significant hypertension, or recurrent ischemia. Dihydropyridines may cause reflex tachycardia, with resultant worsening of angina. These agents should not be used in the absence of concurrent beta blockade. There are no data to show mortality benefit or MI prevention associated with calcium channel blockers (17).

THROMBOLYTIC THERAPY

Because of the recognized role of thrombus formation in UAP, it would seem logical to assume that thrombolysis would be appropriate therapy. However, data from the TIMI IIIB (Thrombolysis in Myocardial Ischemia) randomized trial of 1,473 patients showed no difference in the major outcomes (death or MI) or in the secondary outcomes (evidence of residual ischemia by Holter or exercise tests) between patients with UAP randomized into either a tissue-plasminogen activator (t-PA) or a placebo arm (18). Based on the absence of clinical benefit, a higher incidence of MI, and risk of intracranial hemorrhage, it is recommended that thrombolytic therapy with t-PA not be used routinely in patients with UAP.

Clinical Course

Most patients with UAP will respond to the medical therapy outlined in this chapter and then can be evaluated for extent of disability with the diagnostic tests outlined in Chapter 8. The history, examination, 12-lead ECG, and serum markers help stratify patients into categories of low, intermediate, and high short-term risk of death or nonfatal ischemic events.

Low-risk patients and those that are free of angina, congestive heart failure, or other high-risk features can be evaluated by noninvasive testing. Standard exercise testing without imaging is appropriate for those with normal resting ECG. Exercise or pharmacologic imaging is used in patients with LBBB, LVH, preexcitation, pacemaker, or intraventricular conduction defect. Those who fail to stabilize after initial medical therapy should undergo prompt angiography.

The early management strategy of a conservative approach or an invasive approach has been the focus of several randomized trials. In the TIMI IIIB trial, 1,473 patients with UAP or non–Q wave MI were randomized to early conservative or invasive management. The 1-year and 3-year follow-up data show no significant difference in death or MI between the two groups (18). Critics of this study note that these were generally low-risk patients and that earlier generation PCI was done without stents or IIb/IIIa receptor blockers.

The Veterans Affairs Non–Q-Wave Infarction Strategies in Hospital (VANQWISH) trial showed higher death and MI in the invasive arm compared to the conservative group. It should be noted that mortality was higher (11.6%) among patients undergoing coronary artery bypass graft (CABG) surgery in the early invasive group than in the early conservative group (3.4%) (19). This study also was done before the routine use of stents or IIb/IIIa receptor blockers.

In the FRISC II (Fragmin and Fast Revascularization during InStability in Coronary artery disease) trial, 2,457 patients with UAP or NSTEMI were randomized to an early invasive approach or a noninvasive approach. There was a significant reduction in death or MI in those randomized to early angiography (9.5%) compared to the noninvasive group (12.5%). In the aggressive arm going to CABG surgery, the hospital mortality was 1.2%, and the 30-day mortality was 2.5%. Of the percutaneous transluminal coronary angioplasty (PTCA) group, 60% received stents, and only 10% received IIb/IIIa receptor antagonists (20).

The TACTICS (Treat Angina with Aggrastat and Determine Cost of Therapy with Invasive or Conservative Strategy) trial enrolled 2,200 patients with UAP and MI without ST segment elevation and randomly assigned them to an early invasive strategy or conservative strategy. At 6 months, the primary endpoint composite of death, nonfatal MI, and rehospitalization for ACS was 15.9% for the early invasive strategy and 19.4% for the conservative strategy. The rate of death or nonfatal MI at 6 months was 7.3% versus 9.5%. This latest study done in the stent era with IIb/IIIa receptor antagonists suggests that an early invasive strategy is superior to a conservative approach in reducing the incidence of major cardiac events at 30 days and at 6 months (21).

Unstable Angina Pectoris

A small percentage of patients with UAP will fail to respond to medical management and will proceed to develop MI. Another small percentage will remain unstable with unremitting pain. This latter group has a high incidence of eventual MI with a high mortality, and it is our opinion that aggressive management is indicated as follows:

- Use of intravenous nitroglycerin (5 to 200 µg) to control pain. The goal should be to lower the wedge pressure to 15 to 20 mm Hg without inducing arterial hypotension or an increase in heart rate.

- If aggressive medical therapy is ineffective, intraaortic balloon pumping (IABP) should be tried.
- Urgent coronary arteriography for consideration of angioplasty, coronary stenting, or coronary bypass surgery can be done during IABP support.

Symptoms are relieved in the majority of patients with UAP who undergo angioplasty. However, the rate of restenosis and MI is higher in patients undergoing angioplasty and directional coronary atherectomy acutely (22). The reason for the higher complication rate is unclear, but it probably relates to a stunned myocardium in patients with UAP. Glycoprotein IIB/IIIA platelet receptor blocker therapy has been shown to reduce events of death, MI, and urgent CABG in patients with refractory angina undergoing PTCA or coronary stenting (8).

Debates still will occur as to which patients are to undergo angiography in UAP and NSTEMI and when it should be done. It generally is recommended to do angiography in the following subgroups:

1. Patients who are refractory to medical therapy
2. High-risk subgroups such as those with changing ST segments or elevated troponins
3. Patients with severe ischemia
4. Patients with severe disease and left ventricular dysfunction

REFERENCES

1. Schwartz GG, Karliner JS: Pathophysiology of chronic stable angina. *Atherosclerosis and coronary artery disease.* Philadelphia: J.B. Lippincott, pp. 1389–1400, 1996.
2. Ribeiro PA, Shah PM: Unstable angina: new insights into pathophysiologic characteristics, prognosis, and management strategies. *Curr Prob Cardiol* 21:669, 1996.
3. Haverkate F, Thompson SG, Pyke SD, et al: Production of C-reactive protein and risk of coronary events in stable and unstable angina. European Concerted Action on Thrombosis and Disabilities Angina Pectoris Study Group. *Lancet* 349:462, 1997.
4. Braunwald E, Mark DB, Jones RH, et al: Unstable angina: diagnosis and management: Clinical Practice Guideline, Rockville, MD. Agency for Healthcare Policy and Research and the National Heart, Lung, and Blood Institute. Public Health Service, U.S. Department of Health and Human Services. Agency for Healthcare Policy and Research Publication No. 94–0602:154, 1994.
5. Lewis HD Jr, Davis JW, Archibald DG, et al: Protective effects of aspirin against acute myocardial infarction and death in men with unstable angina. Results of a Veterans Administration Cooperative Study. *N Engl J Med* 309:396, 1983.
6. Balcano F, Rizzon P, Violic F, et al: Antiplatelet treatment with ticlopidine in unstable angina. A controlled, multicenter clinical trial. The Studio della Ticlopidina nell' Angina Instabile Group. *Circulation* 82:17, 1990.
7. Bertrand ME, Rupprecht HJ, Urban P, et al: Double blind study of the safety of clopidogrel with and without a loading dose in combination with aspirin compared with ticlopidine in combination with aspirin after coronary stenting: the Clopidogrel Aspirin Stent International Cooperative Study (CLASSICS). *Circulation* 102:625, 2000.
8. Topol EJ, Byzova TV, Plow EF: Platelet GPIIb-IIIa blockers. *Lancet* 353:227, 1999.

9. Oler A, Whooley MA, Oler J, et al: Adding heparin to aspirin reduces the incidence of myocardial infarction and death in patients with unstable angina. A meta-analysis. *JAMA* 276:811, 1996.

10. Gurfinkel EP, Manos EJ, Mejail RJ, et al: Low molecular weight heparin versus regular heparin or aspirin in the treatment of unstable angina and silent ischemia. *J Am Coll Cardiol* 26:313, 1995.

11. Klein W, Buchwald A, Hillis SE, et al: Comparison of low-molecular-weight heparin with unfractionated heparin acutely and with placebo for 6 weeks in the management of unstable coronary disease. Fragmin in Unstable Coronary Artery Disease study. *Circulation* 96:61, 1997.

12. Comparison of two treatment durations (6 days and 14 days) of a low molecular weight heparin with a 6-day treatment of unfractionated heparin in the initial management of unstable angina or non-Q wave myocardial infarction: FRAX.I.S. (FRAxiparine in Ischaemic Syndrome). *Eur Heart J* 20:1553, 1999.

13. Antman EM, Cohen M, Radley D, et al: Assessment of the treatment effect of enoxaparin for unstable angina/ non-Q-wave myocardial infarction: TIMI IIB-ESSENCE meta-analysis. *Circulation* 100:1602, 1999.

14. Yusuf S, Wittes J, Freidman L: Overview of results of randomized clinical trials in heart disease. 11. Unstable angina, heart failure, primary prevention with aspirin, and risk factor modification. *JAMA* 260:2259, 1988.

15. ISIS-4: a randomised factorial trial assessing early oral captopril, oral mononitrate, and intravenous magnesium sulphate in 58,050 patients with suspected acute myocardial infarction. ISIS-4 (Fourth International Study of Infarct Survival) Collaborative Group. *Lancet* 345: 669, 1995.

16. GISSI-3: Effects of lisinopril and transdermal glyceryl trinitrate singly and together on 6-week mortality and ventricular function after acute myocardial infarction. Gruppo Italiano per lo Studio della Sopravvivenza nell'infarto Miocardico. *Lancet* 343:1115, 1994.

17. Held PH, Yusuf S, Furberg CD: Calcium channel blockers in acute myocardial infarction and unstable angina: an overview. *Br Med J* 299:1187, 1989.

18. Effects of tissue plasminogen activator and a comparison of early invasive and conservative strategies in unstable angina and non-Q-wave myocardial infarction. Results of the TIMI IIIB Trial. Thrombolysis in Myocardial Ischemia. *Circulation* 89:1545, 1994.

19. Boden WE, O'Rourke RA, Crawford MH, et al: Outcomes in patients with non-Q-wave myocardial infarction randomly assigned to an invasive as compared to a conservative management strategy. Veterans Affairs NON-Q-Wave Infarction Strategies in Hospital (VANQWISH) Trial Investigators. *N Engl J Med* 338:1785, 1998.

20. Invasive compared with non-invasive treatment in unstable coronary-artery disease: FRISC II prospective randomised multicentre study. FRagmin and Fast Revascularisation during InStability in Coronary artery disease Investigators. *Lancet* 354:708, 1999.

21. Cannon CP, Weintraub WS, Demopoulos LA, et al: Comparison of early invasive and conservative strategies in patients with unstable coronary syndromes treated with the glycoprotein IIb/IIIa inhibitor tirofiban. *N Engl J Med* 344(25):1879–1887, 2001.

22. Abdelmeguid AE, Ellis SG, Sapp SK, et al: Directional coronary atherectomy in unstable angina, *J Am Coll Cardiol* 24:46–54, 1994.

PART B. MYOCARDIAL INFARCTION

Coronary arteriography within 6 hours of myocardial infarction (MI) has demonstrated a thrombus occluding the infarct-related coronary artery in approximately 85% of cases. Although this thrombotic occlusion may be the result of multiple interacting factors (hemorrhage into a plaque, plaque rupture, platelet aggregation with release of vasoconstrictive substances, and/or coronary spasm), it occurs in the setting of significant underlying coronary atherosclerosis in more than 90% of cases (1). The remaining small number of infarctions without coronary atherosclerosis has been attributed to coronary embolism, isolated coronary spasm, arteritis, trauma, congenital abnormalities, and hematologic disorders.

SYMPTOMS

The major symptom of an acute myocardial infarction (AMI) is chest pain, classically described as a substernal squeezing or pressure sensation, often radiating into the neck or down the arms (usually the left) and lasting 15 to 30 minutes or longer. At times, the pain may be atypical and described as burning, dull-aching, or sharp. It even may be localized just to the arms or neck without associated chest pain. Other symptoms may include shortness of breath, weakness, diaphoresis, and nausea (2). Studies have provided data regarding the relationship between the specific characteristics of the patient's symptoms and the likelihood of acute infarction (3). These are summarized in Table 9b.1.

Two important findings from the Framingham study deserve mention: (a) only 23% of first MIs were preceded by a history of angina and (b) one out of every five MIs was clinically silent or unrecognized (i.e., the pain was atypical in nature or other complaints, such as fatigue or shortness of breath, predominated so that the possibility of an MI was not considered) (4). Unrecognized MI is more frequent in women, people with diabetes, and the elderly (5–7). Certainly, some patients tend to deny or minimize their symptoms, leading to diagnostic difficulties.

SIGNS

Physical findings in patients with AMI vary; however, some generalizations can be made, assuming that pulmonary edema and/or cardiogenic shock is not present (2):

Appearance: normal to diaphoretic, pale, anxious

Vital signs: mild to moderate increase in heart rate (bradyarrhythmias commonly occur with inferior MI), blood pressure (BP) usually is elevated, and respirations may be increased. Fever is common and rarely exceeds 103° F or persists beyond the 8th day post-MI.

Lungs: if left ventricular (LV) dysfunction is present, rales or overt pulmonary edema may be seen. Otherwise, the lungs are clear.

Table 9b.1.   Pain characteristics and acute myocardial infarction

Characteristic	Probability of acute MI %
Description of pain pressure, tightness, crushing burning	24
Indigestion	23
Ache	13
Sharp, stabbing	5
Pleuritic or positional	1
Radiation to jaw, neck, left arm, left shoulder	19
Reproducibility with chest wall palpation	
Partially	6
Fully	5
Combination of variables	
Sharp or stabbing; no history of angina or MI; pain pleuritic/positional or reproducible	0

MI, myocardial infarction.

Heart: S1 is usually of normal intensity, but may be soft. New systolic murmurs may be heard (see later in this chapter). The apical impulse may become diffuse and paradoxic (outward during systole). Paradoxic splitting of S2 may be heard because of a prolonged LV ejection time. An S4 commonly is noted, and occasionally, a soft S3 is present (as a result of ischemia-induced decrease in ventricular compliance).

A friction rub secondary to pericarditis (usually associated with a transmural MI) may be heard. A friction rub usually consists of two or three components (systolic, early and late diastolic) and may occur within hours of acute infarction. Generally, the rub is intermittent, is transient, lasts hours to days, and can be heard in almost every patient with a transmural MI if listened for.

New systolic murmurs may occur and should be listened for carefully and documented accurately. Such murmurs result from the following:

1. Mitral regurgitation secondary to transient ischemia or infarction of the base of the papillary muscle leading to papillary muscle dysfunction (8). This murmur can be early, mid, late or holosystolic in character. Pulmonary edema is a rare complication.
2. Mitral regurgitation secondary to papillary muscle rupture, as opposed to the murmur of papillary muscle dysfunction described earlier, is always hemodynamically significant and generally leads to pulmonary edema (8) (see section on complications).
3. Ventricular septal defect secondary to rupture of the septum (9) (see section on complications).

DIAGNOSTIC TESTS

Electrocardiogram

The electrocardiographic diagnosis of an AMI depends on serial electrocardiogram (ECG) tracings because it is not uncommon in the first few hours of an infarction to have absent or indeterminate ECG findings. Moreover, a classical history and a high index of suspicion should not be influenced by the initial lack of ECG findings. Patients with left bundle branch block (LBBB) or artificially paced rhythms present difficulties in electrocardiographic diagnosis because of secondary ST-T wave changes, but serial tracings may demonstrate changes (2).

Acute inferior, anterior, or lateral **transmural myocardial ischemic injury is associated with ST segment elevation** (i.e., a "subepicardial injury pattern") in those leads that reflect the affected area of the heart (see Chapter 1). The **T wave** in those leads initially is upright, may be very tall or peaked, and subsequently inverts as Q waves develop with infarction/necrosis.

A **posterior transmural MI** is represented by an ST segment vector that is directed posteriorly and reflected as an **ST segment depression on the ECG in leads V1 and V2.** The T wave initially is inverted, but it usually becomes upright (positive) in these leads as a 40-msec R wave develops, representing unopposed anterior depolarization.

The T waves in a so-called **non–ST segment elevation myocardial infarction, non–Q wave myocardial infarction (NQMI)** or subendocardial MI become symmetrically inverted within minutes to hours after the acute event and remain inverted for at least 24 to 48 hours. They may remain inverted indefinitely but, on many occasions, eventually return to normal. The ST segment may be depressed within minutes to hours of the acute event and usually returns to baseline after several days. Q waves do not develop, and there is no distinct change in the R wave. The persistence of these changes for more than 24 hours distinguishes a NQMI from a prolonged ischemic episode without infarction.

Cardiac Enzymes

More than two dozen muscle-associated proteins have been identified as potential markers for AMI (10). The majority are of limited value in the diagnosis of AMI because of lack of specificity, whereas some have proved difficult to assay reliably. Historically, the three serum enzymes most commonly used to diagnose AMI are creatine phosphokinase (CPK, or CK) and its isoenzyme CK-MB, aspartate serum transaminase (AST, or SGOT), and lactic dehydrogenase (LDH). AST and LDH rarely are used because of their limited specificity (these enzymes are found in many other tissues) and the ready availability of more specific serum markers. The efficacy of other markers such a myoglobin, cardiac troponin T (cTnT), and cardiac troponin I (cTnI) has been confirmed. cTnI and cTnT have become the assays of choice in the risk stratification of patients with chest pain and suspected acute cardiac ischemia (11,12). The following is a brief summary of the most frequently used enzymes in diagnosing AMI (Table 9b.2).

Table 9b.2.   Serum markers in acute myocardial infarction

Serum marker	Earliest increase	Peak level	Normalize
Total CK	6 hours	24–30 hours	3–4 days
CK-MB	4–6 hours	18–24 hours	36–48 hours
Myoglobin	1–3 hours	8–12 hours	24–36 hours
Troponin I	4–8 hours	12–16 hours	7–10 days
Troponin T	3–4 hours	12–16 hours	7–14 days

Troponin

The newer markers such as cTnT and cTnI have very high specificity for cardiac injury—greater than that of CK-MB (13). However, cTnT frequently is elevated in patients with uremia. Serum levels of the troponins increase about the same time after the onset of AMI as CK-MB, but they remain elevated for a substantially longer period. If cTnI is performed serially at 0, 6, and 12 hours and levels do not rise above 0.4 ng/mL, it is unlikely myocardial necrosis has occurred. A level between 0.4 to 1.5 ng/mL suggests MI, and a level greater than 1.5 ng/mL strongly suggests an AMI. The cardiac troponins are highly specific and remain elevated for more than 24 hours.

Creatine Kinase

Creatine kinase is a ubiquitous enzyme and is released with skeletal or cardiac muscle injury or trauma. Three CK isoenzymes have been identified: CK-MM (specific for skeletal muscle), CK-BB (specific for brain tissue), and CK-MB (specific for cardiac muscle). Thus, the specificity of an elevated CK improves in myocardial injury by measuring the CK-MB isoenzyme. Detecting elevated levels of CK-MB in the serum has been the gold standard for the diagnosis of AMI for many years (14). Elevated enzyme levels can occur, however, under a variety of circumstances. These include skeletal muscle crush injury, electrical injury, dermatomyositis, hypothyroidism, chronic renal failure (as a result of decreased excretion), rhabdomyolysis, strenuous exercise, cardiac surgery, and defibrillation/cardioversion. When both the CK-MB (ng/mL) and the CK (u/L) are elevated, a relative index is calculated (CK-MB/CK $\times$ 100); a value greater than 2.5 is suggestive of MI.

Aspartate Serum Transaminase

AST lacks specificity, being found in high concentrations in liver and skeletal muscle. It has, thus, fallen out of favor as a marker for MI.

Lactic Dehydrogenase

Elevated in muscle, liver, and hematologic disorder, LDH is nonspecific. The five isoenzymes of LDH provide a means of improving specificity over that of total LDH activity. Myocardium is the only tissue in which LDH1 is the most abundant isoenzyme; in normal serum and in tissue other than the heart, LDH2 activity exceeds that of LDH1. In cardiac injury, the normal LDH1:LDH2 ratio (usually less than 1.0) is more than 1. Elevated levels of LDH can remain elevated up to 7 to 10 days.

Myoglobin

Myoglobin is a heme protein ubiquitous in cardiac and skeletal muscle. It is abnormally elevated in the serum within 2 hours of an AMI and is cleared rapidly. Its rapid clearance explains the rising and falling (staccato pattern) values observed in some patients (15). Therefore, a solitary negative myoglobin level does not exclude acute infarction. It should not be used as a cardiac marker if the patient has suffered noncardiac trauma or has chronic renal or skeletal muscle disease.

None of the current tests are perfect, and serial testing is still necessary to rule out MI. The sensitivity of a given marker in detecting AMI is dependent upon the time it is measured after the onset of symptoms. It is imperative to understand that not even the most specific serum marker of myocardial damage can exempt the physician from careful clinical assessment of patients who presents with chest pain.

Radionuclide Scanning

In the majority of AMIs, the clinical history, ECG, and pattern of enzyme changes will establish the diagnosis without difficulty, and radionuclide scanning will add little useful information. However, in certain situations where the clinical history, ECG, and/or enzyme pattern is confusing or not available, a properly timed radionuclide scan can be helpful in establishing the diagnosis. Patients with LBBB, those with paced ECGs, those who have delayed evaluation of their chest pain beyond the time range in which troponin determinations are useful, those with non–Q wave infarctions, and patients who have had previous infarctions are particularly good candidates for radionuclide imaging. Several techniques using technetium pyrophosphate and thallium-201 are available (16,17) (see Chapter 5).

Echocardiography

Echocardiography may be valuable in evaluating patients with AMI and complications. Wall motion abnormalities such as hypokinesis, akinesis, and dyskinesis can be identified and help the clinician in determining the degree of functional impairment. LV ejection fraction can be calculated, which is useful in determining prognosis. LV thrombus formation can be detected; if the thrombus is large and "shaggy," anticoagulation may be indicated. Complications of mitral regurgitation with papillary muscle rupture, ventricular septal defect, right ventricular (RV) infarction, LV aneurysm, and pericardial effusion can be identified (18).

PROGNOSTIC FACTORS

Infarct Size

The amount of damaged myocardium and resultant LV dysfunction is the principal determinant of outcome following MI. Infarct size varies from minimal loss of myocardial muscle mass (less than 5% in-hospital mortality) to loss of approximately 40% of the LV muscle mass and resultant cardiogenic shock (in-hospital mortality often is more than 80%). No perfect method of infarct size assessment is available; however, clinicians make general estimates based on clinical status, enzyme values, ECGs, nuclear ventriculography, two-dimensional echocardiography, and abnormalities during invasive hemodynamic monitoring (19–21). Limiting infarct size has been attempted using agents that decrease the oxygen demands of the myocardium (nitroglycerin, beta blockers, calcium blockers, etc.) and/or by increasing supply (thrombolytic therapy, IIb/IIIa glycoprotein inhibition, angioplasty, stenting, and coronary bypass surgery) (22). Studies assessing the benefit of interventions designed to limit infarct size must be interpreted cautiously in view of the imprecise methods of quantitation. Research techniques using positron emission tomography and magnetic resonance imaging may prove to be of value.

Infarct Site

The site of the infarct is an important variable in determining outcome. Anterior MIs generally result from occlusion of the left anterior descending coronary artery. They tend to be larger infarcts and therefore are associated with a higher mortality. These infarcts are more prone to expansion, rupture, mural thrombus, and aneurysm formation. Occlusion of the circumflex coronary artery results in lateral infarction. When the circumflex is a dominant artery (10% of cases), the infarct may involve the posterior and inferior walls.

Right coronary artery occlusion may result in inferior or inferoposterior infarction. Although right coronary occlusion usually causes less loss of critical myocardium than obstruction of the left anterior descending branch, the spectrum of clinical presentation varies widely from a "benign" event to major hemodynamic consequences (RV infarction, rupture of the posteromedial papillary muscle) and significant arrhythmias (bradycardia, heart block, and ventricular fibrillation).

Severity of Coronary Artery Disease

Another factor affecting outcome of MI is the presence of coexistent coronary artery disease in vessels supplying noninfarcted myocardium. Of patients with AMI, 75% have at least two major vessels with critical lesions and 50% have triple vessel disease. It thus follows that angina may develop early after infarct (within 7 to 10 days) in approximately 25% of patients with AMI and often is associated with poor prognosis. Patients with angina from "ischemia at a distance" (outside the zone of infarct) now are recognized as having a high mortality at 6 months (75%).

ACUTE INTERVENTION–REPERFUSION THERAPY

Prior to 1980, treatment of AMI was largely expectant or prophylactic in character or directed toward the management of complications. Overwhelming evidence now exists that reperfusion in the setting of AMI improves survival, decreases symptoms of heart failure, and increases LV function. There are two primary methods available to achieve reperfusion: thrombolytic therapy or primary (direct) coronary angioplasty.

Intravenous Thrombolytic Therapy

Intravenous (IV) thrombolytic therapy is the most accepted interventional strategy for treatment of patients with AMI (23,24). The IV thrombolytic agents presently used and available in the United States are streptokinase (SK), recombinant tissue plasminogen activator (rt-PA), alteplase, tenecteplase, and reteplase. All have demonstrated a remarkable capacity to establish blood flow by dissolving occlusive thrombi, especially when given within the first 6 hours of AMI. Each agent has been shown to reduce in-hospital mortality and improve LV function when compared to placebo.

It is believed that thrombolytic therapy is underused and that only about 50% of eligible patients actually receive lytic therapy. Because of published exclusion criteria in many large, highly publicized trials, there has been confusion about who should or should not be treated. Several strategies have been implemented to increase the number of patients who receive therapy. These strategies include raising the upper age limit of therapy, treating patients beyond 4 hours after the onset of symptoms, and disregarding the site of the infarct. Support for widening inclusion criteria has been provided via a meta-analysis of large thrombolytic trials (25).

Eligibility for thrombolytic therapy in AMI has been simplified:

- Ischemic chest pain of longer than 30 minutes and less than 12 hours in duration
- ST segment elevation of more than 1.0 mV in two continuous ECG leads indicative of AMI
- New left bundle branch pattern on ECG

Exclusion criteria include the following:

- Systolic BP higher than 180 mm Hg and diastolic BP higher than 110 mm Hg
- History of bleeding disorder
- Significant gastrointestinal bleed within preceding 5 months
- Major surgery, organ biopsy, or significant trauma within preceding 3 months
- History of central nervous system (CNS) malignancy or arteriovenous malformation
- History of stroke or transient ischemic attack
- Warfarin therapy with an international normalized ratio of more than 1.4 (prothrombin time longer than 14 seconds)
- Cardiopulmonary resuscitation for longer than 10 minutes

Many trials have studied the various thrombolytic agents in an attempt to define which is the best. There have been a number of trials looking at different endpoints, such as early patency rate, late patency rates, and early survival, and trials comparing different thrombolytic agents, various regimens of anticoagulation, and adjunctive therapy [e.g., angiotensin converting enzyme (ACE) inhibitors]. This has led to enormous confusion for the clinician in translating trial results to clinical practice. Other studies such as the GISSI-II (Gruppo Italiano per lo Studio dell soprevvivenza nell'Infarcto Miocardico), ISIS-3 (Third International Study of Infarct Survival), and GUSTO-1 (Global Utilization of Streptokinase and Tissue Plasminogen Activator for Occluded Coronary Arteries) trials have simpler designs and less rigid entry criteria and focus on endpoints of mortality and morbidity. In these statistically powerful studies, there was no advantage of one lytic agent over another when comparing mortality rates. In the ISIS-3 trial, all three agents (SK, t-PA, and APSAC) had a 10% mortality rate. In the GISSI-II and GUSTO-1 trials, there was no difference in mortality between SK and t-PA (26–28).

The GUSTO trial did show an advantage for accelerated t-PA over streptokinase in addition to conventionally used concomitant treatment. The 30-day mortality was 6.3% with t-PA and 7.3% with streptokinase (28). Analysis of subgroups in this study showed that those who benefited most from t-PA were patients with large infarctions, those with anterior MI, those presenting within 6 hours, and those younger than 75 years of age. Because of this, it has been recommended that patients with late treatment (more than 6 hours after pain onset), those with small MIs, and those with increasing risk of stroke (age older than 75 years, female, and low body weight) be treated with streptokinase. An important observation of the GUSTO trial is that survival after infarction even as early as the first day is critically limited to the establishment of complete antegrade flow [Thrombolysis in Myocardial Infarction (TIMI) grade 3 flow] in the infarct-related vessel.

GUSTO-1 showed that accelerated tissue plasminogen activator, or t-PA (alteplase) demonstrated a ceiling of reperfusion in the 60% range. Newer agents have the advantage of ease of administration but have not been shown to increase efficacy. These newer agents include reteplase given as a double bolus and tenecteplase administered as a single bolus (29,30).

Evidence has demonstrated that disordered microvasculature function and inadequate myocardial tissue perfusion often are present despite artery patency and are related to worse clinical outcome (31). Optimal reperfusion extends beyond epicardial reperfusion and focuses on preserving microvascular integrity and function, preventing inflammation, and improving myocardial tolerance to ischemia.

There are several limitations of thrombolytic therapy for AMI:

- Less than half of patients with AMI actually receive thrombolytic therapy.
- Regardless of agent or dose, patency rate is 60%, and only 40% to 50% of vessels achieve normal TIMI 3 flow.
- Patients who receive thrombolytic therapy have a 15% to 30% incidence of recurrent ischemic events, and there is a 0.5% to 2.0% incidence of intracranial bleeding.
- Reocclusion of the culprit artery occurs in 5% to 10% of patients.
- There are no clinical markers that accurately predict clot lysis and reperfusion.

COMBINATION THERAPY—FIBRINOLYTIC THERAPY AND GLYCOPROTEIN IIB/IIIA INHIBITORS

Combination therapy hopes to break through the "lytic ceiling" by achieving more rapid and complete coronary and optimal tissue perfusion without compromising safety. The concept has been promoted by the understanding of the central role of the platelet in addition to fibrin in arterial thrombosis.

Several small trials show that combination therapy has promise without increase in major bleeding. The TIMI 14 trial compared alteplase alone to alteplase plus abciximab, looking at 90-minute TIMI 3 perfusion rates: lytic alone achieved 62%, whereas the combination achieved 77% (32). The SPEED (Strategies for Patency Enhancement in the Emergency Department) trial showed lytic alone reperfusion rate to be 47% versus 61% for combination of low-dose reteplase and abciximab (33). The INTRO-MI (Integrilin and Reduced Dose of

Thrombolytic in Acute Myocardial Infarction) study revealed a 40% reperfusion rate for lytic alone versus a 56% for the combination of reduced dose alteplase and eptifibatide at 60 minutes (34). Several ongoing trial are testing coronary patency with combination therapy; these include the FASTER (Fibrinolytic and Aggrastat for ST Elevation Resolution) (35) trial (tenecteplase alone versus TNK and tirofiban), the INTEGRITI (Integrilin + TNK-t-PA in AMI) (36) trial (TNK alone versus TNK and eptifibatide), and the ENTIRE (Enoxaparin and TNK-t-PA with or without Glycoprotein IIb-IIIa Inhibitor as Reperfusion Strategy in ST Elevation MI) (37) trial (TNK alone versus TNK and abciximab, plus heparin versus enoxaparin). The GUSTO V trial studied 16,588 patients with AMI comparing reteplase alone versus half dose reteplase and abciximab. The 30-day mortality was 5.9% in the reteplase-alone group versus 5.6% in the combination arm. Reinfarction was 3.5% versus 2.3%, and intracranial bleeding was 1.1% versus 2.1%. This trial did not prove superiority of combination therapy; the conclusion was that combination therapy was not inferior to lytic alone (38).

ST segment resolution has become a tool to assess new reperfusion as a measure of myocardial tissue perfusion. There is a threefold to sevenfold increase in risk of death with less than 30% ST segment resolution compared with complete (more than 70%) resolution 3 hours after onset of therapy. The TIMI-14, SPEED, and INTRO-MI trials all showed a higher percentage of patients with more than 70% ST segment resolution in the combination therapy arm versus lytic alone (32–34).

COMBINATION THERAPY—FIBRINOLYTIC THERAPY AND LOW–MOLECULAR-WEIGHT HEPARIN

Low–molecular-weight heparins (LMWHs) have several advantages over unfractionated heparin, such as less inhibition by circulatory proteins, no monitoring requirement, more stable anticoagulation, and ease of use. Several trials have addressed the combined use of thrombolytic therapy and LMWH as compared to lytic plus unfractionated heparin. The HART II (Randomized Comparison of Low Molecular Weight Heparin and Unfractionated Heparin Adjunctive to t-PA Thrombolysis and Aspirin) trial has shown that alteplase with enoxaparin achieved slightly higher 90-minute patency (53% LMWH versus 48% heparin), lower reocclusion, (5.9% versus 9.8%), and similar rates of bleeding (3.6% versus 3.0%) (39).

The ASSENT-plus (Assessment of the Safety and Efficacy of New Thrombolytic Regimens) trial studied 400 patients treated with alteplase and dalteparin versus unfractionated heparin. Dalteparin appeared to be safe (major bleeding, 3.6% versus 5.2% with heparin) and resulted in less reocclusion (1.4% versus 5.4%) The ASSENT-3 trial studied 6,116 patients with acute ST segment MI. The data showed the lowest ischemic events in the TNK plus enoxaparin arm. There was a harmful effect in the elderly with half TNK enoxaparin and abciximab (40).

ANGIOPLASTY IN ACUTE MYOCARDIAL INFARCTION

Primary (Direct) Percutaneous Transluminal Coronary Angioplasty

Primary (direct) angioplasty refers to the use of primary (direct) percutaneous transluminal coronary angioplasty (PTCA) without prior thrombolytic therapy. Primary angioplasty during AMI was first applied in 1982 and subsequently has been used with increasing frequency over the last 15 years. One limiting factor of this approach has been that only 20% of U.S. hospitals have catheterization facilities; thus, the main nationwide strategy has been to administer immediate IV thrombolytic therapy. Other limiting factors include set-up time, cost, and need for skilled personnel. Despite these factors, primary angioplasty has been shown to be a remarkably valuable therapy for patients undergoing MI (41). It is the most effective method of confirming the diagnosis and establishing high-risk subsets by obtaining coronary artery anatomy and LV function data. Opening of the infarct-related artery is confirmed angiographically; this a major advantage over having to estimate vessel patency with the IV lytic approach. Another benefit is that adjunctive therapies such as intraaortic balloon pumping (IABP), pacing, and hemodynamic monitoring can be applied at the time of the procedure. The direct PTCA approach is applicable to nearly all patients with MI including those who have been excluded in most thrombolytic trials [elderly, previous coronary artery bypass graft (CABG), recent surgery or trauma, cerebrovascular accident or CNS damage, active bleeding, etc.]. Direct PTCA approaches a 99% success rate (42), and there is a decreased incidence of recurrent ischemic events and risk of hemorrhagic stroke.

The first randomized trial comparing direct angioplasty to thrombolytic therapy was not available until 1993 (43). Patients were randomized to rt-PA (200 patients) or to primary PTCA (195 patients), with both groups having closely matched baseline characteristics. All patients were treated with acetylsalicylic acid (ASA) 325 mg/day, IV heparin for 3 to 5 days, and IV nitroglycerin for 24 hours. The in-hospital mortality rate was 2.6% for the direct PTCA group and 6.5% for the rt-PA group. At 6 months, reinfarction or death had occurred in 16.8% of the rt-PA group and only 8.5% of the PTCA group. Recurrent ischemia occurred in 10% of the PTCA group versus 28% in the rt-PA group.

Two other randomized single-center trials were published in 1993 (44,45). Meta-analysis of the three randomized trials has shown an in-hospital death rate for PTCA of 2.2% versus 5.8% for the thrombolytic group. In-hospital reinfarction rate was 1.9% for the PTCA group and 7.6% for the thrombolytic group. In those randomized to PTCA, there was less recurrent ischemia, and early and late patency rates were greater with lower residual stenosis. More than 90% of the PTCA groups showed TIMI-3 flow, which is the strongest predictor of improved ejection fraction and survival at 30 days.

Several subsets of patients with infarction are particularly well served by direct angioplasty. Those patients with cardiogenic shock who are treated successfully with direct PTCA and IABP have a much better survival rate (more than 70%) than those treated with thrombolytics or conventional medications (less than 25%) (46). Patients with MI who have had prior CABG usually are better treated with mechanical intervention than thrombolytic treatment. Contemporary thrombolytic agents are less efficacious in saphenous vein grafts than in native occlusions. Thrombus-laden saphenous vein grafts are associated with the risk of distal embolization regardless of the method of reperfusion (46).

Despite the large-scale development of thrombolytic agents during the last decade and expanded indications for their use, a large percentage of thrombolytic-ineligible patients (estimated 35% to 65% of all infarcts) still present to large community hospitals throughout the country (47). This high-risk subset (usually older with more chronic diseases) has an 18% mortality risk and is best treated with direct PTCA (48).

Advantages of Primary Percutaneous Transluminal Coronary Angioplasty in Acute Myocardial Infarction

- Can treat patients ineligible for IV thrombolytic agents
- Early and sustained high percentage of TIMI grade 3 flow
- Lower incidence of recurrent ischemia
- Lower incidence of intracranial hemorrhage
- Better LV function
- Less expensive when compared to accelerated t-PA regimens
- Immediate availability of coronary anatomy with catheterization

Direct Percutaneous Transluminal Coronary Angioplasty/ Stenting in Acute Myocardial Infarction

Even with the advances made by primary PTCA in AMI, there are still limitations with this approach. Of patients, 10% to 15% will have recurrent ischemia, 3% to 6% will have reinfarction, 40% to 50% will have late restenosis, and nearly 20% require repeat PTCA or CABG.

Stents were tried in the AMI setting with the rationale that they would prevent recoil and abrupt closure, as well as reduce the restenosis rate. Despite concerns that thrombus would be a negative factor in MI and stenting, initial trials demonstrated that thrombus was not a major limitation. Initial trials mostly were done with the Palmaz-Schatz stent and showed high success rates and better angiographic results. The PAMI (Primary Angioplasty in Myocardial Infarction) stent pilot trial demonstrated a 98% success rate and lower adverse events when compared to standard balloon. Death was 0.8% for the stent arm versus 2.7% for the standard PTCA arm; rate of CABG was 5.2% versus 6.0%, and reocclusion was 5.6% versus 10% to 14% (49).

The combined results of the PAMI STENT trial and six registries have shown the primary success rate to be 98%, stent thrombosis 1.8%, death 0.9%, reinfarction 1.3%, CABG 1.8%, and repeat PTCA 2.1%. It is clear that stenting has improved results, has reduced ischemia and reclosure, and is safe and effective. Stenting also may facilitate early discharge and appears to be cost neutral.

In the STOPAMI (Stent versus Thrombolysis for Occluded coronary arteries in Patients with Acute Myocardial Infarction) trial, coronary stenting plus platelet glycoprotein IIb/IIIa blockade was compared to t-PA in AMI. Coronary stenting plus abciximab resulted in more myocardial salvage and better clinical outcomes than with t-PA. The incidence of death, reinfarction, or stroke at 6 months was 8.5% in the stent group versus 23.2% in the lytic group (50). The STAT (Stenting versus Thrombolysis in Acute myocardial infarction Trial) trial compared primary stenting to t-PA; primary stenting reduced the composite endpoint at 6 months of death, reinfarction, stroke, or repeat target vessel revascularization for ischemia compared to accelerated t-PA (24.2% versus 55%) (51).

The Facilitated Approach

One major limitation of percutaneous intervention and acute mechanical reperfusion is the 2 hours or more average delay from hospital arrival until the artery is open. The approach of combining early pharmacologic reperfusion therapy followed by mechanical reperfusion has been termed "facilitated angioplasty." This approach involves the immediate use of a low-dose fibrinolytic, IIb/IIIa glycoprotein inhibitors, LMWH followed as soon as possible by angioplasty/stenting. The FINESSE (Facilitated Intervention with Enhanced reperfusion Speed to Stop Events) trial is randomizing 2,700 patients with ST segment elevation MI to half-dose reteplase and abciximab immediately before percutaneous intervention (52).

Immediate Angioplasty

Immediate angioplasty in AMI refers to the use of PTCA immediately after thrombolysis. The theoretic advantages of combining thrombolysis with immediate PTCA include achieving a higher reperfusion rate than lytic agents alone, addressing the underlying residual stenosis that is not affected by lysis alone, and potentially eliminating flow-limiting stenosis and improving function and recovery. This combination of medical and mechanical intervention has been the subject of several clinical trials including the Thrombolysis and Angioplasty in Myocardial Infarction (TAMI) study (53), the TIMI 2A (54), and the European Cooperative Study Group (ECSG) trial (55). Each tested the strategy of immediate angiography and PTCA after thrombolytic therapy versus the alternative strategy of deferred angiography and PTCA after 48 hours to 10 days or indefinitely if stress testing showed no provocable ischemia. When the endpoint of LV function was evaluated, no benefit was shown with immediate PTCA over the deferred strategy. In-hospital mortality was higher in the immediate strategy, and emergency CABG surgery was required more commonly in the immediate strategy. There was also a substantially higher incidence of bleeding complications and blood transfusions in the immediate strategy.

Rescue Angioplasty

Rescue (salvage) angioplasty refers to PTCA after failed thrombolysis. Patients with an occluded infarct artery (TIMI 0–1 flow) 90 minutes after thrombolytic therapy have worse LV function and an increased early mortality (56). Rescue PTCA is indicated in this group to establish reperfusion, salvage myocardium, and improve healing. Patients requiring rescue PTCA to achieve patency had an increased reocclusion rate in several trials (57). With new understanding of the importance of aspirin, heparin, and activated clotting time (ACT) monitoring, reocclusion rates in the GUSTO angiographic substudy appear to be decreasing (58). Unfortunately, the mortality rate in patients who fail rescue PTCA is high (more than 30%).

Deferred Angioplasty

Delayed angioplasty refers to angioplasty performed electively 1 to 7 days after thrombolysis. PTCA commonly has been used for post-MI angina or ischemia after thrombolytic therapy. The DANAMI (Danish multicenter randomized study of invasive versus conservative treatment in patients with inducible ischemia following thrombolysis in acute myocardial infarction) study enrolled 1,008 patients who had post-MI angina or an abnormal exercise test after thrombolysis (59). Patients were randomized to receive a mechanical intervention (n = 503) versus conservative therapy (n = 505). Major events with the interventional approach were diminished (MI 5.6% versus death 3.6%). It is recommended that patients with post-MI angina or ischemia undergo catheterization and mechanical revascularization if indicated.

Emergency Bypass Surgery

Emergency coronary bypass has the potential value of myocardial salvage if difficult logistics can be overcome within the first 4 hours of MI. Surgery should be considered in patients whose coronary anatomy previously has been assessed with angiography and who develop ischemia while in the hospital awaiting surgery or in those who develop the onset of MI while undergoing routine angiography or coronary angioplasty. Bypass of diseased, but noninfarct-related, arteries at the time of surgery could have additional value. However, the usual delay in clinical presentation of the patient who develops MI out of the hospital and the time required for clinical evaluation, angiography, assembling the surgical team, and placing the patient on cardiopulmonary bypass generally will preclude this intervention in most patients.

PHARMACOLOGIC ADJUNCTS TO REPERFUSION THERAPY

Multiple pharmacologic adjuncts to reperfusion have been studied. These generally fall into two categories: those that stabilize platelet-fibrin plaques, such as aspirin and heparin, and those that promote tissue recovery, such as nitrates and beta-blockers, by improving the myocardial oxygen supply/demand ratio.

Antiplatelet/Antithrombin Agents

Platelet activation is a key step in acute arterial thrombosis. **Aspirin** irreversibly inhibits the cyclooxygenase enzyme responsible for the synthesis of eicosanoids. In platelets, aspirin prevents the formation of thromboxane A_2, a substance that induces platelet aggregation. Because platelets are unable to generate new cyclooxygenase, inhibition of the enzyme lasts for the lifetime of the cell (about 10 days). In vascular endothelial cells, aspirin prevents the synthesis of prostacyclin, which inhibits platelet aggregation. However, because endothelial cells can recover cyclooxygenase synthesis, this inhibitory effect of aspirin may be of shorter duration. Aspirin is absorbed rapidly in the stomach and upper gastrointestinal tract, causing platelet inhibition in approximately 60 minutes (60). The different effects of various doses of aspirin (20 to 1,500 mg/day) on platelet and vessel-wall eicosanoid synthesis have been investigated extensively. Doses of 80 to 325 mg/day are used most commonly in the management of coronary artery disease.

Antiplatelet therapy is effective in secondary prevention of MI. A meta-analysis of data from six randomized, placebo-controlled, double-blind trials in patients surviving MI demonstrated that platelet inhibitors reduce vascular mortality rate by 13%, the nonfatal reinfarction rate by 31%, and the nonfatal stroke rate by 42%. No statistically significant differences among the various antiplatelet regimens used were found (61). It currently is recommended that all survivors of AMI be treated indefinitely with aspirin at a dose of 160 to 325 mg/day (62).

The importance of aspirin therapy early in the course of AMI was highlighted by the ISIS-2 trial (63). In this study, the clinical efficacy of streptokinase alone, aspirin alone, or the combination of both agents was assessed. The mortality rate for patients treated with aspirin alone was 21% lower than that for the placebo group. This reduction was only slightly less than that achieved with streptokinase alone. However, when both aspirin and streptokinase were administered, the reduction on mortality was increased dramatically. Aspirin (160 to 325 mg) should be administered as soon as the diagnosis of AMI (or unstable angina) is considered, regardless of whether a thrombolytic agent is used or not.

Thienopyridines (ticlopidine and clopidogrel) are more potent antiplatelet agents than aspirin. These agents block adenosine diphosphate and inhibit binding of fibrinogen to the platelet glycoprotein IIb/IIIa receptor. Combined ASA and ticlopidine has a synergistic effect in reducing coronary platelet deposition (64). When direct PTCA results in stenting, clopidogrel commonly is used with a loading dose of 300 mg followed by 75 mg/day for 2 weeks to a month after the intervention (65).

Glycoprotein IIb/IIIa receptor antagonist agents block the glycoprotein IIb/IIIa receptor and lead to a dose-dependent inhibition of platelet aggregation (66). Reports of reduced acute and 6-month ischemic events in the EPIC (Evaluation of c7E3 for Prevention of Ischemic Complications) trial using c7E3, a monoclonal antibody, are promising, but the beneficial effects have to be weighed against the increased risk of major bleeding (14% versus 7% control) and the high cost ($1,300/dose) (67). The TAMI 8 pilot study reported improved coronary artery patency and a trend to fewer ischemic events with 7E3 (added to aspirin and heparin) following thrombolytic therapy for MI (68).

The IMPACT-AMI (Integrilin to Manage Platelet Aggregation to Combat Thrombosis-Acute Myocardial Infarction) trial concluded that integrelin, when combined with alteplase, aspirin, and heparin, accelerated the speed of reperfusion, but this was not associated with an improved in-hospital outcome (69). The PARADIGM (Platelet Aggregation Receptor Antagonist Dose Investigation and Reperfusion Gain in Myocardial Infarction) trial combined the platelet glycoprotein IIb/IIIa inhibitor lamifiban with thrombolysis in 353 patients with AMI; lamifiban given as an adjunct to the thrombolytic hastened ECG evidence of reperfusion but did not result in clear clinical benefits (70).

The RAPPORT (ReoPro And Primary PTCA Organization and Randomized Trial) is a randomized, placebo-controlled trial of platelet glycoprotein IIb/IIIa blockade with primary angioplasty for AMI. Although abciximab given during primary PTCA did not alter the primary endpoint of elective revascularization procedures at 6 months, it did decrease the incidence of death, reinfarction, and urgent revascularization (71).

Commercial **heparin** is a heterogenous mixture of polysaccharides, not all of which are active in inhibiting the coagulation cascade. Heparin requires the plasma protein cofactor antithrombin III to express anticoagulant activity. This occurs by heparin binding both antithrombin III and activated coagulation proteases, such as thrombin, to catalyze the protease inhibition by antithrombin III (72). Despite numerous clinical trials, the role of heparin after reperfusion still is debated (73). Early administration of heparin combined with a lytic agent does not appear to hasten reperfusion, but heparin may play an important role in preventing reocclusion, especially when used in conjunction with rt-PA (71,72). Several large-scale trials have used subcutaneous heparin combined with thrombolytic therapy, which has led to considerable confusion in defining the role of heparin in AMI. The GISSI-2 and the ISIS trials (collectively involving more than 20,000 patients) failed to show a clinical or survival benefit associated with delayed subcutaneous heparin (73,74). The GUSTO trial demonstrated the importance of systemic IV heparinization when t-PA is used as the thrombolytic agent, and IV heparin is strongly recommended for patients receiving t-PA (62) with the continuous infusion rate being guided by determination of partial thromboplastin time (45 to 75 seconds). With direct PTCA, high-dose heparin to achieve an ACT between 350 to 400 seconds often is used. Little is known about the optimal dose and duration of heparin infusion after PTCA for AMI. There are no data to support IV heparin use for more than 24 to 48 hours. Several studies have suggested that IV heparin should not be stopped abruptly because of the risk of a rebound hypercoagulable state and increased risk of reinfarction (75,76). Based on these data, tapering the heparin infusion rate to one-half of the therapeutic dose for 12 hours prior to discontinuation appears prudent.

LMWH has multiple advantages over unfractionated heparin, such as subcutaneous administration, no need for monitoring, less stimulating of platelets, and a lower incidence of heparin-induced thrombocytopenia. The FRAMI (Fragmin in Acute Myocardial Infarction) trial randomized LMWH (dalteparin) in prevention of LV thrombus formation and arterial embolism after AMI. Dalteparin was effective in preventing LV thrombus in patients with first anterior AMI but was associated with an increased risk of bleeding (major bleeding with dalteparin 2.9% versus 0.3% in the placebo arm (77). The exact role of this drug in AMI still is unresolved, but there are encouraging data suggesting clinical benefits especially in the combination drug trial previously outlined.

Direct thrombin inhibitors, such as hirudin and Hirulog, are not dependent on antithrombin III, are better specific inhibitors of fibrin-bound thrombin than heparin, and are being investigated actively in the management of acute ischemic heart disease (69).

Beta-Adrenergic Blockade

Beta-blocker therapy reduces heart rate, BP, and myocardial contractility, which results in a decrease in myocardial oxygen consumption. Experimental models have shown that beta-blockers decrease myocardial ischemia and reduce infarct size. These observations provided the rationale for clinical studies that can be divided into two main categories: "early" administration (beginning at the time of acute presentation) and "late entry" (after the evolution of the infarct is complete, which is usually after 4 days). Most of the "late entry" trials were completed before the widespread use of thrombolytic therapy.

Five large, multicenter, prospective randomized trials with more than 11,500 patients have evaluated late beta-blocker therapy in MI. Included in this group are the Norwegian Multicenter Study Group (timolol, 20 mg/day) (78), the Beta Blocker Heart Attack Trial (propanolol, 180 to 240 mg/day) (79), and the Goteborg Trial (metoprolol, 200 mg/day) (80). These studies have demonstrated that beta-blocker therapy reduces mortality by about 25% when compared to placebo controls (81). It is postulated that much of the benefit in the beta-blocker–treated patients is the result of a reduction in the risk of sudden cardiac death (i.e., an antiarrhythmic effect resulting from inhibition of adrenergic stimulation). It is difficult to separate this effect from the antiischemic effect.

A meta-analysis of data from 32 randomized trials, which included a total of about 29,000 patients, showed a 13% relative reduction in overall mortality among patients receiving IV beta-blocker therapy initiated within 24 hours of signs and symptoms of MI (82).

In the TIMI-IIB trial, patients who received early IV metoprolol combined with t-PA had a lower incidence of nonfatal reinfarction (2.3% versus 4.5%) and recurrent ischemic events (15.4% versus 21.2%) when compared to patients receiving delayed administration of oral metoprolol (80). Because of contraindications such as hypotension, bradycardia, and reactive airway disease, only about 30% to 40% of patients receiving IV thrombolytics will be eligible for beta-blocker therapy. The ultrashort-acting beta-blocker esmolol has been shown to be effective in lowering heart rate and BP in acute ischemia, and its ability to be titrated may broaden its clinical usefulness in the current era of reperfusion therapy. It currently is recommended that all patients without a contraindication to beta-blocker therapy receive these drugs within 12 hours of onset of infarction, irrespective of administration of concomitant thrombolytic therapy (62).

Contraindications to beta-blocker therapy include the following:

- Heart rate less than 50 beats/minute
- Systolic BP less than 90 mm Hg
- Severe LV failure
- Signs of peripheral hypoperfusion
- Atrioventricular (AV) conduction abnormalities: PR interval more than 0.22 seconds, 2° AV block, or complete heart block (CHB)
- Severe bronchospastic pulmonary disease

Nitrates

Nitrates have been shown in both clinical and experimental infarction to improve LV function, increase cardiac output, and reduce filling pressures. Nitrates also reduce peripheral resistance and relief coronary spasm. Nitrates have the potential for adverse effects if hypotension or reflex tachycardia increases myocardial oxygen consumption.

The clinical efficacy of IV nitroglycerin in AMI has been the subject of at least seven randomized trials. Taken separately, these individual trials have been too small to provide a reliable estimate of the effects of treatment on mortality, but collectively, they show evidence of benefit. The mortality for the pooled group allocated to IV nitroglycerin was 12% (51/426) versus 20.5% (86/425) in the controls (83). IV nitroglycerin currently is recommended for the first 24 to 48 hours in patients with AMI and congestive heart failure (CHF), large anterior infarction, persistent ischemia, or hypertension. Its use in other patients with MI is not well established (62). IV nitroglycerin usually is started at an infusion rate of 10 mcg/minute and is increased by 10 mcg/minute at 10-minute intervals to achieve relieve of chest pain, a 10% reduction in systolic pressure, a systolic pressure of 95 mmHg, or a maximal dose of 200 mcg/minute. After 2 days, a decision regarding a long-term therapy should be made depending on LV function and residual ischemia.

Calcium Channel Blockers

As a group, the **calcium blockers** have failed to demonstrate significant benefits in patients with Q wave infarctions. Nifedipine and verapamil have been shown to be of no benefit or deleterious in this setting (83–86). Coadministration of lytic agents and calcium blockers has yet to demonstrate any benefit but will be the subject of further trials. Diltiazem has been shown to reduce cardiac events after non–Q wave MI in the absence of pulmonary congestion (87, 88). Verapamil or diltiazem may be given to patients in whom beta-blockers are ineffective or contraindicated for relief of continuing ischemia or for rapid control of ventricular response rate if atrial fibrillation complicates AMI (62).

Angiotensin Converting Enzyme Inhibitors

Angiotensin converting enzyme inhibitors have both cardioprotective properties and vasculoprotective properties that are unrelated to their blood–pressure-lowering effect. ACE inhibitors appear to have a role in reducing myocardial and vascular hypertrophy, progression of atherosclerosis, plaque rupture, and thrombosis.

The combined results of the CONSENSUS II (Cooperative New Scandinavian Enalapril Survival Study II) (89), ISIS-4 (90), GISSI-III (91), and the Chinese Cardiac Study (92), in addition to 11 small trials, show that ACE inhibitors started early in AMI will save 5 lives per 1,000 treated in the first month. The ISIS-4 trial demonstrated that the benefit of only 1 month of early ACE-inhibitor treatment seemed to persist for at least 1 year and the benefit was greater in patients at higher risk (90). The AMI trials generally have shown ACE inhibitor therapy to be very safe, even when added to other agents that lower BP. There also appears to be a benefit of long-term ACE inhibitor treatment started days to weeks post-MI in patients with LV dysfunction with or without overt heart failure. In the SOLVD (Studies Of Left Ventricular Dysfunction) and SAVE (Survival And Ventricular Enlargement) trials, an additional two lives per 1,000 were saved during each later month of treatment (93–96). It currently is recommended that ACE inhibitor therapy be initiated within 24 hours in patients with suspected AMI who meet ST segment elevation criteria or in those patients with clinical heart failure in the absence of significant hypotension or known contraindications to use of ACE inhibitors. Patients with MI and a LV ejection fraction of less than 40% or patients with symptomatic heart failure on the basis of systolic pump dysfunction are most likely to benefit from such therapy (62). In patients without complications and no evidence of symptomatic or asymptomatic LV dysfunction at 6 weeks post-MI, ACE inhibitors can be discontinued.

THE 10 COMMANDMENTS OF MYOCARDIAL INFARCTION TREATMENT

1. Reperfusion therapy should be given to as many patients as possible with MI (including those with LBBB); benefits exist up to 12 hours from the onset of symptoms.
2. If thrombolysis is chosen for reperfusion, accelerated t-PA should be given when the time frame is 0 to 4 hours, with an anterior MI, and when the age is younger than 75 years. Streptokinase is preferred if the patient is older than 75 years old, when the MI is smaller, and when there is an increased risk of hemorrhagic stroke.
3. Primary angioplasty is superior to thrombolytic therapy. Stenting is safe and effective. Facilitated percutaneous coronary intervention (PCI) is an emerging new strategy.
4. Aspirin and beta-blockers should be given at the onset of treatment. ACE inhibitors should be given early (within first 24 hours), especially in those with larger infarcts.
5. Nitrates are not necessary in the ongoing therapy of AMI. There is no effect on mortality, LV function, or infarct size.
6. IV heparin should be given to those who are treated with t-PA; there is no evidence of improved outcome if IV heparin is used with streptokinase.
7. Platelets play a major role in MI. Glycoprotein IIb/IIIa inhibitors are safe and most effective when combined with PCI.
8. Avoid prophylactic lidocaine (see later).
9. Avoid calcium channel blockers.
10. Cardiac catheterization should be performed in patients with post-MI ischemia.

COMPLICATIONS OF ACUTE MYOCARDIAL INFARCTION

Cardiac Rhythm Disturbances

Prompt recognition and treatment of arrhythmias is important to minimize their deleterious hemodynamic effects (reduced cardiac output and increased myocardial oxygen demand—MVO_2) and their tendency to lead to more serious electrical instability. Recognition and management of common arrhythmias is discussed in Chapter 2. This section is limited to selected rhythm disturbances and management issues in the setting of AMI.

Supraventricular Arrhythmias

1. Sinus tachycardia: This rhythm is detrimental in the setting of myocardial ischemia as a result of the increase in MVO_2 in the presence of a fixed blood supply. With adequate pain control, appropriate sedation, no fever, and no clinical evidence of LV failure, sinus rates of more than 110 may need investigation with a pulmonary artery flotation catheter to determine the underlying etiology: hypovolemia, subclinical LV failure, or hyperadrenergic state. Therapy should be directed at correcting the underlying abnormality. Beta-blockers may be used for the control of sinus tachycardia in isolated hyperadrenergic states [normal pulmonary capillary wedge pressure (PCWP), increased cardiac output, increased heart rate]. Decreased preload (low PCWP) can be corrected with volume infusions using normal saline or a colloid solution.

2. Sinus bradycardia: Bradycardia may be transient or persistent and may be associated with hypotension. The combination of hypotension and bradycardia usually represents a vasovagal reaction (Bezold-Jarisch reflex) and is a common occurrence in acute inferior MI. Therapy is not required unless the patient is symptomatic or the bradycardia is accompanied by premature ventricular contractions (PVCs) or escape rhythms.

3. Atrial fibrillation: Atrial fibrillation complicates the clinical course of AMI in approximately 10% of patients and is associated with a higher early mortality. In the setting of AMI, it usually is encountered in patients with extensive infarction resulting in LV failure; in patients with atrial infarction; or, occasionally, in patients with post-MI pericarditis. About 90% of episodes will occur within the first 48 hours and usually persist for more than 24 hours. Electrical cardioversion is for patients with severe hemodynamic compromise or intractable ischemia. IV beta-blockers can be used to control ventricular response rate in patients without contraindications to their use. IV diltiazem or verapamil can be used to slow the ventricular response rate if beta-blockers are contraindicated.

Ventricular Arrhythmias

Before 1992, prophylactic lidocaine was in widespread use because of its ability to reduce the incidence of primary ventricular fibrillation in limited clinical studies (97). However, randomized control trials have not demonstrated any significant mortality effect with prophylactic lidocaine (98). In addition, lidocaine may be harmful to some patients who are treated prophylactically but who later are found not to have suffered AMI. Meta-analysis of 14 randomized controlled trials with lidocaine suggests there may be some negative mortality effect, as well as reports of several life-threatening lidocaine-related events (sinus arrest, marked bradycardia, and seizures) (99). Based on these data, routine use of lidocaine for PVC suppression is no longer recommended in the setting of AMI.

1. PVCs. The management of PVCs after AMI has been the subject of intense interest and clinical trials. At present, no strong data show a benefit from treating asymptomatic complex ventricular ectopy after AMI. The highly publicized CAST (Cardiac Arrhythmia Suppression Trial) study has shown a twofold to threefold increase in mortality when the class 1C agents flecainide and encainide were tested in comparison to placebo controls (100). Pooled data with class 1A and 1B agents also show a higher mortality in the treated group (101). These data have underscored the need for caution when using any oral antiarrhythmic after AMI. Patients with ejection fractions less than 40%, late potentials on signal-averaged ECGs, and complex ventricular ectopy may benefit from suppression of the PVCs provided the drug is well tolerated (see Chapter 14).

a. Amiodarone: The loading dose is initiated with 150 mg infused over 10 minutes (15 mg/minute) followed by 360 mg over the next 6 hours (1 mg/minute). In cardiac arrest resulting from shock-refractory ventricular fibrillation or pulseless ventricular tachycardia, the initial dose should be 300 mg IV push as recommended by the 2000 Advanced Cardiac Life Support guidelines. The maintenance infusion is 540 mg over the remaining 18 hours (0.5 mg/minute).

b. Lidocaine: The loading dose is 1.0 to 1.5 mg/kg intravenously.

Additional doses of 0.5 to 0.75 mg/kg can be given at 5 to 10-minute intervals to a maximum of 3 mg/kg total loading dose. A constant infusion (with an infusion pump) of 2 mg/minute should be started with the first dose. The maximum infusion rate is 4 mg/minute. The loading dose and infusion rate should be reduced by half in the presence of CHF, shock, or liver disease or in a patient 70 years of age or older. The infusion can be stopped (not tapered) at 36 hours in the absence of ventricular arrhythmias. If ventricular ectopy develops with cessation of the infusion, lidocaine should be restarted and continued for another 24 to 36 hours. If complex ventricular ectopy (i.e., multiform, runs or pairs, or frequent PVCs (more than 5/minute) develops when the infusion is stopped, oral antiarrhythmics may be necessary. Almost all patients will have PVCs during the acute phase of MI. Complete or nearly complete suppression of ventricular ectopy in the acute phase of an infarction is the goal of therapy.

c. Procainamide: 20 to 30 mg/minute loading infusion up to 12 to 17 mg/kg is recommended. Monitor BP and ECG closely because hypotension and conduction disturbances (prolonged QRS and QT interval) can occur if dose is given too rapidly. After loading is completed, a constant infusion at 1 to 4 mg/minute should be started.

d. A combination of procainamide and lidocaine may be used but can result in neurotoxicity (altered mental status, seizures) because the two drugs have additive CNS effects; combined infusion rate should not exceed 5 mg/minute.

e. Bretylium: 5 to 10 mg/kg can be administered intravenously over 10 minutes, followed by a constant infusion of a rate of 1 to 2 mg/minute. After an initial increase in BP, hypotension may occur as a result of the blocking of the efferent limb of the baroreceptor reflex. Initial sinus tachycardia may be the result of catecholamine release. Bretylium should not be used in patients with a fixed cardiac output (e.g., severe aortic stenosis). Postural hypotension is a common complication.

2. Ventricular tachycardia. This rhythm is defined as more than three consecutive PVCs at a rate of 120/minute or greater. Therapy is dictated by the clinical status of the patient. If transient or sustained without clinical evidence of hypoperfusion, IV amiodarone or lidocaine may be used (see earlier). Synchronized countershock at 50 to 400 W/sec should be used if the rhythm is sustained and associated with hemodynamic deterioration.

3. Accelerated idioventricular rhythm. This rhythm may be the result of enhanced automaticity of an ectopic ventricular pacemaker or the result of variable exit block of a focus of ventricular tachycardia. The wide ectopic QRS complexes occur at regular intervals, resulting in AV dissociation when the prevailing supraventricular rhythm slows below the intrinsic rate of the idioventricular pacemaker (60–90/minute). It is usually benign and does not result in ventricular fibrillation. Close monitoring for 24 hours is advisable because of a rare association with ventricular tachycardia. If the rhythm is not hemodynamically tolerated, suppression with lidocaine, procainamide, or atropine (by increasing the sinus rate) can be used. Overdrive atrial pacing is also effective. Treatment is infrequently necessary.

Atrioventricular Block and Myocardial Infarction

The incidence of progression to high-degree AV block, without previous ECG evidence of conduction disturbance, is approximately 6%. The onset of CHB is different, depending on the site of infarction.

Inferior Myocardial Infarction

CHB is the result of increased vagal tone or ischemia of the AV node. CHB rarely occurs suddenly. Progression from first-degree block to various degrees of second-degree AV block usually precedes CHB. During CHB, the heart rate is generally 50 beats/minute, and QRS commonly is narrow. Treatment ranges from observation in the stable patient to using IV atropine in the hemodynamically unstable patient (dosage of 0.5 mg IV up to 2 mg IV).

Anterior Myocardial Infarction

Caused by ischemia or infarction of the His bundle or both bundle branches, CHB frequently develops suddenly and results in wide, bizarre QRS complexes and bradycardia. Pacemaker therapy may be necessary. Any patient who develops permanent or transient high-degree AV block associated with bundle branch block (BBB) during an MI should have a permanent pacemaker implanted.

Indications for temporary pacing (transcutaneous or transvenous) in AMI include the following:

- Marked symptomatic bradycardia (sinus bradycardia or type-I, second-degree AV block) unresponsive to atropine
- Unresponsive type-II, second-degree AV block or CHB when the patient is unstable
- Bilateral BBB—alternating BBB, or right bundle branch block (RBBB) and alternating left anterior superior hemiblock (LASH), left posterior inferior hemiblock (LPIH)
- Newly acquired or age indeterminate LBBB or RBBB with LASH or LPIH
- New RBBB or LBBB and first-degree AV block

Recurrent Chest Pain

Recurrent chest pain during and after the first 24 hours is not unusual and often is relieved with nitrates alone. Nitroglycerin should be used in small doses (0.4 mg sublingual) in normotensive patients. If chest pain persists or recurs, consider the following:

1. A combination of sublingual nitroglycerin tablets and parenteral morphine (in incremental 2-mg IV doses). Adequate sedation usually is achieved with morphine.

2. If the pain persists or recurs and hypotension is not present, start topical nitroglycerin ointment or nitroglycerin patches.

3. If the previous two listed are ineffective, start IV nitroglycerin—40 mg in 250 cc of 5% dextrose in water at 5 cc/hour. IV nitroglycerin can be administered safely to hemodynamically stable patients without pulmonary artery (PA) pressure monitoring. The usual range of nitroglycerin needed for pain control is 10 to 200 mcg/minute. In invasively monitored patients, fluids should be administered if PCWP falls below 15 mm Hg and is associated with a significant drop in BP or cardiac output. If clinical evidence of hypoperfusion occurs in a patient without PA-pressure monitoring in the low-dose range, fluids should be given judiciously and a PA catheter should be considered. IV nitroglycerin is an arterial vasodilator, as well as a venodilator; therefore, attempts to maintain BP by volume challenge may not always be successful. The rationale of IV nitroglycerin therapy is reduction of MVO_2, coronary vasodilation, promotion of collateral supply, and reversal of any coronary spasm.

4. If pain recurs or persists despite maximal IV nitroglycerin, IV propranolol or metoprolol may be used if PCWP is less than 18 and the cardiac index (CI) is greater than 2.4 L/minute/M². Propanolol can be given in 1-mg doses every 10 to 15 minutes to a total dose of 0.05 to 0.1 mg/kg. Metoprolol can be given in 5-mg boluses at 5-minute intervals to a total dose of 15 mg. In the setting of an AMI, beta-blocking agents may affect the myocardium unpredictably and their use must be monitored closely. If acutely effective and tolerated, beta-blockers then can be given orally.

5. Calcium channel blockers should be used with caution in the setting of AMI (see earlier) but may be of value if recurrent or persistent chest pain is unresponsive to nitrates and beta-blockers.

6. Recurrent chest pain may not be the result of ongoing myocardial ischemia. Postinfarction pericarditis should be considered and can be treated with additional aspirin or nonsteroidal antiinflammatory drugs.

7. If low BP, low CI, or a high PCWP prohibit the use of beta blockers or calcium channel blockers or they are not effective, IABP (see later) and continued IV nitroglycerin may result in pain relief.

Coronary arteriography and coronary revascularization (PTCA or bypass surgery) should be considered if the previously listed measures fail to control symptoms.

Hemodynamic Dysfunction

An AMI almost always causes some degree of acute LV dysfunction. Whether this dysfunction becomes clinically apparent or important depends on the amount of myocardium damaged; a loss of myocardium greater than 40% generally leads to cardiogenic shock. Several classifications have been developed that correlate LV dysfunction during an AMI to in-hospital mortality. The Killip Classification (based on clinical data prior to reperfusion therapy) is one of the most frequently quoted and is based entirely on clinical findings (Table 9b.3) (102).

A clinical, noninvasive evaluation of the patient with an AMI has significant limitations in that it will overestimate CI in 25% of patients and it will underestimate PCWP in 15% of patients. Therefore, in high-risk mortality groups (Killip Classes III and IV) or in a patient with a confusing clinical picture, a PA catheter should be considered so that therapeutic decisions can be based upon hemodynamic findings.

Table 9b.3.   Killip classification

		Incidence %	Mortality %
I.	No heart failure	33	6
II.	Mild failure (bibasilar rales)	38	17
III.	Frank pulmonary edema	10	38
IV.	Cardiogenic shock (hypotension with blood pressure of <90 mm Hg, peripheral vasoconstriction, oliguria, and pulmonary vascular congestion)	19	81

Indications for Balloon Flotation Right-Heart Monitoring in Acute Myocardial Infarction

Indications for balloon flotation right-heart monitoring in AMI include the following (46):

- Severe or progressive CHF or pulmonary edema
- Cardiogenic shock or progressive hypotension
- Suspected mechanical complications (see later)
- Hypotension that does not respond promptly to fluid administration in a patient without pulmonary congestion

It should be noted, however, that the value of right-heart monitoring in AMI and in other critically ill patients has not been well established (103). A classification that correlates clinical signs with invasive hemodynamic data and that is helpful in planning treatment is that of Forrester and colleagues (104) shown in Fig. 9b.1.

Subset or groups of patients (noted by Roman numerals) are defined based on the measurement of pulmonary capillary pressure (wedge pressure) (mm Hg) and CI (L/minute/M^2).

Subset I: uncomplicated. No specific therapy indicated. Mortality is approximately 3%.

Subset II: mild to moderate CHF. A major problem is elevated PCWP. Treatment involves reduction of preload with either diuretics or nitrates. In evaluating therapeutic response, it should be remembered that there is a "lag period" between normalization of PCWP and disappearance of rales and radiographic resolution. Mortality is approximately 9%.

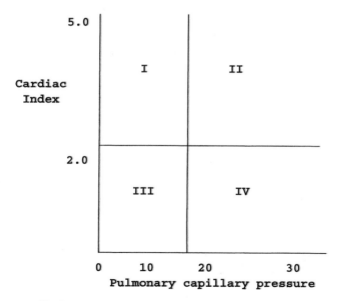

Fig. 9b.1. Hemodynamic subsets in acute myocardial infarction.

Subset III. Low cardiac output in the setting of a "normal" PCWP. This group would include patients with an inappropriately low wedge pressure in the setting of acute infarction (optimal in AMI is 14 to 18 mm Hg) and those patients with RV infarction (see later). Management should be directed toward optimizing preload with fluid administration. Mortality is approximately 20%.

Subset IV: Cardiogenic shock. The major problem is a markedly reduced CI, usually less than 2.2 L/minute/M^2 and an elevated pulmonary pressure. Mortality is approximately 60% to 80%.

The systolic pressure primarily will dictate the therapeutic approach:

1. If the systolic pressure is more than 100 mm Hg, increase CI through afterload reduction with very cautious vasodilator therapy.

2. With moderately severe hypotension (systolic BP 75 to 90 mm Hg), dobutamine may improve CI and BP. Dopamine may be added to increase BP if dobutamine alone fails to do so.

3. With significant hypotension (systolic pressure less than 75 mm Hg), use a pressor agent (e.g., dopamine) because rapid attainment and maintenance of an adequate BP (systolic 90–100) is of prime importance in treating cardiogenic shock. Dobutamine may be added for its effect on cardiac output, but usually it will not raise the BP enough to be used without a pressor. A combination of dobutamine and dopamine may be most effective (105).

Intraaortic Balloon Pump in Cardiogenic Shock

Ideal candidate criteria for IABP include early in course (less than 6 hours postinfarction), younger patients, first MI, absence of any terminal disease, and no aortic insufficiency.

Indications for intraaortic balloon counterpulsation include the following:

- Cardiogenic shock not quickly reversed with pharmacologic therapy as a stabilizing measure for angiography and prompt revascularization
- Acute mitral regurgitation or ventricular septal defect complicating MI as a stabilizing intervention before angiography and repair/revascularization
- Recurrent intractable ventricular arrhythmias with hemodynamic instability
- Refractory post-MI angina as a bridge to angiography and revascularization
- Signs of hemodynamic instability, poor left heart function, or persistent ischemia in patients with large areas of myocardium at risk

Hemodynamic effects of IABP: Afterload is reduced, and diastolic pressure is increased, thereby improving coronary perfusion pressure and cardiac output. Overall effect is to improve myocardial metabolism and decrease LV size.

Course: Of AMI patients with cardiogenic shock, 20% recover to be weaned off IABP and discharged home. The remainder usually improves but continues to be IABP dependent. Heart catheterization and cardiac surgery may be beneficial. Surgery is most successful in patients with a correctable mechanical defect (i.e., ventricular septal defect, aneurysm, or ruptured papillary muscle) in addition to bypassable coronary artery obstructions (106).

Complications of IABP: There is a 15% to 30% incidence of complications. These include (a) rupture of balloon; (b) emboli from balloon to kidneys or lower extremities; (c) dissection of the aorta; (d) leg ischemia resulting in neuropathy, myopathy or amputation; (e) groin infections; (f) thrombocytopenia and anemia; and (g) leg claudication. Embolic phenomena are markedly decreased by the use of anticoagulation with heparin during IABP therapy.

Right Ventricular Infarction

Right ventricular infarction almost exclusively is associated with acute inferior infarction. Of inferior infarctions, 19% to 43% are complicated by RV involvement, but only 3% to 8% of these have clinical findings suggestive of RV dysfunction, such as neck-vein distention or arterial hypotension (107). The syndrome of hypotension and low cardiac output associated with an RV infarction is attributed to the inability of the infarcted right ventricle to maintain adequate LV filling.

Confirm the diagnosis by the following:

ECG: An ECG sign of RV infarct is the presence of ST elevation in the right precordial leads, especially V4R (108)
Swan-Ganz catheter: Elevated mean right atrial pressures (12 to 20 mm Hg), which is equal to or greater than the PCWP (107)
Gated cardiac blood pool scan: Poor RV function (107)

Therapy includes (a) plasma expanders to increase the filling pressure in the right heart, favoring increased passive flow through the lungs to the left heart (follow PCWP as a guide to fluid therapy), and (b) afterload reduction of the left heart to increase cardiac output and decrease left atrial pressure, encouraging passive filling from the right heart (107).

Cardiogenic shock as a result of predominant RV dysfunction is uncommon; however, this is an important entity to recognize because it represents a treatable subset of cardiogenic shock with a survival of better than 50% compared to 10% to 15% survival in shock resulting from LV wall infarction.

MECHANICAL DEFECTS CAUSING DECOMPENSATION

Certain mechanical defects cause decompensation (109). They include ruptured papillary muscle and ventricular septal rupture.

1. Ruptured Papillary Muscle

Clinical picture: Sudden appearance of an apical systolic murmur associated with abrupt clinical LV failure. Course may be less severe if only papillary head and not the entire body of the muscle is ruptured.
Incidence: Incidence is 1% to 5% among patients dying of an AMI. Occurs 2 to 10 days post-MI, primarily involves the posterior side of the papillary muscle, and is associated with inferior–posterior MI.
Mortality: 70% within 24 hours; 90% within 2 weeks.
Diagnosis: Large V waves on PCWP tracing (see Figure 11.3B). Two-dimensional ECG may show the ruptured papillary muscle. Doppler echocardiography will demonstrate severe mitral regurgitation.

Therapy

a. Afterload reduction and inotropic support; if ineffective, consider IABP.
b. If stabilized medically, surgery in weeks to months. If unstable and in need of IABP, cardiac catheterization is indicated and possibly immediate surgery.

2. Ventricular Septal Rupture

Clinical picture: Very similar to ruptured papillary muscle. Sudden onset of harsh systolic murmur along the left sternal border associated with hemodynamic deterioration.

Incidence: Incidence is 0.5% to 1%, accounting for approximately 2% of deaths following an infarction. Usually associated with an anteroseptal infarction occurring 9 to 10 postinfarction. Rupture commonly involves the apical anterior muscular septum.

Mortality: 24% within 24 hours; 87% within 2 months.

Diagnosis: Oxygen saturation step-up in the pulmonary artery as compared to right atrium in blood samples drawn from the Swan-Ganz catheter. Echocardiography may demonstrate the defect in the interventricular septum. Doppler echocardiography will show flow from left to right across the defect.

Therapy: Same as for ruptured papillary muscle.

EMBOLIC COMPLICATIONS

Pulmonary Embolism

With the advent of early ambulation in patients with AMI, incidence of pulmonary embolism seemingly has decreased. Predisposing factors include LV failure, arrhythmias, old age, obesity, and varicose veins. Low-dose heparin (5,000 units subcutaneously bid) markedly reduces the incidence of deep-vein thrombosis in patients with AMI and, therefore, should reduce the incidence of pulmonary emboli.

Arterial Embolism

Older studies (prior to 1973) have quoted a 2.5% to 4.9% incidence of arterial emboli to the brain, kidneys, or limbs, supposedly from intraventricular mural thrombus overlying the infarction. There are no current figures; clinically, the incidence seems less. Recommendations regarding the use of prophylactic anticoagulation therapy vary among institutions. Therapeutic recommendations include anticoagulation in patients with echo or nuclear scan documented new ventricular aneurysms or mural clots.

HYPERTENSION

Hypertension is not uncommon in the early phase of an AMI. It has many possible causes, including underlying essential hypertension, CHF, or elevated catecholamines secondary to chest pain or anxiety. Hypertension causes an increase in intraventricular pressure, which results in an increased MVO_2 via Laplace's law. This may worsen ischemia and even cause extension of the MI. If the patient is seen early in the infarction period (less than 6 hours after the onset of pain) or has evidence of ongoing ischemia (recurrent chest pain), cautious but aggressive management of hypertension is recommended in hopes of modifying infarct size. Attempt to adequately control chest pain with nitrates and/or morphine.

Sedation can be used if the patient is anxious. If BP remains elevated, continue the use of nitrates and beta-blockers and consider the cautious use of low doses of diuretics. If the BP remains significantly elevated, the use of IV medication is warranted. With mild cases, IV nitroglycerin is recommended, but with a markedly elevated BP, IV antihypertensive agents in the form of beta blockers (labetalol) or ACE inhibitors should be given.

REINFARCTION

Recurrent chest pain and sudden deterioration of functional status, as well as secondary elevation of plasma troponins, are the clues that reinfarction has occurred. Of reinfarctions, 85% occur during the initial hospitalization (between the third and tenth hospital day). The overall incidence is 25% of cases, with an incidence of 10% in transmural MIs and 42% in non–ST elevation MIs. Along with recurrent chest pain and the clinical setting of non–ST elevation MI, other predictors of extension of MI are female gender and obesity. Early reinfarction carries with it a high mortality (25%) in the first 3 weeks.

LOW-LEVEL EXERCISE TESTING

Under close supervision of trained personnel, a slow, gradual increase in activity levels is started in the coronary care unit and then continued throughout the hospital course. A low-level stress test may be performed just before discharge to determine a safe level of home activity and a safe exercise prescription for outpatient cardiac rehabilitation and to identify patients at high risk for future cardiac events. Patients with a positive low-level stress test have a significant risk of cardiac-related mortality over the subsequent year (110). This subgroup should have close observation and possibly early heart catheterization and bypass surgery, PTCA, or other interventional procedure.

CARDIAC REHABILITATION

One of the goals of a comprehensive rehabilitation program is to encourage risk-factor modification such as cessation of smoking, dietary counseling, and treatment of hypertension and diabetes. Exercise training is also a significant component of cardiac rehabilitation and should focus on improving work capacity and reducing symptoms. The positive training effects of a lower heart rate and BP reduce myocardial oxygen consumption and thus help relieve symptoms. Attention also should be given to vocational status and psychosocial manifestations of the illness. Unfortunately, cardiac rehabilitation patients have not been shown to have significant reduction in mortality after MI.

REFERENCES

1. Fuster V, Badimon L, Badimon JJ, et al: The pathogenesis of coronary artery disease and the acute coronary syndromes. *N Engl J Med* 326:310, 1992.
2. Reeder GS, Gersh BJ: Modern management of acute myocardial infarction. *Curr Prob Cardiol* 21:591, 1996.
3. Gaspoz JM, Lee TH, Goldman L: Emergency room evaluation and triage strategies for patients with acute chest pain: lessons from the pre-thrombolytic era. In: Califf RM, Mark DB, Wagner GS, eds.

Acute coronary care, 2nd ed. Philadelphia: Mosby-Year Book, pp. 255–263, 1995.

4. Kannel WB, Feinleib M: Natural history of angina pectoris in the Framingham study. *Am J Cardiol* 29:154, 1972.

5. Kannel WB, Abbott RD: Incidence and prognosis of unrecognized myocardial infarction. An update on the Framingham study. *N Engl J Med* 311:1144, 1984.

6. Chiariello M, Indolfi C: Silent myocardial ischemia in patients with diabetes mellitus. *Circulation* 93:2089, 1996.

7. Duncan AK, Vittone J, Fleming KC, et al: Cardiovascular disease in elderly patients. *Mayo Clin Proc* 71:184, 1996.

8. Tcheng JE, Jackman JD, Nelson CL, et al: Outcome of patients sustaining acute ischemic mitral regurgitation during myocardial infarction. *Ann Intern Med* 117:18, 1992.

9. Pohjola-Sintonen S, Muller JE, Stone PH, et al: Ventricular septal and free wall rupture complicating acute myocardial infarction: experience in the Multicenter Investigation of Limitation of Infarct Size. *Am Heart J* 117:809, 1989.

10. Puleo PR, Roberts R: An update on cardiac enzymes. *Cardiol Clin* 6:97, 1988.

11. Ohman EM, Armstrong PW, Christenson RH, et al: Cardiac troponin T levels for risk stratification in acute myocardial ischemia. *N Engl J Med* 335:1333, 1996.

12. Antman EM, Tanasijevic MJ, Thompson B, et al: Cardiac-specific troponin I levels to predict the risk of mortality in patients with acute coronary syndromes. *N Engl J Med* 335:1342, 1996.

13. Adams JE 3rd, Abendschein DR, Jaffe AS: Biochemical markers of myocardial injury: is MB creatine kinase the choice for the 1990s? *Circulation* 88:750, 1993.

14. Guest TM, Jaffe AS: Rapid diagnosis of acute myocardial infarction. *Cardiol Clin* 13:283, 1995.

15. Keffer J: Myocardial markers of injury. Evolution and insights. *Clin Chem* 105:305, 1996.

16. Zaret BL, Wackers FJ: Nuclear cardiology (Part 1). *N Engl J Med* 329:775, 1993.

17. Gersh BJ: Noninvasive imaging in acute coronary disease. A clinical perspective. *Circulation* 84(Suppl I):I-140, 1991.

18. Feigenbaum H: Role of echocardiography in acute myocardial infarction. *Am J Cardiol* 66:17H, 1990.

19. Moss AJ, Benhorin J: Prognosis and management after a first myocardial infarction. *N Engl J Med* 322:743, 1990.

20. O'Rourke RA: Risk stratification after myocardial infarction. Clinical overview. *Circulation* 84(Suppl I):I-177, 1991.

21. Reeder GS, Gibbons RJ: Acute myocardial infarction: risk stratification in the thrombolytic era. *Mayo Clin Proc* 70:87, 1995.

22. Mehta JL: Emerging options in the management of myocardial ischemia. *Am J Cardiol* 73:18A, 1994.

23. Anderson HV, Willerson JT: Thrombolysis in acute myocardial infarction. *N Engl J Med* 329:703, 1993.

24. Gossage JR: Acute myocardial infarction. Reperfusion strategies. *Chest* 106:1851, 1994.

25. Fibrinolytic Therapy Trialists' (FTT) Collaborative Group: Indications for fibrinolytic therapy in suspected acute myocardial infarction: collaborative overview of early mortality and major morbidity

results from all randomized trials of more than 1000 patients. *Lancet* 343:311, 1994.

26. Gruppo Italiano per lo Studio dell soprevvivenza nell'Infarcto Miocardico: GISSI-2: A factorial randomized trial of alteplase versus streptokinase and heparin versus no heparin among 12,490 patients with acute myocardial infarction. *Lancet* 336:65, 1990.

27. ISIS-3: A randomised comparison of streptokinase vs tissue plasminogen activator vs anistreplase and of aspirin plus heparin vs aspirin alone among 41,299 cases of suspected acute myocardial infarction. ISIS-3 (Third International Study of Infarct Survival) Collaborative Group. *Lancet* 339:753, 1992.

28. The GUSTO Investigators: An international randomized trial comparing four thrombolytic strategies for acute myocardial infarction. *N Engl J Med* 329:673, 1993.

29. Cannom CP, Gibson CMM, McCabe CH, et al: TNK-tissue plasminogen activator compared with front loaded alteplase in acute myocardial infarction: results of the TIMI 10B trial. Thrombolysis in Myocardial Infarction (TIMI) 10 B Investigators. *Circulation* 98:2805, 1998.

30. Den Heijer P, Vermeer F, Ambrosioni E, et al: Evaluation of a weight adjusted single-bolus plasminogen activator in patients with myocardial infarction: a double-blind, randomized angiographic trial of lanoteplase versus alteplase. *Circulation* 98:2117, 1998.

31. Roe MT, Ohman EM, Maas AC, et al: Shifting the open-artery hypothesis downstream: the quest for optimal reperfusion. *J Am Coll Cardiol* 37:9, 2001.

32. Antman EM, Guiliamo RP, Gibson CM, et al: Abciximab facilitates the rate and extent of thrombolysis: results of the Thrombolysis in Myocardial Infarction (TIMI) 14 Trial *Circulation* 99:2720, 1999.

33. Trial of abciximab with and without low-dose reteplase for acute myocardial infarction. Strategies for Patentcy Enhancement in the Emergency Department (SPEED) Group. *Circulation* 101:2788, 2000.

34. Brener SJ, Adgey JA, Zeymer U: Combination low-dose t-PA and eptifibatide for acute myocardial infarction-final results of the Intro-AMI Study. *Circulation* 102: 11: 599, 2000.

35. FASTER trial—to be published.

36. INTEGRETI trial—to be published.

37. Antam EM, Louwerenburg HW, Baars HF, et al: Enoxaparin as adjunctive antithrombin therapy for ST-elevation myocardial infarction: results of the ENTIRE-Thrombolysis in Myocardial Infarction (TIMI) 23 Trial. *Circulation* 105(14):1642–1649, 2002.

38. Topol EJ: Reperfusion therapy for acute myocardial infarction with fibrinolytic therapy or combination reduced fibrinolytic therapy and platelet glycoprotein IIb/IIIa inhibition: the GUSTO V randomised trial. *Lancet* 357:1905, 2001.

39. Ross AM, Moelbeck P, Lundergan C, et al: Randomized comparison of enoxaparin, a low-molecular weight heparin, with unfractionated heparin adjunctive to recombinant tissue plasminogen activator thrombolysis and aspirin: second trial of heparin and aspirin reperfusion therapy (HART—II). *Circulation* 104:648, 2001.

40. Efficacy and safety of tenecteplase in combination with enoxaparin, abciximab or unfractionated heparin: the ASSENT-3 randomised trial in acute myocardial infarction. *Lancet* 358:605, 2001.

41. O'Keefe JH Jr, Rutherford BD, McConahay DR, et al: Early and late

results of coronary angioplasty without antecedent thrombolytic therapy for acute myocardial infarction. *Am J Cardiol* 64:1221, 1989.

42. Horrigan MC, Ellis SG: Primary angioplasty for myocardial infarction. *J Invasive Cardiol* 7(Suppl F):47, 1995.

43. Grines CL, Browne KF, Marco J, et al: A comparison of immediate angioplasty with thrombolytic therapy for acute myocardial infarction. *N Engl J Med* 328:673, 1993.

44. Gibbons RJ, Holmes DR, Reeder GS, et al: Immediate angioplasty compared with the administration of a thrombolytic agent followed by conservative treatment for acute myocardial infarction. *N Engl J Med* 328:685, 1993.

45. Zijlstra F, de Boer MJ, Hoorntje JCA, et al: A comparison of immediate coronary angioplasty with intravenous streptokinase in acute myocardial infarction. *N Engl J Med* 328:680, 1993.

46. Belli G, Topol E: Coronary angioplasty in acute MI. *Advances in cardiovascular medicine*, vol 1(2). pp 1–8, 1994.

47. Rodgers WJ, Bowlby LJ, Chandra NC, et al: Treatment of myocardial infarction in the United States (1990 to 1993). Observations from the National Registry of Myocardial Infarction. *Circulation* 90:2103, 1994.

48. Fan T, Mueller HS: Recent trends in thrombolytic therapy. *Advances in cardiovascular medicine* 2:1, 1995.

49. Grines CL, Cox DA, Stone GW, et al: Coronary angioplasty with or without stent implantation for acute myocardial infarction. *N Engl J Med* 341:1949, 1999.

50. Schomig A, Kastrati A, Dirschinger J, et al: Coronary stenting plus platelet glycoprotein IIb/IIIa blockade compared with tissue plasminogen activator in acute myocardial infarction. Stent versus Thrombolysis for Occluded Coronary Arteries in Patients with Acute Myocardial Infarction Study Investigators. *N Engl J Med* 343:385, 2000.

51. Le May MR, Labiraz M, Davies RF, et al: Stenting vs. thrombolysis in acute myocardial infarction trial (STAT). *J Am Coll Cardiol* 37:985, 2001.

52. Hermann HC, Kelly MP, Ellis SG: Facilitated PCI: rationale and design of the FINESSE trial. *J Invasive Cardiol* 13(Suppl A):10, 2001.

53. Topol EJ, Califf RM, George BS, et al: A randomized trial of immediate versus delayed elective angioplasty after intravenous tissue plasminogen activator in acute myocardial infarction. *N Engl J Med* 317:581, 1987.

54. Rodgers WJ, Baim DS, Gore JM, et al: Comparison of immediate invasive, delayed invasive, and conservative strategies after tissue-type plasminogen activator. Results of the Thrombolysis in Myocardial Infarction (TIMI) Phase II-A Trial. *Circulation* 81:1457, 1990.

55. Simoons ML, Arnold AER, Betriu A, et al: Thrombolysis with tissue plasminogen activator in acute myocardial infarction: no additional benefit from immediate percutaneous coronary angioplasty. *Lancet* 1:197, 1988.

56. Ellis SG, Vande Weft F, DaSilva ER, et al: Present status of rescue angioplasty: current polarizations of opinion and randomized trials. *J Am Coll Cardiol* 19:681, 1992.

57. Gibson CM, Cannon CP, Piana RN, et al: Rescue PTCA in the TIMI 4 trial. *J Am Coll Cardiol* 1A:225A, 1994.

58. Ross AM, Reiner JS, Thompson MA, et al: Immediate and follow-up procedural outcome of 214 patients undergoing rescue PTCA in

the GUSTO trial: no effect of the lytic agent. *Circulation* 88(Suppl I):I-410, 1993.

59. Grande P, Madsen JK, Saunamaki K, et al: The Danish multicenter randomized study of invasive vs. conservative treatment in patients with inducible ischemia following thrombolysis in acute myocardial infarction (DANAMI). A multivariate analysis. *Circulation* 94(Suppl I):I-29, 1996.

60. Fuster V, Dyken ML, Vokonas PS, et al: Aspirin as therapeutic agent in cardiovascular disease. *Circulation* 87:659, 1993.

61. Antiplatelet Trialists' Collaboration: Secondary prevention of vascular disease by prolonged antiplatelet treatment. *Br Med J* 296:320, 1988.

62. Ryan TJ, Anderson JL, Antman EM, et al. ACC/AHA Guidelines for the management of patients with acute myocardial infarction: executive summary. *Circulation* 94:2341, 1996.

63. ISIS-2 Collaborative Group: Randomized trial of intravenous streptokinase, oral aspirin, both, or neither among 17,187 cases of suspected acute myocardial infarction (ISIS-2). *Lancet* 2:349, 1988.

64. Turpie A: Anticoagulant therapy after acute myocardial infarction. *Am J Cardiol* 65:20C, 1990.

65. Mehta SR, Yusuf S, Peters RJ, et al. Effects of pretreatment with clopidogrel and aspirin followed by long-term therapy in patients undergoing percutaneous coronary intervention: the PCI-CURE study. *Lancet* 358:527, 2001.

66. Schafer AI: Antiplatelet therapy. *Am J Med* 101:199, 1996.

67. Use of a monoclonal antibody directed against the platelet glycoprotein IIb/IIIa receptor in high risk coronary angioplasty. The EPIC Investigation. *N Engl J Med* 330:956, 1994.

68. Kleiman NS, Ohman ME, Califf RM, et al: Profound inhibition of platelet aggregation with monoclonal antibody 7E3 Fab following thrombolytic therapy: results of the TAMI 8 pilot study. *J Am Coll Cardiol* 22:381, 1993.

69. Ohman EM, Kleiman NS, Gacioch G, et al: Integrelin to manage platelet aggregation to combat thrombosis. *Circulation* 95:846, 1997.

70. Combining thrombolysis with the platelet glycoprotein IIb/IIIa inhibitor lamifiban: results of the Platelet Aggregation Receptor Antagonist Dose Investigation and Reperfusion Gain in Myocardial Infarction (PARADIGM) trial. *J Am Coll Cardiol* 32:2003, 1998.

71. Brener SJ, Barr LA, Burchenal JE, et al: Randomized, placebo-controlled trial of platelet glycoprotein IIb/IIIa blockade with primary angioplasty for acute myocardial infarction. ReoPro And Primary PTCA Organization and Randomized Trial (RAPPORT) Investigators. *Circulation* 98(8):734–741, 1998.

72. Rodgers GM: Novel antithrombotic therapy. *West J Med* 159:670, 1993.

73. Ridker PM, Hebert PR, Fuster V, et al: Are both aspirin and heparin justified as adjuncts to thrombolytic therapy for acute myocardial infarction? *Lancet* 341:1574, 1993.

74. Delanty N, Fitzgerald DJ: Subcutaneous heparin during coronary thrombolysis. Too little, too late. *Circulation* 86:1636, 1992.

75. Granger CB, Miller JM, Bovell EG, et al: Rebound increase in thrombin generation and activity after cessation of intravenous heparin in patients with acute coronary syndromes. *Circulation* 91:1929, 1995.

76. Flather M, Weitz J, Campeau J, et al: Evidence for rebound activation of the coagulation system after cessation of intravenous anticoagulant therapy for acute MI. *Circulation* 92(Suppl I):I-485, 1995

77. Kontny F, Dale J, Adildgaard U, et al: Randomized trial of low molecular weight heparin (dalteparin) in prevention of LV thrombus formation and arterial embolism after anterior myocardial infarction: the fragmin in acute myocardial infarction (FRAMI) study. *J Am Coll Cardiol* 30:962, 1997.

78. Timolol-induced reduction in mortality and reinfarction in patients surviving acute myocardial infarction. *N Engl J Med* 304:801, 1981.

79. A randomized trial of propranolol in patients with acute myocardial infarction. I. Mortality results. *JAMA* 247:1707, 1982.

80. Hjalmarson A, Elmfeldt D, Herlitz J, et al: Effect on mortality of metoprolol in acute myocardial infarction: a double-blind randomized trial. *Lancet* 2:823, 1981.

81. Koch-Weser J: Beta-adrenergic blockade for survivors of acute myocardial infarction. *N Engl J Med* 310:830, 1984.

82. Held PH, Yusuf S: Effects of beta-blockers and calcium channel blockers in acute myocardial infarction. *Eur Heart J* 14(Suppl F): 18, 1993.

83. Yusuf S, Collins R, MacMahon S, et al: Effect of intravenous nitrates on mortality in acute myocardial infarction: an overview of the randomized trials. *Lancet* 1:1088, 1988.

84. Muller JE, Morrison J, Stone PH, et al: Nifedipine therapy for patients with threatened and acute myocardial infarction: a randomized double-blind, placebo-controlled comparison. *Circulation* 69: 740, 1984.

85. Wilcox RG, Hampton JR, Banks DC, et al: Trial of early nifedipine in acute myocardial infarction: the TRENT study. *Br Med J* 293: 1204, 1986.

86. Verapamil in acute myocardial infarction. Danish Multicenter Study Group on Verapamil in Myocardial Infarction. *Am J Cardiol* 54:24E, 1984.

87. The effect of diltiazem on mortality and reinfarction after myocardial infarction. The Multicenter Diltiazem Postinfarction Trial Research Group. *N Engl J Med* 319:385, 1988.

88. Gibson RS, Boden WE, Theroux P, et al: Diltiazem and reinfarction in patients with non-Q wave myocardial infarction. Results of a double-blind, randomized, multicenter trial. *N Engl J Med* 315:423, 1986.

89. Swedberg K, Held P, Kjekshus J, et al: Effects of the early administration of enalapril on mortality in patients with acute myocardial infarction. Results of the Cooperative New Scandinavian Enalapril Survival Study II (CONSENSUS II). *N Engl J Med* 327:678, 1992.

90. ISIS-4 (Fourth International Study of Infarct Survival) Collaborative Group: ISIS-4: A randomized factorial trial assessing early oral captopril, oral mononitrate, and intravenous magnesium sulphate in 58,050 patients with suspected acute myocardial infarction. *Lancet* 345:669, 1995.

91. Gruppo Italiano per lo Studio della Soprovvivenza nell'Infarcto Miocardico: GISSI-3: Effects of lisinopril and transdermal glyceryl trinitrate singly and together on 6-week mortality and ventricular function after acute myocardial infarction. *Lancet* 343:1115, 1994.

92. Chinese Cardiac Study Collaborative Group: Oral captopril versus placebo among 13,634 patients with suspected acute myocardial

infarction: interim report from the Chinese Cardiac Study (CCS-1). *Lancet* 345:686, 1995.

93. The SOLVD Investigators: Effect of enalapril on survival in patients with reduced left ventricular ejection fractions and congestive heart failure. *N Engl J Med* 293:641, 1991.

94. The SOLVD Investigators: Effect of enalapril on mortality and the development of heart failure in asymptomatic patients with reduced left ventricular ejection fractions. *N Engl J Med* 327:685, 1991.

95. Pfeffer MA, Braunwald E, Moye LA, et al: Effect of captopril on mortality and morbidity in patients with left ventricular dysfunction after myocardial infarction: results of the Survival and Ventricular Enlargement Trial. *N Engl J Med* 327:669, 1992.

96. Rutherford JD, Pfeffer MA, Moye LA, et al: Effects of captopril on ischemic events after myocardial infarction. Results of the Survival and Ventricular Enlargement Trial. *Circulation* 90:1731, 1994.

97. Harrison DC: Should lidocaine be administered routinely to all patients after acute myocardial infarction? *Circulation* 58:581, 1978.

98. MacMahon S, Collins R, Peto R, et al: Effects of prophylactic lidocaine in suspected acute myocardial infarction. An overview of results from the randomized, controlled trials. *JAMA* 260:1910, 1988.

99. Hine LK, Laird N, Hewitt P, et al: Meta-analytic evidence against prophylactic use of lidocaine in acute myocardial infarction. *Arch Intern Med* 149:2694, 1989.

100. Echt DS, Liebson PR, Mitchell B, et al: Mortality and morbidity in patients receiving encainide, flecainide, or placebo. The Cardiac Arrhythmia Suppression Trial. *N Engl J Med* 324:781, 1991.

101. Teo KK, Yusuf S, Furberg CD: Effects of prophylactic antiarrhythmic drug therapy in acute myocardial infarction. An overview of results from randomized controlled trials. *JAMA* 270:1589, 1993.

102. Killip T III, Kimball JT: Treatment of myocardial infarction in a coronary care unit: a two-year experience with 250 patients. *Am J Cardiol* 20:457, 1967.

103. Connors AF, Speroff T, Dawson NV, et al: The effectiveness of right heart catheterization in the initial care of critically ill patients. *JAMA* 276:889, 1996.

104. Forrester JS, Diamond G, Chatterjee K, et al: Medical therapy of acute myocardial infarction by application of hemodynamic subsets. Part 1. *N Engl J Med* 295:1356, 1976.

105. Richard C, Ricome JL, Rimailho A, et al: Combined hemodynamic effects of dopamine and dobutamine in cardiogenic shock. *Circulation* 67:620, 1983.

106. Goldenberg IF: Nonpharmacologic management of cardiac arrest and cardiogenic shock. *Chest* 102(Suppl 2):596S, 1992.

107. Kinch JW, Ryan TJ: Right ventricular infarction. *N Engl J Med* 330:1211, 1994.

108. Robalino BD, Whitlow PL, Underwood DA, et al: Electrocardiographic manifestations of right ventricular infarction. *Am Heart J* 118:138, 1989.

109. Chatterjee K: Complications of acute myocardial infarction. *Curr Prob Cardiol* 18:7, 1993.

110. Pitt B: Evaluation of the postinfarct patient. *Circulation* 91:1855, 1995.

CONGESTIVE HEART FAILURE

DEFINITION

Congestive heart failure (CHF) is not a single disease but a symptom complex with many different presentations and etiologies. CHF can be defined in hemodynamic terms as a pathophysiologic state in which impaired cardiac performance is responsible for the inability of the heart, at normal filling pressures, to increase cardiac output (CO) in proportion to the metabolic demands placed on the circulation. In clinical terms, CHF is a pathophysiologic condition in which ventricular dysfunction is accompanied by reduced exercise capacity. The latter definition incorporates less severe forms of ventricular dysfunction (1).

OVERVIEW

CHF is a common clinical entity that affects nearly 5 million people in the United States. Approximately 1 million Americans will be hospitalized with CHF per year. This represents a significant economic burden on society, consuming an estimated $60 billion annually. Of CHF cases, 75% have antecedent hypertension. Approximately one-fourth of male myocardial infarction (MI) cases and one-half of female MI cases will develop CHF in 5 years. The 5-year mortality for CHF in general is about 50%. For severe class 4 CHF, there is a 50% mortality in 1 year (2).

PATHOPHYSIOLOGY

Because CO = stroke volume (SV) × heart rate (HR), the variables that regulate these determinants play a role in the etiology and therapy of CHF. Heart rate is a reflection of the interaction between sympathetic and parasympathetic tone. Stroke volume is determined by three factors: preload, contractility, and afterload. These factors actually relate to isolated muscle strip performance and, therefore, cannot be measured accurately in the clinical setting. However, the terms are used widely in clinical practice in the following contexts (3):

1. **Preload.** This term refers to the passive stretch of myocardial fibers and is approximated by the left ventricular end-diastolic volume (LVEDV). **Clinically, it often is equated with the pulmonary capillary wedge pressure (PCWP).** It is important to recognize that *the left ventricular end-diastolic pressure (LVEDP) or PCWP is inversely related to the compliance of the ventricle.* As shown in Fig. 10.1, the ventricle becomes stiffer (less compliant) with ischemia or hypertrophy; therefore, an increase or decrease in PCWP in a given patient may reflect changes in volume, compliance, or both.

2. **Contractility.** Contractility refers to a reflection of the force-velocity-length relationship of the myocardium, independent of ventricular load or volume. It often is **equated with the rate of rise of ventricular pressure (dp/dt).**

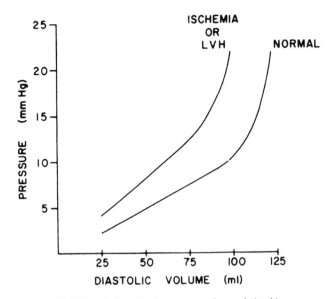

Fig. 10.1.   Left ventricular pressure-volume relationship.

3. **Afterload.** This term refers to the load or resistance encountered by the contracting myocardium, often **clinically approximated by the aortic pressure or the systemic vascular resistance.** It should be recognized that (a) afterload is related directly to the left ventricular (LV) wall tension and is, therefore, higher in a larger ventricle and (b) preload directly alters afterload. A stenotic aortic valve or systemic hypertension greatly increases LV afterload.

When added work is imposed on the heart (i.e., hypertension, valvular disease), three principle **compensatory mechanisms** may function to help maintain CO (4,5).

1. **The Frank-Starling curve.** A myocardial muscle strip will contract with greater force if stretched to a greater resting or presystolic length. Clinical application of this principle requires substituting LVEDV or LVEDP (approximated by PCWP) for fiber length and stroke work, SV, or CO for force. Frank-Starling curves relating preload (LVEDP) to force CO in the normal heart and in progressive LV dysfunction are shown in Fig. 10.2. **An impaired or failing LV requires a higher filling volume or pressure to perform the same work as does a normal ventricle.** It can be appreciated from Fig. 10.2 that as the need for increased cardiac work occurs, the increase in filling pressure may exceed the pulmonary capillary oncotic pressure (approximately 25 mm Hg) and pulmonary edema may ensue. Diuretics, nitrates (nitroglycerin), arterial vasodilators, and inotropic agents (digoxin, dopamine) alter the LVEDP-CO relationship and are useful in the acute and chronic management of CHF (see later).

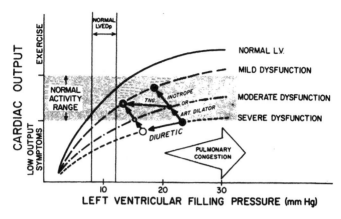

Fig. 10.2.   Frank-Starling curves.

2. **Ventricular hypertrophy.** Hypertrophy, or an increased muscle mass, is stimulated by both pressure and volume overload states.
Although hypertrophy potentially provides a beneficial increase in
contractile elements, the benefits are counterbalanced by decreasing
ventricular compliance, which is reduced further by ischemia when
the oxygen demand exceeds supply.

3. **Sympathetic nervous system.** The heart is richly innervated
by sympathetic fibers, and the increased release of endogenous catecholamines increases contractility and heart rate.

CLINICAL SIGNS AND SYMPTOMS

There is a wide spectrum of patients who present with CHF. The
acute, severely decompensated patients with CHF are primarily cold
and wet, implying low cardiac output and clinical congestion. The
vast majority of patients with CHF fall into an intermediate severity
category. These patients are frequently clinically congested but do
not exhibit signs of low cardiac output. As CHF develops, there is a
progressive increase in vasoconstrictor substances (norepinephrine,
angiotensin II, aldosterone, endothelin, and vasopressin) as well as
a decrease in endogenous vasodilators (atrial and B-type natriuretic
peptides, nitric oxide, prostacyclin, and bradykinin).

The major clinical manifestations of CHF can be divided arbitrarily
into two categories: those resulting from fluid retention [right heart
failure (RHF)] and those resulting from pulmonary vascular congestion [left heart failure (LHF)] (6,7). This division is clinically useful
but can be misleading because the right and left heart are intimately
associated with each other; moreover, the most common cause of
RHF is LHF.

Left Heart Failure

Basic abnormality: Increased left atrial pressure, resulting from
an elevation in LVEDP or from mitral valve disease, is transmitted
to the pulmonary vascular bed and is reflected clinically by an increased PCWP. If this pressure elevation exceeds the colloid osmotic

pressure of the pulmonary vascular bed, fluid accumulation within the interstitial spaces (seen as Kerley A and B lines on the chest x-ray) will result. Progression of this pathologic process subsequently will result in the accumulation of fluid within the alveolar spaces (pulmonary edema), leading to poor oxygen exchange and hypoxia.

Symptoms: Decreased exercise tolerance, dyspnea, cough, orthopnea, and/or paroxysmal nocturnal dyspnea may occur.

Signs: Tachycardia and inspiratory rales (beginning at the base of the lungs and heard progressively higher as the severity of LHF increases) are signs. Expiratory wheezes resulting from bronchospasm (cardiac asthma) are not infrequent.

Laboratory: Arterial blood gas analysis may reveal hypoxemia and hypocarbia. Chest x-ray may demonstrate prominent upper lobe vessels ("reversal of flow"), Kerley's lines, the classic "butterfly" pattern of alveolar pulmonary edema, and/or pleural effusions (see later).

Right Heart Failure

Basic abnormality: Physiologic hormonal and renal responses occur to compensate for chronically decreased CO. These adaptive mechanisms lead to sodium and water retention in an effort to increase intravascular volume and (by means of the Starling mechanism) CO.

Symptoms: Dyspnea on exertion and fluid retention occur.

Signs: Increased central venous pressure, hepatojugular reflux, hepatomegaly, ascites, and peripheral or sacral edema may be seen.

Laboratory: Abnormal liver function tests may occur (elevated transaminases, elevated bilirubin, prolonged prothrombin time). Pleural and pericardial effusions are not uncommon. Hyponatremia with a low urinary sodium (less than 20 mEq/L) ("dilutional hyponatremia") and an elevated blood urea nitrogen are frequent and reflect a decrease in renal perfusion.

RADIOGRAPHY OF CONGESTIVE HEART FAILURE

Irrespective of the underlying cause of CHF in an individual patient, the diagnosis of CHF must be confirmed before the initiation of any therapy. The physical examination may be very helpful, especially in RHF, but may be less helpful in diagnosing LHF because inspiratory rales may be associated with chronic lung abnormalities. Thus, the chest x-ray then becomes of clinical importance in diagnosing CHF.

Different **radiographic stages** reflecting the severity of CHF have been described, but the classical radiographic progression is not always seen. Moreover, the appearance and resolution rates of CHF on the chest x-ray are variable. The chest x-ray may not correlate temporally with the patient's immediate condition (i.e., there may be as much as a 12-hour diagnostic lag with the onset of CHF and a posttherapeutic lag of up to 4 days after the clinical resolution of CHF).

1. **Pulmonary venous congestion and redistribution of flow.** Normally, more blood flow occurs to the dependent portions of the lungs. When the PCWP is elevated from 12 to 18 mm Hg, flow to the lower lung fields is reduced as a result of vasoconstriction, whereas flow to the upper lung fields is increased. Recognition of flow distribution will be dependent on the quality of the upright chest x-ray

and usually is seen only in cases of chronic elevation of the PCW, such as in mitral stenosis.

2. **Interstitial pulmonary edema.** This is probably the most common radiographic sign of LHF. Fluid that accumulates in the interstitial spaces within the lung is seen as Kerley B lines (found in the lower lung fields peripherally and usually extending to the pleural surface). Fluid also can accumulate in the lobular septa, which form the framework of support for the lung and is seen as Kerley A lines (found emanating from the hila outward to the lung parenchyma). The pulmonary vessels typically are enlarged somewhat, and their radiographic shadows are blurred. A PCWP of 18 to 25 mm Hg is usually present.

3. **Alveolar edema.** As the severity of the LHF increases and the PCWP rises acutely higher than 25 mm Hg, actual filling of the alveolar spaces with fluid (i.e., pulmonary edema) can occur. This is recognized by the classic butterfly pattern of bilateral perihilar infiltrates.

IMPORTANT QUESTIONS IN CONGESTIVE HEART FAILURE ASSESSMENT

What is the Underlying Cardiac Disorder?

CHF itself is not a diagnosis—it is only a symptom complex. Two different classifications of the etiology of CHF follow.

Functional Classification of Congestive Heart Failure

1. Disorders of contractility (e.g., ischemic heart disease, cardiomyopathy)
2. Diastolic mechanical inhibition of cardiac performance (e.g., mitral stenosis, left atrial myxoma, pericardial tamponade); abnormalities of LV relaxation (as a result of hypertrophy, fibrosis, ischemia, infiltrative disorders)
3. Systolic mechanical ventricular overload (pressure: aortic stenosis, hypertension; volume: aortic insufficiency, mitral regurgitation)

Anatomic Classification of Congestive Heart Failure

1. Valvular
2. Systemic hypertension
3. Pulmonary hypertension
4. Pericardial disease
5. Myocardial disease
6. Congenital
7. High output states
8. Traumatic (acute aortic insufficiency)

What Is the Precipitating Cause of the Congestive Heart Failure?

Knowing the precipitating cause(s) of CHF may aid greatly in the management of the disorder. Common precipitating factors include the following:

1. Infection
2. Pulmonary embolus
3. Lack of medications
4. Arrhythmias

5. MI
6. Physical stress
7. Increased sodium intake
8. Sodium-retaining drugs
9. Anemia
10. Thyroid diseases
11. Bacterial endocarditis

PULMONARY EDEMA

Clinical Presentation

The end result of LHF may be acute pulmonary edema, which is associated with considerable morbidity and mortality if not recognized quickly and treated appropriately. Because the identification of the underlying abnormality producing CHF is just as important as making the clinical diagnosis of CHF, some comments on the physical examination, electrocardiogram (ECG), and chest x-ray in regard to this end in a typical patient may be helpful.

1. **Feel the carotid arteries carefully.** The quality of the upstroke may be helpful in identifying pathologic conditions (i.e., aortic stenosis) because its rate of increase is related to LV function. The carotid pulse also serves as an invaluable tool in helping to correctly identify and time any murmurs heard on auscultation of the heart.

2. **Auscultate the heart.** Do not let the presence of adventitious breath sounds limit your attempt to correctly identify heart sounds and murmurs. Listen for signs of mitral stenosis (a loud first heart sound, an opening snap best heard at the apex, and an apical diastolic rumble). Appreciation of these findings may be hindered by atrial fibrillation with a rapid ventricular response rate. A loud middiastolic crescendo-decrescendo murmur should alert one to the possibility of acute aortic insufficiency. This murmur, at times, is so loud that house staff consistently call it a systolic murmur, failing to properly time it with the carotid upstroke. A midsystolic murmur and loud S4 gallop in the presence of sinus rhythm should alert one to the possibility of acute mitral regurgitation.

3. **Examine the ECG.** Evidence of an old or new MI may be present. Atrial fibrillation in combination with large fibrillatory waves in the anterior precordial leads (V1) suggests mitral valvular disease with left atrial enlargement.

4. **Examine the chest x-ray.** This is used to confirm a clinical diagnosis. Clear lung fields in the presence of a large cardiac silhouette in a patient with dyspnea suggests pericardial tamponade (see Chapter 14).

Therapy of Acute Pulmonary Edema

Therapy for acute pulmonary edema involves the following (6):

1. **Identify and eliminate any aggravating factors.**

2. **High-flow oxygen** is best tolerated if administered by nasal prongs. Pulse oximetry may be helpful in determining the response to supplemental oxygen administration.

3. **Morphine sulfate** should be used in doses of 3 to 5-mg slow intravenous (IV) push. This drug is beneficial in several ways:
Venous dilatation rapidly decreases preload.
Sedative effect relieves extreme anxiety.

Hyperventilation is decreased by directly depressing the respiratory center.

The venodilatation does not become prominent until higher doses are reached. At high doses, respiratory depression may occur before venodilatation. IV Lasix and the nitrates are more potent venodilators and should be used initially.

4. **Diuretics.** Rapidly acting loop diuretics (furosemides) are usually effective in doses of 40 to 80-mg IV push. Venous dilatation ensues quickly and decreases preload. An increase in urinary output will occur later (7). If no clinical response is noted after 15 to 30 minutes, double the diuretic dose and administer again.

5. **Bronchodilators** are useful if substantial bronchospasm is present (cardiac asthma). β-2 selective inhaled bronchodilators such as albuterol sulfate can be administered via a handheld nebulizer. Aminophylline has been used in the past but may precipitate arrhythmias, nausea, and vomiting. Bronchospasm is usually brief and frequently will diminish or resolve with the use of oxygen and diuretics.

6. **Endotracheal intubation** and artificial airway control are indicated if uncontrollable and excessive secretions, marked hypoxemia, excessive work of breathing, and/or severe respiratory acidosis occur.

7. **Inotropic agents. Dopamine** and **dobutamine** are potent cardiac inotropes that can be given intravenously and titrated to clinical response in the acute setting. The usual effective dose range is 5 to 15 mg/kg/minutes. These agents are also chronotropes and may produce arrhythmias. **Digitalis** does not produce consistent beneficial hemodynamic effects in acute CHF. It is a weaker inotropic agent compared with dopamine or dobutamine, and thus, it is not the drug of choice for inotropic support in pump failure complicating acute myocardial infarction (AMI). Digitalis therapy, because of its late onset of action (6 to 8 hours), is also of limited value in the acute setting for the control of atrial fibrillation with a rapid ventricular response. **Amrinone** and **milrinone** are phosphodiesterase inhibitors and are additional potent inotropic drugs with a different hemodynamic profile. Both agents increase cardiac cAMP (cyclic adenosine monophosphate) and increase contractility while producing vasodilation (decreased afterload). Amrinone is used at an initial dose of 0.75 mg/kg followed by a maintenance infusion of 5 to mcg/kg/min. Milrinone is about 15 times more potent than amrinone but has fewer side effects.

8. **Nitrates.** Pulmonary venous pressure decreases promptly with acute nitrate administration; sublingual nitrates can be very effective in relieving congestive symptoms in the immediate treatment of pulmonary edema. With **IV nitroglycerin,** the arterial pressure decreases slightly, the heart rate remains unchanged, and cardiac output may show a modest increase. These beneficial effects progressively decline with continuous use. After 24 hours, most of the hemodynamics return to control levels; this appears to be the result of nitrate tolerance.

9. **Nitroprusside** (10 to 200 micrograms/min) can be used in patients with hypertension or patients with aortic or mitral regurgitation who do not respond to diuretics and nitroglycerin. Caution must be used because of the reflex tachycardia that can exacerbate ischemia. With prolonged use and in the setting of renal dysfunction,

thiocyanate, a metabolite of nitroprusside, may accumulate and cause lactic acidosis.

10. **Intraaortic balloon counterpulsation.** In the setting of AMI, acute mitral regurgitation, or acute rupture of the interventricular septum following infarction, intraaortic balloon counterpulsation augments diastolic coronary blood flow and helps to decrease afterload. This device usually is placed in the cardiac catheterization laboratory but can be inserted at the bedside if the patient is being treated at a facility without catheterization facilities. Contraindications include aortic regurgitation and aortic dissection, which, if suspected, can be diagnosed by transesophageal echocardiography.

11. **Pulmonary artery catheterization.** Placement of a pulmonary artery balloon catheter can be useful in patients who are in cardiogenic shock or who have pulmonary edema and who are not responding to pharmacologic therapy. Additionally, this is a valuable diagnostic tool in determining if pulmonary edema is of noncardiac origin. The optimal PCWP is 14 to 18 mm Hg.

The pneumonic **"UNLOAD ME"** is helpful in the treatment of acute pulmonary edema:

U—head of the bed upright
N— nitrates (sublingual or IV)
L— Lasix
O— oxygen
A— albuterol (if needed for bronchospasm)
D— dopamine or dobutamine
M— morphine
E— electrical cardioversion for tachyarrhythmias (atrial fibrillation or ventricular tachycardia)

MANAGEMENT OF CHRONIC CONGESTIVE HEART FAILURE

The treatment of CHF is guided best by knowledge of the etiology and pathophysiology of the underlying cardiac abnormality. The most common cause of both acute and chronic heart failure is systolic dysfunction, usually resulting from ischemic heart disease, hypertension, and idiopathic dilated cardiomyopathy (a diagnosis of exclusion). However, up to 30% of patients with heart failure have normal systolic function, defined as an ejection fraction of more than 55%, and have evidence of diastolic dysfunction echocardiographically (see Chapter 4). Diastolic dysfunction can precede, and commonly occurs together with, systolic dysfunction. Common causes for diastolic dysfunction include ischemic heart disease, ventricular hypertrophy (usually secondary to systemic hypertension or aortic stenosis), diabetes, and the aging process. Echocardiography is the noninvasive diagnostic test of choice in defining ventricular function. The importance of a correct diagnosis is emphasized by the differing treatments (8–10).

Treatment of Patients with Congestive Heart Failure and Systolic Dysfunction

In patients with signs and symptoms of chronic CHF, medical therapy is necessary to maintain a near optimal LVEDP (15 to 20 mm Hg) to maximize CO, thereby preventing pulmonary vascular congestion. The mainstays of medical therapy consist of the following (11):

1. **Restriction of physical activity.** Bed rest sometimes may be required in patients with decompensated heart failure (American Heart Association Class IV). In stable compensated patients, skeletal muscle conditioning may play a role in the exercise capacity of patients with heart failure. Although mild to moderate dynamic exercise may be beneficial, isometric exercise (such as weight training) can cause an acute increase in afterload and may be detrimental (12).

2. **Low-sodium diet.** In patients on an extremely low-sodium diet (1 g), free water restriction also may be necessary to prevent symptomatic hyponatremia. Low-sodium diets are difficult to comply with and extensive dietary counseling often is required (12).

3. **Diuretics.** The **loop diuretics** (furosemide, ethacrynic acid, bumetanide, torsemide) are most effective in doses titrated to the desired clinical effort without inducing hypotension or azotemia. For patients who do not respond to a loop diuretic alone, the addition of a **thiazide** diuretic (hydrochlorothiazide or metolazone) that works at a different nephron site (the early distal tubule) may be helpful (13). After the initiation of diuretic therapy, serum electrolyte monitoring should be performed because clinically significant electrolyte abnormalities may occur, specifically hypokalemia. If hypokalemia becomes a chronic problem, the use of **potassium-sparing diuretics** such as triamterene, spironolactone, or amiloride may be helpful. Magnesium depletion commonly occurs with chronic diuretic therapy and can worsen potassium loss. Nonsteroidal antiinflammatory drugs, because of their effects on prostaglandin metabolism, can block the effectiveness of diuretics as well as promote fluid retention.

4. **Digoxin.** Digoxin therapy is unlikely to be of benefit in all patients with chronic CHF (14–16). Minimal or no benefit is seen in patients with mild heart failure and relatively well-preserved LV systolic function. In patients with more severe heart failure with significantly reduced LV ejection fraction, digoxin therapy combined with diuretics and vasodilators should be considered. Clinical studies indicate that digoxin can increase ejection fraction, increase exercise tolerance, and decrease the compensatory sympathetic activity that accompanies a chronic decrease in CO. However, digoxin has not been shown to improve 5-year mortality in patients with CHF. A reduced daily dose of digoxin usually is required in patients with renal failure. Digitalis toxicity is more likely to occur in (a) elderly patients; (b) patients with renal failure; (c) patients with a small body size; (d) patients with chronic obstructive pulmonary disease; (e) patients with hypokalemia; or (f) patients taking digoxin in combination with quinidine, verapamil, or the macrolide antibiotics. The most frequent symptoms of digitalis toxicity are anorexia and nausea. Serum digoxin levels may be helpful in documenting toxicity but should not be overused and should be drawn at least 6 hours after the last dose. Patients with chronic atrial fibrillation may require higher than normal "therapeutic levels" to control the ventricular rate but may not be clinically toxic. Digoxin-specific Fab antibody fragments are the recommended therapy in the management of life-threatening digitalis toxicity. Approximately 75% of patients will exhibit a clinical response within 60 minutes of antibody administration (17).

5. **Vasodilator therapy.** One often assumes that reflex compensatory mechanisms for maintaining CO and blood pressure in the face of acute or chronic CHF will produce a favorable effect. Unfortunately, this is not always true. The increase in systemic vascular resistance, which usually occurs when CO decreases, may have a deleterious effect on the heart by increasing the afterload or wall tension of the left ventricle.

Vasodilator drugs frequently can alter the vicious circle of increasing systemic vascular resistance leading to decreased CO by decreasing total peripheral vascular resistance and impedance to LV ejection. Hemodynamic improvement is the result of the following:

Improved ejection fraction, which decreases LVEDP and pulmonary congestion

Decreased pressure work of the failing ventricle

Reduced wall tension and decreasing myocardial oxygen demand

Mechanism of Action

Nitrates. This class of drugs have their most pronounced effect on venous capacitance (venodilatation leading to a decrease in preload) and a variable effect an arterial resistance (decreased afterload). Nitrates also may cause dilatation of the coronary arteries and possible redistribution of blood flow to the subendocardium in ischemic heart disease. Nitrates have no direct effect on myocardial contractility. Sublingual, oral, and topical preparations may be used. Long-term therapy frequently is complicated by nitrate tolerance, which can be minimized by appropriate dosing (18).

Hydralazine. An effective arterial vasodilator, hydralazine usually is administered orally in combination with diuretics and/or long-acting nitrates. Used alone, hydralazine has little effect on preload; it is predominantly an arteriolar vasodilator and increases cardiac output. The combined regimen of hydralazine and nitrates provides substantial advantage in CHF by combining the increase in cardiac output with a decrease in PCWP. In the Veterans Administration Cooperative Study, the combination of hydralazine (300 mg/day) and isosorbide dinitrate (160 mg/day) was shown to decrease mortality of patients with mild to moderately severe CHF by approximately 25% compared to the placebo group who received digitalis and diuretics. This combination has been effective in improving symptoms and exercise tolerance (19). Lower doses of hydralazine and nitrates do not improve mortality. The combination of hydralazine and oral nitrates most commonly is reserved for those patients who are unable to tolerate angiotensin converting enzyme (ACE) inhibitor therapy.

ACE inhibitors. It has been shown that the renin-angiotensin system (RAS) is stimulated in patients with CHF, resulting in elevated levels of angiotensin II, plasma renin, and aldosterone (20). Angiotensin-mediated vasoconstriction results in increased systemic vascular resistance, and the increased renin and aldosterone contribute to sodium and water retention. Some local autocrine-paracrine RAS have been described in many tissues, including blood vessels, heart, kidney, and adrenals. These may participate in the pathophysiology of CHF.

The principal action of the ACE inhibitors is the blockade of the conversion of angiotensin I to angiotensin II in the serum, as well as at local tissues. Data suggest that the acute effect of ACE inhibitors occurs in the circulation and that the chronic effect is related to the inhibition at the tissue level (20).

ACE inhibitors have been shown to improve hemodynamics, enhance diuresis, reduce symptoms, improve exercise capacity, and prolong survival of patients with CHF. The main hemodynamic effects include systemic vasodilation, reduced blood pressure, increased cardiac output, and reduced filling pressures. A total of 70% to 80% of patients report symptomatic improvement, compared to 25% of placebo controls. The most compelling case for the use of ACE inhibitors is the data on improved survival (21). The Cooperative North Scandinavian Enalapril Survival Study (CONSENSUS) showed that enalapril significantly reduced mortality (by 31%) compared to placebo at the end of 1 year (22). Similar positive results were reported in the Captopril Multicenter Research Group study (23). At the present time, ACE inhibitors should be given preference to other vasodilators in the management of chronic CHF. These drugs have emerged as the most important advance in CHF therapy in recent years.

Asymptomatic patients with LV systolic dysfunction also benefit from the use of ACE inhibitors. In the Studies of Left Ventricular Dysfunction (SOLVD) trial, enalapril reduced the incidence of symptomatic heart failure and rate of hospitalization for heart failure compared with a placebo group. There was also an overall trend toward decreased cardiovascular mortality in the enalapril treatment group (24). In the Survival and Ventricular Enlargement (SAVE) trial, patients with asymptomatic LV dysfunction (LVEF less than 40%) who received captopril after MI had an improvement in survival and a reduction in morbidity and as a result of cardiovascular events (25). Two other large, multicenter controlled trials, GISSI-3 (Gruppo Italiano per lo Studio dell soprevvivenza nell'Infarcto Miocardico) and ISIS 4 (Fourth International Study of Infarct Survival), also support the use of ACE inhibitors in patients with and without heart failure after MI (26,27). However, IV administration of enalapril followed by oral therapy after infarction has not been shown to improve survival (28). All patients who have an ejection fraction of less than 35% to 40% should receive an ACE inhibitor, if tolerated, after MI.

All patients with CHF as a result of LV systolic dysfunction should receive an ACE inhibitor unless they are unable to tolerate treatment with these agents. ACE inhibitors in the setting of CHF are recommended to improve symptoms, improve clinical status, reduce hospitalization, and decrease the risk of death.

Adverse effects of ACE inhibitors include marked hypotension, bradycardia, skin rash, impaired renal function, and occasional cases of immune complex glomerulonephritis. Cough occurs in 1% to 5% of patients. Taste disturbance occurs in about 5% of patients. Proteinuria occurs in 1% of all patients but is more common in patients with azotemia (2.1% to 2.5%). Hypotension usually is encountered only with the first several doses, and it is seldom that the drug needs to be withdrawn because of hypotension (0% to 6%). Attenuation of this hypotensive effect occurs rapidly, and clinical symptoms of hypotension during maintenance therapy are rare. Hydralazine and isosorbide dinitrate should be considered for those patients who cannot tolerate ACE inhibitors.

Angiotensin-receptor-blockers (ARBs). ARBs are more effective inhibitors of the RAS than are ACE inhibitors. However, clinical testing was done to test whether more intense inhibition of the RAS would offer morbidity and mortality benefits in CHF. The ELITE II trial showed equivalent effect on mortality and morbidity between losartan and captopril (29). The conclusion was that losartan was not superior to captopril. The Val Heft trial showed additive benefits of valsartan when added to standard treatment with ACE inhibitors, diuretics, and digitalis in patients with CHF (30). The CHARM trial will elucidate the clinical utility of candesartan in patients with CHF whose LV ejection fraction is greater than 40% (31).

It has been assumed that ARBs are an effective treatment for CHF (i.e., superior to placebo), although there are little data to support this assumption. Several conclusions can be reached at the present time:

1. ARBs may be used as an alternative to an ACE inhibitor in the patient who is truly tolerant of an ACE inhibitor.
2. ARBs may be used in addition to an ACE inhibitor.
3. "Triple neurohumoral blockade" with an ACE inhibitor, ARB, and beta blocker is not advised presently.

Beta-Adrenergic Blockers

With decreasing LV performance, the body releases hormones such as norepinephrine. Although these hormones help the heart pump better in the short run, over time the heart will weaken faster. Activation of both the adrenergic and renin-aldosterone systems results in salt and water retention and peripheral vasoconstriction. Beta blockers are known to turn off mediators of a vicious cycle of disease progression associated with salt and water resorption, cardiac remodeling, myocyte death, loss of contractility, and impaired cardiac metabolism.

Based on placebo-controlled trials of more than 10,000 patients, the 1999 Heart Failure Consensus Recommendations stated that all patients with stable New York Heart Association Class II or III heart failure resulting from LV systolic dysfunction should receive a beta blocker (in addition to an ACE inhibitor) unless they have a contraindication to its use or cannot tolerate treatment with the drug (32). Treatment with a beta blocker should not be delayed until the patient is found to be resistant to treatment with other drugs (33).

Both second-generation beta blockers such as metoprolol or bisoprolol and third-generation nonselective beta blockers such as carvedilol reduce mortality and morbidity in mild to moderate CHF. The key mechanics of action of these beta blockers are prevention and partial reversal of adrenergically-mediated myocardial dysfunction and remodeling and blocking the cytotoxic and growth-promoting effects of norepinephrine mediated by the B1, B2, and a1 cardiac receptors.

The pharmacology of the third-generation carvedilol differs from the second-generation compound metoprolol. Carvedilol is a nonselective blocker of B1 versus B2 receptors and blocks a1 receptors(which accounts for its vasodilatory properties). Carvedilol has the potential for greater cardioprotection from harmful adrenergic stimuli by blocking all three receptors and lowering cardiac adrenergic activity. Compared with patients treated with metoprolol, patients treated with Carvedilol have a greater improvement in functional class and a greater improvement in stroke volume and LV ejection fraction (34).

Positive Inotropic Drugs

Dopamine was introduced in the 1970s and largely has replaced toxic agents such as epinephrine and isoproterenol. Dopamine has both α and β effects. At low doses (1 to 5 μg/kg/minute), it dilates mesenteric and renal vessels producing increased renal blood flow. At 5 to 10 μg/kg/minute, β stimulation increases cardiac output with relatively little tachycardia. At higher doses (more than 10 μg/kg/minute), tachycardia and α stimulation occur.

Dobutamine is a synthetic analogue of dopamine that stimulates B1, B2, and a receptors. It increases cardiac contractility by virtue of the B1 effect but does not increase peripheral resistance because of the balance between α-mediated vasoconstriction and B2-mediated vasodilation. Tachyarrhythmia is a major adverse side effect.

Milrinone is a phosphodiesterase-inhibiting agent that has both inotropic and vasodilator properties. This inhibition reduces the breakdown of intracellular cAMP, resulting in enhanced calcium entry into the cell and increased force of contraction. A significant limiting factor can be the development of tachycardia and ventricular arrhythmias. The drug is valuable for seriously ill, decompensated heart failure (35).

Levosimendan is a positive inotropic drug that is available in Europe. It increases the sensitivity of the myofilaments (specifically troponin-C) to intracellular calcium. Its actions are independent of cAMP. It also has a vasodilating effect mediated through inhibition of phosphodiesterase-III and by activation of potassium-dependent adenosine triphosphate channels. Ventricular arrhythmias and tachycardia are noted at higher doses (36).

Toborinone is a positive inotropic and has vasodilating properties through its inhibition of phosphodiesterase-III. Short-term benefits include increasing cardiac output, reducing filling pressures, and reducing systemic vascular resistance. It does not appear to increase heart rate (37).

Tezosentan is a short-acting, dual endothelin receptor antagonist. Positive responses to the drug include reduction in PCWP and systemic vascular resistance as well as significant increase in cardiac output. There is no tachycardia or proarrhythmic effect (38).

Nesiritide, a recombinant human B-type natriuretic peptide, has been shown to produce favorable hemodynamics (including balanced vasodilation) associated with a rapid improvement in clinical symptoms. This hormone is secreted naturally in response to CHF. The actions of the endogenous natriuretic peptides partially counteract the harmful effects of renin, aldosterone, and norepinephrine. Hemodynamic benefits include reducing filling pressures, lowering systemic resistance, and increasing stroke volume. Nesiritide is not associated with an increase in heart rate or proarrhythmia (39).

The import role of brain natriuretic peptide (BNP) in the setting of CHF has emerged. BNP is a neurohormone similar to atrial natriuretic peptide. It is produced by ventricular myocytes in response to stretch. There is a correlation between elevated BNP blood levels and NYHA classification, LVEDP, and mortality. There is now a rapid assay that can provide BNP levels within 15 minutes. A relationship between the severity of the decompensated heart failure and BNP values has been demonstrated; as the severity of the heart failure increases, the median concentration of BNP increases. A BNP cut-off level of 80 pg/mL has a sensitivity of 96% and a positive predictive value of 95% (40).

Cardiac transplantation. In patients with disabling symptoms of CHF or unacceptable risk of cardiac death and no contraindications to the procedure, heart transplantation remains an option. Unfortunately, there are far too many patients who need transplants compared to the number of donor hearts available. LV assist devices are experimental but provide a bridge to transplantation in selected patients. Contraindications include excessive age, active infection, active peptic ulcer disease, chronic seizure disorder, severe peripheral vascular disease, insulin-dependent diabetes, renal failure, liver failure, severely elevated pulmonary vascular resistance (unless a combined heart–lung transplant is considered), alcoholism or drug abuse, psychiatric instability, or risk of medical noncompliance.

TREATMENT OF PATIENTS WITH DIASTOLIC HEART FAILURE

Patients with diastolic dysfunction have abnormal LV relaxation because of a noncompliant left ventricle. This discussion will exclude the diastolic abnormalities seen in mitral stenosis, pericardial constriction, and hypertrophic cardiomyopathy. Symptoms usually are related to elevated filling pressures with pulmonary congestion and dyspnea. The goal of therapy is to reduce filling pressures without lowering cardiac output (8–10). Diuretics and nitrates are the mainstay of therapy, although calcium channel blockers and beta blockers have been used with the intention of increasing the diastolic filling period and relaxing the ventricle. However, studies have not shown these agents to be effective. There is no role for digoxin in diastolic heart failure. ACE inhibitors may help if the patient has diastolic heart failure as a result of LV hypertrophy from untreated hypertension. Coronary revascularization may be beneficial in patients who have a noncompliant LV as a result of ischemic heart disease.

REFERENCES

1. Ventura HO, Murgo JP, Smart FW, et al: Current issue in advanced heart failure. *Med Clin N Amer* 76:1057, 1992.
2. American Heart Association: *2001 heart and stroke statistical update.* Dallas, TX, 2000.
3. Arai AE, Greenberg BH: Medical management of congestive heart failure. *West J Med* 153:406, 1990.
4. Burkart F, Kiowski W: Circulatory abnormalities and compensatory mechanisms in heart failure. *Am J Med* 90(Suppl 5B):19S, 1994.
5. LeJemtel TH, Sonnenblick EH: Heart failure: adaptive and maladaptive processes. *Circulation* 87(Suppl VII):VII-1, 1993.
6. Karon BL: Diagnosis and outpatient management of congestive heart failure. *Mayo Clin Proc* 70:1080, 1995.
7. Report of the American College of Cardiology/American Heart Association Task Force on Practice Guidelines (Committee on Evaluation and Management of Heart Failure): Guidelines for the evaluation and management of heart failure. *Circulation* 92:2764, 1995.
8. Bonow RO, Udelson JE: Left ventricular diastolic dysfunction as a cause of congestive heart failure. Mechanisms and management. *Ann Intern Med* 117:502, 1992.

9. Goldsmith SR, Dick C: Differentiating systolic from diastolic heart failure: pathophysiologic and therapeutic considerations. *Am J Med* 95:645, 1993.

10. Vasan RS, Benjamin EJ, Levy D: Congestive heart failure with normal left ventricular systolic function. Clinical approaches to the diagnosis and treatment of diastolic heart failure. *Arch Intern Med* 156:146, 1996.

11. Cohn JN: The management of chronic heart failure. *N Engl J Med* 335:490, 1996.

12. Dracup K, Baker DW, Dunbar SB, et al: Management of heart failure. II. Counseling, education, and lifestyle modifications. *JAMA* 272: 1442, 1994.

13. Cody RJ, Kubo SH, Pickworth KK: Diuretic treatment for the sodium retention of congestive heart failure. *Arch Intern Med* 154:1905, 1994.

14. Jaeschke R, Oxman AD, Guyatt GH: To what extent do congestive heart failure patients in sinus rhythm benefit from digoxin-therapy? A systematic overview and meta-analysis. *Am J Med* 88:279, 1990.

15. Smith TW: Digoxin in heart failure. *N Engl J Med* 329:51, 1993.

16. The Digitalis Investigation Group: The effect of digoxin on mortality and morbidity in patients with heart failure. *N Engl J Med* 336:525, 1997.

17. Antman EM, Wenger TL, Butler VP, et al: Treatment of 150 cases of life-threatening digitalis intoxication with digoxin-specific Fab antibody fragments. Final report of a multicenter study. *Circulation* 81: 1744, 1990.

18. Abrams J, ed.: A symposium: Third North American Conference on Nitroglycerin Therapy. *Am J Cardiol* 70:1B, 1992.

19. Cohn JN, Archibald DG, Ziesche S, et al: Effect of vasodilator therapy on mortality in chronic congestive heart failure. Results of a Veterans Administration Cooperative Study (V-HeFT). *N Engl J Med* 314:1547, 1986.

20. Gavras H: Angiotensin-converting enzyme inhibition and the heart. *Hypertension* 23:813, 1994.

21. The SOLVD (Studies of Left Ventricular Dysfunction) Investigators: Effect of enalapril on survival in patients with reduced left ventricular ejection fractions and congestive heart failure. *N Engl J Med* 325: 293, 1991.

22. The CONSENSUS Trial Study Group: Effects of enalapril on mortality in severe congestive heart failure. *N Engl J Med* 316:1429, 1987.

23. Captopril Multicenter Research Group: A placebo-controlled trial of captopril in refractory congestive heart failure. *J Am Coll Cardiol* 2: 755, 1983.

24. The SOLVD Investigators: Effect of enalapril on mortality and the development of heart failure in asymptomatic patients with reduced left ventricular ejection fractions. *N Engl J Med* 327:685, 1992.

25. Pfeffer MA, Braunwald E, Moye LA, et al: Effect of captopril on mortality and morbidity in patients with left ventricular dysfunction after myocardial infarction. Results of the Survival and Ventricular Enlargement Trial. *N Engl J Med* 327:669, 1992.

26. GISSI-3: Effects of lisinopril and transdermal glyceryl trinitrate singly and together on 6-week mortality and ventricular function after acute myocardial infarction. *Lancet* 343:1115, 1994.

27. ISIS-4: A randomised factorial trial assessing early oral captopril, oral mononitrate, and intravenous magnesium sulphate in 58,050 patients with suspected acute myocardial infarction. *Lancet* 345:669, 1995.

28. Swedberg K, Held P, Kjekshus J, et al: Effects of the early administration of enalapril on mortality in patients with acute myocardial infarction. Results of the Cooperative New Scandinavian Enalapril Survival Study II (Consensus II). *N Engl J Med* 327:678, 1992.

29. Pitt B, Pool-Wilson PA, Segal R, et al: Effect of losartan compared with captopril on mortality in patients with symptomatic heart failure; Randomized trial-the losartan heart failure survival study ELITE II. *Lancet* 355:1582, 2000

30. Cohn JN, Tognoni G, Glazer RD, et al: Rationale and design of the valsartan heart failure trial: a large multinational trial to assess the effects of valsartan, an ARB, on morbidity and mortality in chronic congestive heart failure. *J Card Fail* 5:155, 1999.

31. Swedberg K, Pfeffer M, Granger C, et al: Candesartan in heart failure-assessment of reduction in mortality and morbidity (CHARM): rationale and design. *J Card Fail* 3:276, 1999.

32. Vantrimpont P, Rouleaue JL, Wun CC, et al: For the SAVE Investigators. Additive beneficial effects of beta-blockers to angiotensin-converting enzyme inhibitors in the Survival and Ventricular Enlargement (SAVE) Study. *J Am Coll Cardiol* 292:229, 1997.

33. Consensus recommendations for the management of chronic heart failure. *Am J Cardiol* 83 (Suppl 2A):1A, 1999.

34. Bristow MR: Beta-adrenergic receptor blockade in chronic heart failure. *Circulation* 101:558, 2000.

35. Slawsky MP, Colucci WS, Gottlieb SS, et al: Acute hemodynamic and clinical effects of levosimendan in patients with severe heart failure. *Circulation* 102:2222, 2000.

36. Mager G, Cocke RK, Kux A, et al: Phosphodiesterase 111 inhibition or adrenoreceptor stimulation: milrinone as an alternative to dobutamine in the treatment of severe heart failure. *Am Heart J* 121:1974, 1991.

37. Young J: New therapeutic choices in the management of acute congestive heart failure. *Rev Cardiovasc Med* 2:519, 2001.

38. Torre-Amione G, Young JB, Durand JB, et al: Hemodynamic effects of tezosentan, an intravenous dual endothelin receptor antagonist in patients with heart failure. *Circulation* 103:973, 2001.

39. Rayburn B, Bourge R: Nesiritide: a unique therapeutic cardiac peptide. *Rev Cardiovasc Med* 2:525, 2001.

40. Maisel A: B-Type natriuretic peptide (BNP) levels: diagnostic and therapeutic potential. *Rev Cardiovasc Med* 2:513, 2001.

VALVAR HEART DISEASE

BEDSIDE EVALUATION OF THE PATIENT WITH SUSPECTED VALVE DISEASE

There is a close relationship between cardiovascular physical findings and their underlying hemodynamic parameters, so an understanding of valvar pathophysiology greatly enhances the accuracy of bedside physical diagnosis. An understanding of pathophysiology requires knowledge of normal cardiac physiology (Fig. 11.1). Therefore, this chapter will begin with a review of normal cardiac function and the interaction between cardiac and respiratory function, then cover four common valve lesions, and finish with a review of bedside cardiovascular physical findings.

PHASES OF THE RESPIRATORY CYCLE

Inspiration transiently increases return to the right heart chambers and thus their output and increases the compliance (capacity to store blood) of the pulmonary vasculature. Left heart filling and output therefore are reduced. **Expiration** transiently augments return to, and output from, the left heart chambers while inhibiting inflow to the right heart and lungs. The two circulations reciprocate these "feast and famine" cycles and, in the long term, match their outputs. These intracardiac events are matched by phenomena that either can be observed, palpated, or heard with a stethoscope (Fig. 11.2).

ORIGIN AND TRANSMISSION OF CARDIAC SOUNDS AND MURMURS

Audible events generated by the heart are classified as **sounds** when they are abrupt or short in duration and **murmurs** if they consist of prolonged vibrations. Sounds result from an abrupt cessation of blood flow, whereas murmurs occur when there is disturbed or turbulent high-velocity flow. Abrupt interruption of the momentum of local blood flow normally occurs with closure of the cardiac valves in response to the initiation of retrograde flow, as shown by the arrows in the normal heart cartoons in Fig. 11.3. Opening of normal valves is silent, but commissural fusion in a mobile, stenotic valve will abruptly decelerate a column of blood that has gained momentum as it enters the space provided by the parting leaflets. If the distal mitral valve sleeve has been converted to a funnel, as shown in the cartoons depicting mitral stenosis, the moving blood entering the base of the valve is thwarted by the failure of the mitral sleeve to open, resulting in an **opening snap** that is transmitted principally back toward the source of the moving column of blood. The opening snap is best heard at the base (close to the left atrium), whereas the **murmurs** caused by disturbed inflow are heard only at the apex.

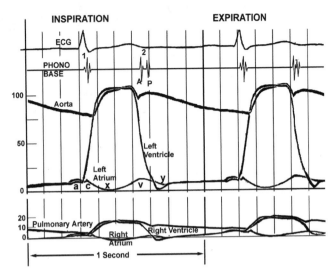

Fig. 11.1. Phases of the normal cardiac cycle. Diastole: 1: isovolumic relaxation (initiated by aortic and pulmonic valve closure and the dicrotic notch), 2: rapid (passive) filling, 3: diastasis, and 4: atrial systole. Systole: 5: isovolumic contraction (initiated by mitral and tricuspid closure) and 6: ventricular ejection. The positive atrial waves result from atrial contraction (*a wave*), atrioventricular valve closure (*c wave*), and atrial filling (*v wave*). The x-descent results from negative atrial pressure related to ventricular ejection, and the y-descent results from passive atrial outflow as atrioventricular valves open. The atrium therefore has four cycles: (6 + 1) a closed compartment (reservoir) during ventricular systole that (2) unloads into the ventricle, (3) a passive conduit, and (4) an active pump. Heart sounds result from atrioventricular (first sound) and semilunar valve closure (second sound). Inspiration increases right heart filling and pulmonary vascular compliance, delaying the pulmonary (*P*) component of the second sound, splitting it away from the aortic (*A*) component.

VALVAR DISEASES

Valve malfunction can result in stenosis, regurgitation, or combinations of both. These forms of malfunction can occur when a valve is structurally normal but subjected to extraordinary perturbations (e.g., severe pressure or volumetric changes), but they more often occur when there is structural damage, which may be congenital and/or acquired.

Aortic Regurgitation

Aortic valve incompetence can result from a number of pathologic processes that affect the valve leaflets and/or the aortic root. Congenital bicuspid valve deformity, with or without superimposed endocarditis, is the leading cause of aortic regurgitation in individuals younger than age 30, whereas aortic root dilation from hypertension often causes the valves to fail to coapt in older individuals. Rheumatic fever, Marfan disease, rheumatoid arthritis, aortitis, trauma, and aortic dissection are additional etiologies.

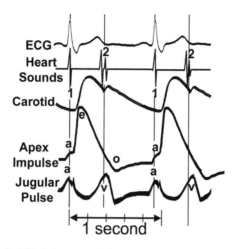

Fig. 11.2. Bedside timing events in the normal cardiac cycle. The **carotid pulse** is monophasic, often visible and readily palpable, and defines the ejection phase of systole. The **jugular venous pulse** is usually biphasic, rarely palpable, and varies in amplitude with respiration, reproducing the right atrial pressure contour. The isovolumic systolic portion of the **apex impulse** is usually palpable as a positive wave that ends with ejection (*e*). Note that the jugular a **wave** occurs at the approximate time of the first heart sound (*1*), and the *v-wave* occurs with the second sound (*2*). These correlated events assist in correct identification of sounds or pulses during bedside examination.

Bedside examination of a patient with significant aortic regurgitation often reveals multiple visible and audible abnormalities that may overwhelm the unprepared examiner (Fig. 11.4). The primary pathophysiologic condition is **backflow** into the left ventricle, which leads to **arterial diastolic collapse,** lowering of the arterial diastolic pressure, and a **decrescendo early diastolic murmur.** Two secondary outcomes are an increase in the systolic stroke volume and turbulent mitral valve inflow. Increased stroke volume and outflow velocity are accompanied by **a midsystolic murmur** emulating that of aortic stenosis. Turbulent mitral inflow causes **middiastolic and presystolic murmurs (Austin Flint murmur)** that emulates mitral stenosis in patients with severe aortic regurgitation.

Prominent **sounds** can be heard as well. The second sound may be **tambour** (like a kettle drum) if the aorta is dilated. The first sound may be perceived as "split" because of the loud **ejection sound.**

The findings in aortic regurgitation can be quite different if the condition is **acute** rather than **chronic,** resulting from endocarditis, trauma, or aortic dissection. The ventricle poorly tolerates the volume load, which rapidly raises the diastolic pressure **preclosing** the mitral valve. Ventricular diastolic pressure may rise to equal aortic pressure, preventing arterial diastolic collapse. The stroke volume is less than in the chronic state, so the pulses are unlike the Corrigan pulse. The early diastolic murmur is truncated by the equilibrating left ventricular and aortic pressures, and the presystolic component

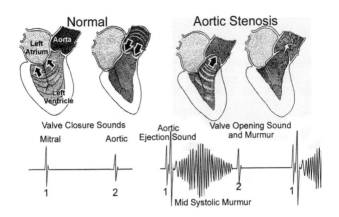

Fig. 11.3. Causation and transmission of cardiac sounds. *Normal*: Cartoons depict the vectors of moving blood (*arrows*) that cause closure of the mitral and aortic valves. The abrupt impact results in the first (*1*) and second (*2*) heart sounds, and shockwaves are transmitted in a direction opposite to the arrows. The first heart sound is best heard at the apex, and the second heart sound is best heard at the base because of wave propagation. *Aortic stenosis*: Commissural fusion prevents the valve from opening fully, halting the momentum of blood moving through the outflow tract (*arrows*), generating an **ejection sound** and sending a shockwave back toward the ventricular apex. Disturbed flow through the restricted orifice causes a crescendo–decrescendo murmur beginning with the ejection sound and ending before the second sound (*2*). The density of the shading in the cardiac chambers in this and subsequent figures indicates their pressure, with darker shading in the aorta representing pressure of more than 60 mm Hg, medium shading indicating pressures from 20–60, and lightest shading indicating pressures of less than 20 mm Hg.

of the Austin Flint murmur and the first heart sound are absent because of mitral valve preclosure. These signs often are associated with other visible, palpable, and audible events that by themselves can point to the correct diagnosis:

1. **Quincke's sign:** pulsatile nail beds (with light pressure)
2. **Musset's sign:** head bobbing
3. **Traube's sign:** pistol shot sounds over brachial or femoral artery
4. **Durozier's sign:** to-and-fro bruits in femoral artery (with light upstream pressure)
5. **Corrigan pulse:** visible bounding, collapsing pulses in neck and arms while sitting
6. **Bisferiens pulse:** two-pronged palpable pulse in carotid arteries
7. **Waterhammer pulse:** Shock wave from pulse with arm extended upward

Clinical Significance and Management

Aortic regurgitation is usually well tolerated for many years because of compensatory mechanisms that can serve to counterbalance the impact of the leaking valve. The principal impact is a **volume overload** on the left ventricle, which, if slowly progressive, can be balanced by four compensatory mechanisms:

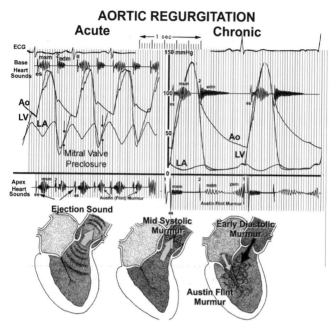

Fig. 11.4. Hemodynamic correlates in aortic regurgitation. The intracardiac pressures in **acute** and **chronic regurgitation** demonstrate important differences. Acute aortic regurgitation finds the ventricle unprepared for the sudden volume overload and, thus, greatly increases the ventricular diastolic pressure. The pressure increase is sufficiently abrupt to **preclose** the mitral valve in middiastole and then buoy up the aortic diastolic pressure, preventing further backflow in late diastole. The relatively normal **aortic pulse pressure**—in this illustration, 50 mm Hg (125/75)—may obscure the expected bounding character of the pulse. **Chronic aortic regurgitation** usually develops gradually over months or years, allowing the ventricular compliance to accept the massive volume overload with a minimal rise in left ventricular diastolic pressure. Aortic runoff into the ventricle lowers the aortic diastolic pressure, and the increased resulting systolic stroke volume raises the systolic pressure, so the resulting pulse pressure may be 100 mm Hg or more.The cartoons illustrate the proposed mechanisms of the sounds and murmurs in **acute** and **chronic** states. The explosive opening of the aortic valve leads to an ejection sound (*es*) that initiates a midsystolic murmur (*msm*) from ejection of the large stroke volume. The incompetent valve begins to leak immediately on closure, yielding an early diastolic murmur (*edm*) that is decrescendo in character as the pressure in the aorta approaches that of the left ventricle; early equilibration of these pressures in acute aortic regurgitation truncates this murmur. The middiastolic (*mdm*) and presystolic murmurs (*psm*), described by Austin Flint, result from the interaction of aortic regurgitation and mitral inflow producing functional mitral stenosis. The presystolic component is absent in the **acute** process because mitral inflow ceases when the valve "precloses."

1. Sinus tachycardia
2. Increased ventricular compliance
3. "Athletic" supernormal systolic function
4. Maintenance of normal or low systemic vascular resistance

Because aortic regurgitation occurs during diastole, the amount of regurgitation is dependent in part on diastolic time (the time between aortic valve closure and the onset of ventricular systole), as well as on the diastole pressure difference between the aorta and the relaxed left ventricle. Many patients with aortic regurgitation will be aware of their rapid, bounding pulse and excessive diaphoresis before any limiting symptoms occur. Bradycardia lengthens diastole and increases the regurgitant volume; tachycardia has the opposite effect. These relationships often permit patients with aortic regurgitation to tolerate exercise quite well, but they develop their earliest symptoms when sleep-induced bradycardia leads to ventricular volume overload with paroxysmal nocturnal dyspnea.

If the ventricle in **chronic** aortic regurgitation is able to progressively increase its compliance (i.e., less pressure response to ventricular diastolic filling), the filling volume may double or triple with only a mild increase in filling pressure, as shown in the illustration of chronic aortic regurgitation (Fig. 11.4), in which the end-diastolic pressure is about 15 mm Hg (normal is 8 to 12). At the same time, the "athleticism" of the chronically exercising ventricle can maintain supernormal systolic function for years.

However, **acute** aortic regurgitation, resulting from endocarditis, deceleration trauma, or aortic dissection can overwhelm the ventricle with only a modest increase in volume, leading to an intolerable increase in filling pressure, as shown in Fig. 11.4, in which the left ventricular pressure equilibrates with aortic diastolic pressure. In this situation the visible signs of aortic regurgitation may be obscured. The pulse pressure may not be increased because the aortic diastolic pressure is buoyed up by equilibration with the left ventricular diastolic pressure, and the stroke volume may not be increased because of the ventricle's inability to accept a significant increase in diastolic filling. Because coronary artery perfusion pressure is comparable to the diastolic pressure difference between aortic and left ventricular pressure, inadequate coronary blood flow renders the overworked ventricle ischemic.

Decompensation in aortic regurgitation occurs when the systolic power of the ventricle declines and is no longer able to bail out the excessive diastolic volume, which sets in motion reflex neural and humoral changes that further burden the left ventricle by increasing blood volume and systemic vascular resistance. Short-term partial relief often can be achieved by arterial dilator and angiotensin converting enzyme (ACE) inhibitor agents, but aortic valve replacement should be undertaken preferably before the end-systolic volume rivals the end-diastolic volume of a normal ventricle.

Echocardiography provides a noninvasive means of monitoring left ventricular function and assessing the severity and impact of aortic regurgitation. Ventricular size and systolic function can be readily assessed, and Doppler interrogation of the regurgitant jet can provide hemodynamic assessment of the left ventricle's ability to tolerate the volume overload, as shown in Fig. 11.5.

Poorly tolerated aortic regurgitation would be suspected if the

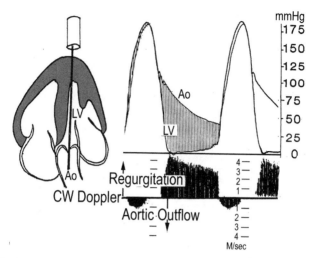

Fig. 11.5. Continuous-wave (CW) Doppler interrogation of aortic regurgitation performed from the left ventricular apex permits a hemodynamic assessment of the volume overload. The magnitude of the Doppler-derived velocity of regurgitant flow toward the apical probe can be converted to mm Hg by the Bernoulli equation: **Pressure difference between Ao (aorta) and LV (left ventricle) = 4 V^2.** The regurgitant velocity initially is about 4.5 M/second (81 mm Hg) and gradually falls to 2.5 M/seconds (25 mm Hg). If the cuff blood pressure is found to be **180/40**, the end-diastolic left ventricular pressure can be estimated to be the following: **40 − 25 = 15**, suggesting that the volume overload is well tolerated by the left ventricle. The small (1.2 M/second) outflow velocity rules out concomitant aortic stenosis because the calculated outflow gradient is less than 6 mm HG.

Doppler velocity were to decline rapidly, indicating that the end-diastolic left ventricular and aortic pressure were approaching the same level.

Maintenance of low arterial impedance with arterial dilators in chronic aortic regurgitation can ameliorate the impact of aortic regurgitation by promoting forward flow and reducing regurgitation. Although digoxin's ability to enhance systolic performance has not been tested for efficacy in aortic regurgitation, it traditionally has been used. Beta blocking agents should be avoided because of their negative inotropic and chronotropic effects: longer diastoles result in more aortic regurgitation.

Aortic valve replacement is required when clinical and noninvasive data indicate that the left ventricle is not tolerating the volume overload or that the systolic function of the left ventricle is declining. In an acute setting, particularly when endocarditis destroys the valve's ability to close competently, urgent surgery is required. The surgeon may be able to debride the infected tissue, including perivalvar abscesses, and affect a bacteriologic cure more effectively than with antibiotics alone.

The choice of prosthetic valve should take into account the patient's age, life expectancy, and ability to maintain and tolerate lifelong anticoagulation. Tissue valves, fashioned from porcine aortic valves or bovine pericardium, permit freedom from anticoagulation, have a functional longevity of approximately 10 years, and should be used for women that may consider future pregnancies. However, modern mechanical valves are unlikely to undergo component failure and should last indefinitely in the absence of infection, thrombosis, or fibrous ingrowth. Mechanical valves' durability greatly exceeds that of tissue valves and should be used if the patient is competent and willing to have frequent assessment of prothrombin time and to maintain therapeutic anticoagulation assiduously.

Homograft cryopreserved (freeze-dried) aortic valves from human cadavers have not always fulfilled predictions of superior durability over xenograft (animal) tissue valves. The "Ross procedure," in which the patient donates his or her own pulmonic valve to the aortic position and has the explanted pulmonic valve replaced with a homograft, requires considerably more surgical complexity but in the hands of experienced surgeons shows promise of durability as well as growth of the living tissue valve. Valvuloplasty, or valve repair without replacement, is only applicable to a small percentage of cases and, as a result, rarely is performed with a realistic expectation of long-term freedom from reoperation.

Aortic Stenosis

Valvar stenosis can be **congenital** or can result from **rheumatic** heart disease or from progressive **calcific** deposits in previously normal valves that may manifest in elderly patients. Progressive calcification also can render a congenitally deformed but nonstenotic valve progressively stenotic by depositions of calcium that thicken and stiffen the leaflets, possibly in reaction to the turbulent outflow through the deformed valve. Calcification also occurs after rheumatic fever distorts the valve leaflets.

Congenital aortic stenosis is usually a result of a bicuspid aortic valve that may be critically stenotic in childhood or may be initially tolerated until the leaflets are rendered progressively immobile over time by deposition of calcium related to the turbulent flow environment. Outflow obstruction from congenital discrete subaortic stenosis and supravalvar aortic stenosis are relatively rare. Rheumatic aortic stenosis usually is combined with other valve pathology, especially mitral valve disease. The most common type of acquired aortic stenosis has been called "senile aortic stenosis" because of its late onset (sixth decade and beyond). There is mounting evidence that this form of aortic stenosis is related to atherosclerosis because the deposits in the valve leaflets are similar to atherosclerotic plaque and young patients with familial hypercholesterolemia develop valve deposits along with premature arterial disease. Progression from aortic sclerosis (stiffened leaflets without obstruction) to calcific aortic stenosis can occur in a few years, and efforts are under way to develop treatment strategies to inhibit this progression. The roles of inflammation and infection also are being explored.

Clinical Significance and Management

Aortic stenosis results in a left ventricular pressure overload, a stimulus to progressive hypertrophy, and fibrous tissue proliferation. The thickened ventricular walls and maintenance of a small ventricular chamber size partially compensate for the high intracavitary pressures by decreasing the wall tension via the Laplace relationship within the left ventricle:

$$\text{Wall tension} = \text{Pressure} \times \text{Radius } 2 \times \text{Wall thickness}$$

The classic triad of symptoms in critical aortic stenosis is **angina, dyspnea, and syncope.** The myocardial oxygen supply/demand balance is difficult to maintain when the ventricle must create more than 200 mm Hg pressure to deliver 100 mm Hg to the aorta, coronary perfusion is compromised when the ratio of capillaries to the myocardial mass is reduced by ventricular hypertrophy, and passage of capillary blood through the myofibers is obstructed by the prolonged systolic compressions. **Ischemia** results when coronary blood flow fails to keep pace with the increased metabolic demands of the left ventricle, further increasing the "stiffness" of the left ventricle and its diastolic filling pressure. The left atrial pressure rises and must compensate for the reduced passive filling by increasing active atrial transport function with a more powerful "atrial kick." The onset of atrial fibrillation deprives the ventricle of its essential "atrial kick" and may cause acute decompensation. The exact cause(s) of **syncope** are not known, but ischemia-induced arrhythmias and excess baroreceptor stimulus in the high-pressure left ventricle have been implicated. **Sudden and unexpected death** may result from prolonged syncope when there is lack of perfusion.

The **length of the harsh outflow murmur** is a rough guide to the magnitude of the outflow pressure gradient (Fig. 11.6). The presence of a **fourth heart sound** and a **sustained apical systolic**

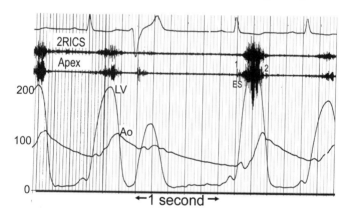

Fig. 11.6. The postextrasystolic beat in aortic stenosis. Recordings from the left ventricle (LV) and aorta and phonocardiograms in a patient with **severe congenital aortic stenosis** demonstrate a **systolic pressure gradient of almost** 100 mm Hg, a **slow rising** (*parvus et tardus*) aortic contour, **prolongation of systolic ejection,** and a **premature ventricular contraction.** There is a prominent **"atrial kick"** before the systolic ventricular pressure rise. An **ejection sound** (*ES*) initiating a long, diamond-shaped **midsystolic murmur** is recorded at the apex and base. The murmur starts after the **first** (*1*) and ends before the **second** (*2*) (*not* holosystolic). The postextrasystolic beat (the next to last beat) generates a gradient of more than 150 mm Hg, and the murmur intensity increases in proportion to the increase in the gradient. Postextrasystolic potentiation of the LV contraction and murmur is a result of an increase in the inotropic state of the ventricle and *not* the "Starling effect" from increased filling. A prominent anacrotic notch is seen in the aortic pressure and is even more prominent in the postextrasystolic beat.

impulse also connotes severity. The murmur, caused by disturbed, high-velocity turbulent flow through the narrow orifice, is harsh, rough, or coarse in character but often is transformed by radiation to the cardiac apex into a pure, blowing, or musical murmur, called the **Gallavardin murmur,** which may be mistaken for a murmur of **mitral regurgitation.** In differentiating the murmurs of mitral regurgitation and aortic stenosis, it should be remembered that the murmur of mitral regurgitation is almost always holosystolic, whereas the murmur of aortic stenosis cannot be holosystolic. Unlike mitral regurgitant flow, aortic outflow neither begins with the onset of ventricular systole nor persists to the time of aortic valve closure because semilunar valve closure results after cessation of forward flow and initiation of retrograde flow in the aorta. Careful auscultation focuses on the separation of the systolic murmur from the second sound ("rup-da") as opposed to the "ruuup" cadence of mitral regurgitation. It should be noted in Fig. 11.5 that the postextrasystolic murmur is greatly augmented compared to the murmur in the preceding normal beats, yet it is still separated from the second sound. Postextrasystolic augmentation is characteristic of outflow murmurs, but it rarely is heard in mitral regurgitation.

The diagnosis usually can be made by cardiac physical examination. A retarded carotid pulse upstroke combined with a midsystolic murmur is strong evidence for outflow obstruction. The severity can be assessed accurately by **Echo-Doppler interrogation** (Fig. 11.7). **Cardiac catheterization** usually is performed to assess the coronary arteries preoperatively or when the noninvasive data are equivocal.

There is no effective medical therapy for aortic stenosis. Congestive failure can be treated with digoxin and cautious diuresis, avoiding dehydration with excessive lowering of left ventricular filling pressure. Aortic valve replacement is the only effective therapy. Percutaneous aortic balloon valvuloplasty has all but been abandoned in adults, but children with flexible bicuspid valves can see improvement with this intervention. Similarly, operative valvuloplasty can confer prolonged relief for some children and young adults with suitable valve architecture.

The choice of valve prosthesis was covered in the section on aortic regurgitation. The 10-year functional life of tissue valves limits their usefulness in younger individuals, except women wishing to have children or those with contraindications to lifelong anticoagulation. The dimensions of the patients' aortic annulus can dictate the choice of valve because the sewing rings of small (less than 20 mm) tissue valves encroach on the available outflow orifice.

Mixed Aortic Stenosis and Regurgitation

The combination of obstruction and incompetence is more poorly tolerated than either isolated valve defect because aortic regurgitation increases ventricular size and forward stroke volume, magnifying both the ventricular wall stress and the aortic pressure gradient. The patient with mixed aortic stenosis and regurgitation illustrated in Fig. 11.8 had an additional hemodynamic burden because of a slow heart rate, facilitating more retrograde filling of the left ventricle and greatly raising the left ventricular filling pressure. **Diastolic mitral regurgitation** was seen by color-flow Doppler studies (not shown).

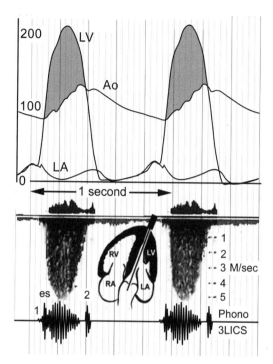

Fig. 11.7.   Hemodynamic and Doppler correlates in valvar aortic stenosis. With Doppler interrogation, the outflow tract pressure gradient (*gray shading*) can be estimated by the Bernoulli equation: Pressure gradient = $4 (V)^2$, or $4 (5)^2 = 100$ mm Hg. The phonocardiogram from the third left intercostal space depicts an ejection sound (*es*) initiating a midsystolic murmur that ends before S2.

Mitral Regurgitation

Mitral valve competence requires integration of structure and function involving the leaflets, annulus, chordae, papillary muscles, and the ventricular myocardium underlying the papillary muscles. Normal mitral valve closure starts with atrial systole, which in turn initiates a progressive sphincteric contraction of the mitral annulus, followed by traction on the chordae by the papillary muscles that maintain the valve leaflets in a competent subannular position to withstand the pressure buildup in the left ventricle. Malfunction of any these factors can result in "functional" mitral regurgitation, whereas "structural mitral regurgitation results from damage or distortion of the component parts listed previously.

Rheumatic fever causes retraction of the leaflets and dilation of the mitral annulus. Rheumatic mitral regurgitation is three times more common in men than in women. Because rheumatic fever is rare in the United States and other industrialized nations, other causes of mitral regurgitation are more prevalent, such as **mitral**

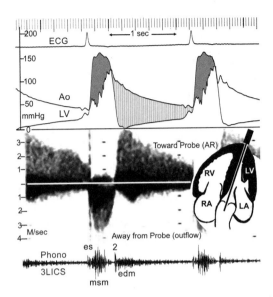

Fig. 11.8. Hemodynamic and Doppler correlates in mixed aortic stenosis and regurgitation. Doppler interrogation indicates bidirectional high-velocity flow detected by a probe at the cardiac apex in a patient with a heart rate of 40. The long diastolic intervals result in a large volume of regurgitation that elevates the left ventricular diastolic pressure and progressively diminishes the aortic/left ventricular pressure difference. The outflow Doppler signal indicates a significant pressure gradient across the aortic valve that is indicated on the pressure tracing by dark gray shading. Compare this systolic pressure gradient and Doppler outflow velocity with the depiction of pure aortic regurgitation in Fig. 11.5.

prolapse, endocarditis, hypertension, ischemic disease, and **the cardiomyopathies**.

Mitral prolapse has been detected in about 5% of the population, but most of this cohort have a benign prognosis because less than 10% progress to significant mitral regurgitation or develop endocarditis. **Antibiotic prophylaxis** for dental procedures has been recommended for most patients with cardiac murmurs to reduce the incidence of endocarditis, but the efficacy of this practice is currently under review by the American Heart Association and may be negated by the time this book is printed.

In **mitral prolapse**, the valve is "floppy" and redundant, with elongation of the leaflets, which inflate during ventricular systole and herniate into the left atrium when their restraints fail to hold them in a competent subannular position (Fig. 11.9). The leaflets' increasing curvature raises the tension because the Laplace relationship (tension = pressure × **radius**) causes the leaflets to prolapse. This tension may cause the leaflets and chordae to stretch further.

The unique findings in mitral prolapse consist of a variably timed systolic click and late systolic murmur. The **click** results from the maximal inflation of the parachutelike leaflets, and the **murmur** results from mitral regurgitation through the poorly opposed leaflets.

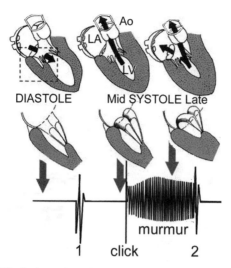

Fig. 11.9. Mitral valve prolapse. Three phases of the cardiac cycle are depicted in cartoons of the left heart chambers. Closeup cutaway views (*in the middle row*) reveal a portion of the posterior leaflet and papillary muscle in **diastole** with the slack leaflet lying flat against the posterior wall of the ventricle as blood flows over it and into the ventricle. After the posterior leaflet has inflated to meet the anterior leaflet to produce the first sound (*1*), the mitral valve is initially competent, but it progressively herniates into the left atrium. The inflating leaflets are halted abruptly by chordal restraint in **midsystole**, which produces a **click.** In **late systole**, the posterior leaflet has lost apposition with the anterior leaflet and mitral regurgitation (*arrow*) ensues, causing a **late systolic murmur** that persists until or through the second sound (*2*). The distance between the annular and papillary muscle attachments of the leaflet shorten during systole, which allows the elongated leaflet to overinflate, lose apposition with the anterior leaflet, and render the valve incompetent.

The **disproportion** between valve and ventricle (valve > ventricle) explains why maneuvers that **decrease venous return** cause the **click to occur earlier** and **increase the length and intensity of the murmur. Standing** and **squatting** can be used to move the click and modulate the murmur (Fig. 11.10). With **squatting,** left ventricular filling and afterload increase, causing later prolapse, a later **click,** and a **shorter murmur.** These sounds and murmurs are best heard over the left midprecordium and cardiac apex.

Postural changes in the timing of the click and murmur are influenced by the left ventricular dimensional changes during systole. As the ventricular size decreases, a hypothetic **prolapse threshold** is traversed and the ventricle can no longer hold the valve in a competent subannular position.

Clinical Significance and Management

Mitral valve prolapse rarely produces significant hemodynamic impairment, except when complicated by chordal rupture or endocarditis. The tension exerted by the ventricle on the billowing valve

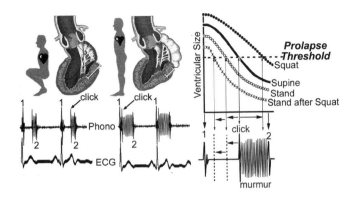

Fig. 11.10. Postural mobility of the click and murmur of mitral prolapse. The click associated with prolapse of the mitral valve will occur earlier in systole when the end-diastolic ventricular volume is reduced and later when the volume is increased. If there is mitral regurgitation associated with the prolapse, the murmur may be affected similarly by starting earlier when the volume is reduced. A profound volume change occurs when the subject stands after squatting, as the filling volume is reduced abruptly. In the panel on the right, a hypothetic **"prolapse threshold"** denotes the ventricular dimensions necessary to facilitate prolapse—the threshold is crossed earlier when standing and later when squatting.

is increased further when ventricular pressure is increased by hypertension or intense isometric exercise (weightlifting), both of which should be avoided. Despite the lack of demonstrable hemodynamic impairment, many patients with this condition are symptomatic, complaining of fatigue, chest pain, and palpitations. These symptoms have not been explained adequately, but they may involve faulty autonomic adjustments to posture and a propensity to arrhythmias. We have found that reassurance and treatment with beta-adrenergic blocking agents often ameliorate symptoms. Antibiotic prophylaxis for "dirty" procedures should be used.

It has been suggested that the volume of ventricular blood contained in the prolapsing leaflets functions as an aneurysmal third space that fills during systole, diminishing the percentage of the stroke volume that would have otherwise been ejected through the aorta. This expanding chamber applies excessive tension on the chordae and their attachments to the papillary muscles and may be responsible for chest pain, autonomic reflexes, and arrhythmias. Spontaneous rupture of chordae almost always occurs on a background of preexisting mitral valve prolapse because the chordae are subjected to increasingly more wall stress as the radius of curvature of the leaflets increases. Chordal rupture often is found at the time of valve surgery. Valve repair, rather than replacement, is often possible when mitral regurgitation warrants operative intervention because of progressive left atrial and ventricular enlargement. When the atrium achieves a diameter (by echocardiographic measurement) of more than 5 cm, the onset of atrial fibrillation is almost invariably predictable, if not already present. The leaflets are usually sufficiently redundant to tolerate resection of one-fourth of the leaflet area (quadrangular resection) combined with reinforcement of the annulus (annuloplasty) to render the valve competent.

Mitral Regurgitation from Other Causes

Other forms of **mitral regurgitation** do not share the previously mentioned responses to postural maneuvers because the valvar/ventricular disproportion is reversed: ventricle > valve (i.e., the leaflet tissue is deficient and not redundant). Perturbations that increase the ventricular volume or impedance to ejection worsen the mitral regurgitation. The volume of mitral regurgitation therefore is responsive to therapy that decreases the loading conditions, both preload and afterload. All regurgitant lesions impose a **volume overload** on the cardiac chambers adjacent to the faulty valve; in mitral regurgitation the left atrium and ventricle must dilate to adapt to the valvar incompetence without excessive pressure rise. Unfortunately, this adaptation that increases tolerance of the volume overload also begets more mitral regurgitation as the annulus stretches and the leaflets coapt less well.

When **mitral regurgitation** is **acute and severe,** as in bacterial endocarditis or chordal rupture, the sudden volume overload leads to a marked elevation in left atrial pressure during ventricular systole (**v waves**) and the ventricle receives an excessive diastolic volume that **raises its filling pressure** (Fig. 11.11). More often, **mitral regurgitation** increases gradually in severity, allowing the adjacent

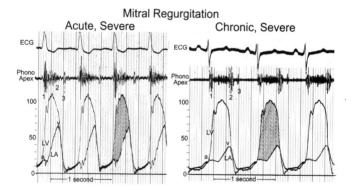

Fig. 11.11. Hemodynamic relationships in chronic and acute mitral regurgitation. Pressure recordings from left heart catheterization combined with phonocardiography in two patients with mitral regurgitation demonstrate the increased magnitude of the v waves in the left atrium, systolic murmur, and third heart sound (*3*) indicative of hemodynamically severe regurgitation. In the **acute** setting, the 70-mm Hg v waves and abbreviation of the systolic murmur reflect the diminished capacity of the left atrium to accept the volume load imposed by the regurgitation. In the **chronic** case, a large pressure difference (*shaded area*) between the left ventricle and left atrium is sustained throughout systole, facilitating holosystolic regurgitation and a holosystolic murmur. The quantity of mitral regurgitation is significantly greater in the patient with chronic mitral regurgitation, but the increased compliance of the chambers adjacent to the mitral valve resulted in a smaller v wave than is seen in the acute case.

cardiac chambers to increase their compliance and accommodate the gradually increasing volume of regurgitation. The volume shifts from the ventricle to the atrium and back, resulting in a modest increase in systolic pressure in the left atrium (the **v wave**) and an exaggerated diastolic rapid filling wave in the ventricle. The large volume entering the ventricle may cause a middiastolic murmur and/or a third heart sound. The **increased compliance** in **chronic mitral regurgitation** permits larger volume shifts with less pressure impact on the two chambers. A **holosystolic murmur** is heard in chronic **mitral regurgitation,** whereas **acute mitral regurgitation** truncates the murmur because the pressure difference driving the regurgitation (left ventricular>left arterial) diminishes in late systole. The shortened systolic murmur of **acute mitral regurgitation** results from the **"ventricularization" of the left atrial pressure** in the previous example.

Mitral competence requires a coordinated effort of the valve leaflets and their support structures. Functional, reversible mitral regurgitation may result from **ischemia** of the left ventricle and papillary muscles, as shown in recordings of left atrial and ventricular pressure illustrated in Fig. 11.12.

Coronary artery disease may also **cause** or **exacerbate** mitral regurgitation through **ischemia** or **infarction** of the **papillary muscles.** These hemodynamic records depict intracardiac pressures in a patient with intermittent "flash" pulmonary edema and document

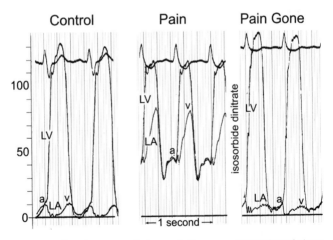

Fig. 11.12.   Transient acute mitral regurgitation reversed by sublingual nitrate administration. A patient with multiple episodes of "flash pulmonary edema" underwent left heart catheterization and had normal pressures initially while asymptomatic (*control*). Shortly thereafter he complained of severe dyspnea and chest discomfort and was noted to have markedly abnormal pressures in the left atrium and ventricle with v waves of 80 mm Hg and left ventricular diastolic pressures of 40 mm Hg. Administration of 15-mg sublingual isosorbide dinitrate restored normal pressures in about 5 minutes. These episodes were attributed to ischemic papillary muscle dysfunction, and the patient later successfully aborted them by self-administration of sublingual nitrates.

the extreme hemodynamic derangement that may be initiated by ischemic **papillary muscle dysfunction.** Note the marked elevation of the **v waves** and the **left ventricular diastolic pressure.** The patient's severe dyspnea and chest pressure were relieved rapidly by administration of isosorbide dinitrate.

Clinical Significance and Management

Chronic mitral regurgitation is often well tolerated for many decades, but it may eventually lead to irreversible chamber enlargement and atrial arrhythmias. As noted earlier, increasing compliance of the left heart chambers often can compensate for the volume overload and therefore avoid the high pulmonary venous pressures present in mitral stenosis. The advent of coronary disease or hypertension may increase the volume of regurgitation and/or render the ventricle less able to cope with the excessive stroke work and wall tension demands. Digoxin and prevention or reversal of hypertension with arterial dilators or ACE inhibitors may be used chronically to improve systolic performance and minimize the regurgitant fraction. These drugs also may be effective in the short term to prepare previously untreated patients for valve replacement surgery.

Standard chest x-rays and echocardiography are useful imaging techniques for following patients with mitral regurgitation. The overall heart size can be followed with radiographs, whereas the dimensions and function of the left atrium and ventricle can be determined by echocardiography. Assigning the degree of mitral regurgitation from color-flow Doppler jets can be misleading, and these signals should be integrated with chamber measurements before reaching a decision. Either an increase in left atrial dimensions to more than 5 cm (normal is 4 cm) or left ventricular diastolic dimension to more than 6 cm (normal is 5 cm) are causes for concern. Once the left atrium reaches or exceeds a dimension of 6 cm, the likelihood of atrial fibrillation or flutter increases markedly.

Repair of rheumatic mitral regurgitation is rarely successful, dictating the need for valve replacement in the vast majority. The choice of tissue versus mechanical valves is predicated on the patients' willingness and/or ability to tolerate lifelong anticoagulation. A female with childbearing potential should have a tissue valve, whereas the durability of mechanical prostheses favors their use in virtually every other setting, especially if there is chronic atrial fibrillation. Mitral valve replacement will be less effective or actually may be harmful if the left ventricle is both markedly dilated (more than 100 mL/ M^2) and poorly contractile (ejection fraction more than 50%). The regurgitation is helping to offload the failing ventricle, acting as a pop-off valve to reduce systolic wall tension and falsely elevate the ejection fraction. This scenario especially applies to conditions in which the mitral regurgitation appears to be secondary to, and not causative of, a dilated cardiomyopathy.

Mitral Stenosis

Mitral stenosis almost always results from **rheumatic fever** and as a result is more prevalent where **group A β hemolytic streptococcal infections** are not readily detected or treated, especially in immigrants from Latin America, Pacific Islands, India, and the Far

East. In the United States, most cases are found in habitants of over-crowded communities. It is more common in women than in men for unknown reasons.

Although relatively rare in members of an affluent population, it often is overlooked as an important cause of **atrial fibrillation, systemic embolism, pulmonary edema, pulmonary hypertension,** and **dyspnea with pregnancy or minimal exertion.** Moreover, if it is not suspected, treatment for "congestive heart failure" using arterial dilators or inotropic drugs can be deleterious. Mitral stenosis should be considered in any woman with severe dyspnea during pregnancy; in anyone with poorly tolerated atrial fibrillation, especially if the first heart sound is loud; or when systemic embolism is suspected. Because the murmur often is missed or its timing is

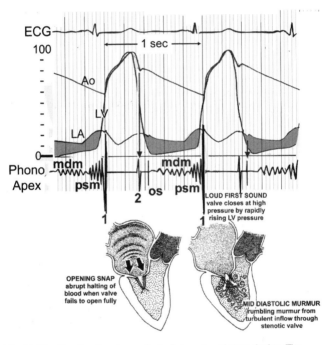

Fig. 11.13. Functional anatomy of mitral stenosis and sinus rhythm. The cartoons demonstrate the valve action during the **opening snap** (*os*) and the **middiastolic murmur** of mitral stenosis. When the early diastolic left ventricular pressure falls below left atrial pressure, blood moves anterograde from the left atrium into the expanding mitral sleeve and gains momentum, only to be thwarted by the failure of the tips of the leaflets to part, abruptly decelerating the column of blood. The resulting shockwave is audible as the os. The disturbed, high-velocity, middiastolic flow through the stenotic orifice causes a rumbling **middiastolic murmur** (*mdm*), followed by a crescendo presystolic murmur (*psm*) that is terminated by a **loud first heart sound.** The elevated end-diastolic left atrial pressure permits anterograde flow through the mitral valve after the onset of left ventricular systole, and the valve closes late, under high pressure that augments the sound intensity.

thought to be "systolic," it is imperative to listen at the apex to the quality of the first sound for a sharp reduplication of the second sound (the opening snap) and to correlate any murmurs with the apical impulse or carotid pulse.

The complete **auscultatory complex** of mitral stenosis is depicted in Figs. 11.13 and 11.14. Shortly after the second sound there is a crisp extra sound, usually best heard at the base or along the left sternal border. The cadence of these sounds at the base can be emulated by saying "lup butter," with the two syllables in "butter" duplicating the usual interval between the second sound and the opening snap. The low-pitched, rumbling middiastolic and presystolic murmur(s) of mitral stenosis often can be heard only at the left ventricular apex, with the stethoscope bell lightly applied. Turning the patient on his or her left side (left lateral decubitus) while listening at the apex will augment the murmur intensity briefly.

Intracardiac pressures are shown along with **heart sounds at the apex** in a patient with mitral stenosis and sinus rhythm. The **mitral valve area is 0.7 cm^2** (normal is 3 to 4 cm^2). The second heart sound is followed by an opening snap, a rumbling middiastolic murmur that blends into a crescendo presystolic murmur that ends with a prominent first sound. The first sound is late and loud, well after the electrocardiogram (ECG) R wave because the left ventricular pressure must exceed pressure in the left atrium, in this case 35 mm Hg, to close the valve. There is a **pressure gradient** of 20 mm Hg (shaded area) across the mitral valve. The **Gorlin formulae** determine the **mitral valve flow** from the time that the valve is open and determine the **mitral valve area** from the flow, the mean pressure gradient, and a gravity-acceleration constant.

An analogy to mitral stenosis can be made with a partially stopped up sink drain; without relieving the obstruction, the outflow rate can be increased only by increasing the inflow, and this will in turn lead

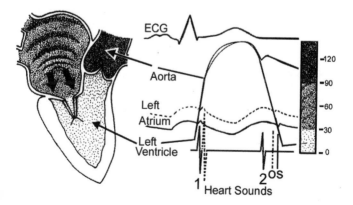

Fig. 11.14. The opening snap (os) occurs earlier when the left atrial pressure rises. Elevation of left atrial pressure (*dotted line*) causes the mitral valve to open earlier, causing the **opening snap** (*os*) to occur closer to the second heart sound (*2*). Perturbations that will predictably raise the left atrial pressure and shorten the interval between the second sound and opening snap are tachycardia, exercise, and pregnancy.

to a rapid backup and an overflowing sink that defeats the original purpose. **Pregnancy, fever,** and **anemia** will affect left atrial pressures in the left atrium in a similar fashion to continuous exercise. Sustained elevation of left atrial pressure higher than 25 mm Hg usually will produce pulmonary edema. The **opening snap** occurs earlier, and the apical diastolic murmur(s) are louder and more sustained when the left atrial pressure increases (Fig. 11.14). The mechanism underlying the earlier appearance of the opening snap is shown in Fig. 11.14.

The **mechanism of the opening snap** can best be understood by imagining a crowd trying to leave a theater hurriedly when the exit doors have been chained. The leading members of the crowd will have gathered momentum as the door partially opens, and then impact against the unyielding door when it abruptly halts their egress. The impact will drive them back into the theater. Similarly, the opening snap is best heard over the left atrium, where the sound of the impact is maximally reflected, as shown by the shock waves in Fig. 11.15. The **density of shading** in Fig. 11.15 designates the approximate **magnitude of pressures** in the various chambers at the time of mitral valve opening, with the aortic pressure highest (darkest) and the left ventricular pressure lowest (lightest). When atrial pressure increases, the opening snap will be earlier and the first heart sound will be later. Disturbed inflow produces a rumbling **middiastolic murmur** that follows the opening snap. The **Gorlin formulae** (Fig. 11.15B) indicate that either an increase in heart rate and/or an increase in cardiac output will increase the **gradient** and, in turn, the left atrial pressure because the mitral valve flow rate will increase.

Clinical Significance and Management

The relationship between the pressure gradient and transvalvar flow, in which the gradient (and left atrial pressure) must quadruple to double the flow, explains the respiratory distress that is experienced by patients with mitral stenosis under circumstances that increase cardiac output and/or shorten diastolic time. Tachycardia, even without an increase in cardiac output, will increase transmitral flow rate by decreasing the time, per minute, that the flow can traverse the valve. When both heart rate and cardiac output increase together, further magnification of the gradient, and the left atrial and pulmonary capillary pressure upstream, occurs. The onset of **atrial fibrillation** often precipitates pulmonary edema because the ventricular rate usually increases and then increases further when respiratory distress triggers an adrenergic response. The loss of "atrial kick" with the onset of atrial fibrillation is of minor hemodynamic significance because atrial systole does not significantly contribute to ventricular filling when the valve is stenotic (note the lack of an a wave in the left ventricular pressure in Fig. 11.16). Atrial fibrillation is a significant complication because the resulting stagnation of the atrial blood pool and the loss of purging by the auricular appendage contribute to the formation of clots and the likelihood of **systemic embolization.**

Significant mitral stenosis is associated with **pulmonary hypertension** because of the elevation of pulmonary venous pressure (Fig. 11.17). The pulmonary hypertension may be **passive,** meaning that it is an obligatory increase in right ventricular and pulmonary artery

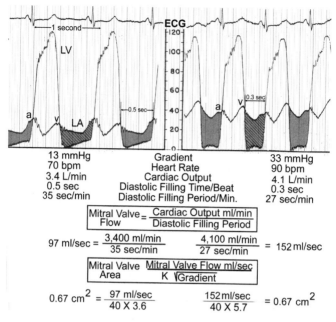

Fig. 11.15. Exercise in mitral stenosis (**top**) and the Gorlin formulae (**bottom**). Left atrial and ventricular pressures at rest (*left*) and exercise (*right*) demonstrate the effect of increasing heart rate and cardiac output on the pressure gradient (*shaded area*). The Gorlin formulae indicate that more heart beats/minute (more systoles) and therefore less diastolic time for mitral inflow (35 to 27 seconds in this example), and the 20% increase cardiac output, must traverse the mitral valve in less time, increasing the mitral valve flow by more than 50%, from 97 to 152 mL/second. The increase in flow rate across the mitral valve requires a marked increase in left atrial pressure and the pressure gradient. It is important to note in the mitral valve area formula, that a doubling of flow (in the numerator) will require an increase of $2^2 = 4$ times the mitral valve gradient (in the numerator, under a square root sign). A normal mitral valve area is more than 3 cm^2, so this valve is less than 25% of normal.

pressure necessary to continue forward flow through a high-resistance circuit. In some patients, most commonly younger patients from developing countries, the degree of pulmonary hypertension is out of proportion to the elevation in pulmonary venous pressure. This reaction results from **pulmonary arteriolar constriction,** a profound pressure overload to the right ventricle, and an inhibition of increases in pulmonary blood flow because of the inability of the right ventricle to overcome the downstream resistance. The physical signs of mitral stenosis may be obscured in this latter subset of patients because of the enlarged right ventricle, tricuspid and pulmonary valvar regurgitation, and insufficient flow through the mitral valve to produce an audible murmur.

Passive and **reactive pulmonary hypertension** are contrasted.

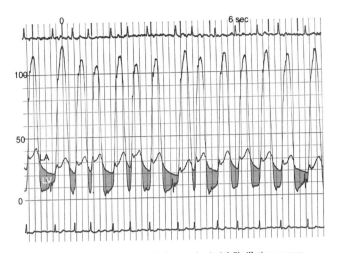

Fig. 11.16. Atrial fibrillation in mitral stenosis. Atrial fibrillation causes variable lengths of diastole and inhibits atrial emptying when diastoles are abbreviated. The average ventricular rate is about 90 (9 cycles in 6 seconds), and the magnitude of the gradients (*shaded areas*) varies inversely with the time available for left atrial emptying. Back-to-back short diastoles are followed by elevation of the subsequent left atrial pressure, whereas long diastolic cycles result in a fall in atrial pressure and a higher left ventricular systolic pressure.

The inability of the right ventricle to overcome downstream resistance prevents an increase in flow that would magnify further the left atrial pressure in **reactive pulmonary hypertension.** Without this protective effect, an increase in flow through the mitral valve requires a marked elevation in left atrial pressure and will cause pulmonary edema.

Lessening of the symptoms of mitral stenosis can be achieved medically by preventing heart rate increases or treating existing sinus tachycardia or rapid response to atrial fibrillation with beta-adrenergic blocking agents. Beta blockers may be given in the presence of pulmonary edema if the heart rate is elevated and can bring rapid relief by allowing the left atrium time to decompress. It should be emphasized that pulmonary edema in mitral stenosis is not the "fault" of the left ventricle; therefore, the negative inotropic properties of beta blockers are outweighed by their ability to slow the heart rate. The use of arterial dilator drugs should be discouraged because they will not help and, in fact, will make matters worse by causing reflex tachycardia and increased flow rate through the stenotic valve. Unless there is a strong contraindication, anticoagulation with warfarin (Coumadin) is recommended in patients with mitral stenosis, especially if intermittent or chronic atrial fibrillation is present. Thromboembolic complications of mitral stenosis are not confined to only those with atrial fibrillation. The presence of echocardiographic "smoke," a hazy swirling pattern of spontaneous echo-dense contrast in the left atrium, is thought to herald an increased likelihood of thromboembolism.

Significant mitral stenosis (mitral valve area of less than 1 cm^2) should be relieved by mechanical means, either catheter-based bal-

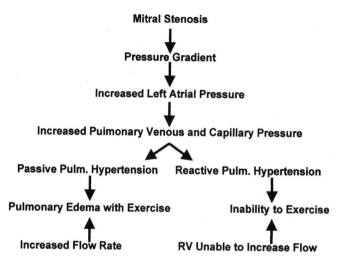

Fig. 11.17. Pulmonary hypertension in mitral stenosis. An elevation in left atrial pressure requires a compensatory rise in right ventricular and pulmonary artery pressure to maintain forward flow, termed **"passive pulmonary hypertension."** The left atrial pressure will rise further with exercise and/or tachycardia, precipitating pulmonary edema because the pulmonary capillary bed is exposed to pressures exceeding the oncotic pressure. In some patients **"reactive pulmonary hypertension"** serves to protect the pulmonary capillary bed from high pressure by active vasoconstriction. In this setting, the flow rate through the pulmonary circuit is prevented from increasing because the right ventricle is unable to generate sufficient pressure to support increases in cardiac output. This pulmonary vasoconstriction is reversible by administration of oxygen or pulmonary vasodilators and usually resolves after successful relief of mitral stenosis.

loon or direct surgical commissurotomy, depending on the characteristics of the stenotic valve and the experience of the operators. A flexible, noncalcific valve with symmetric commissural fusion can be relieved of obstruction equally well by expert percutaneous or surgical means with an expectancy of 10 or more years of improved function. Heavily calcified or immobile valves require replacement. A good-quality transthoracic echocardiogram combined with Doppler interrogation can provide invaluable data regarding the functional anatomy of the valve, the degree of stenosis, and the presence of mural thrombus. Transesophageal echocardiography is a prerequisite for performance of either commissurotomy procedure because of the enhanced ability to screen the atrium for thrombus and the better images of the valve leaflets.

HEART SOUNDS AND MURMURS WITH RELATED PATHOLOGY

The secret to mastering bedside cardiac auscultation (as in real estate) can be summarized in three words: **location, location, and location.** The **precordial location** of an abnormal sound or murmur provides information about its intracardiac origin. Sounds are *reflected back* from the zone of impact (abrupt deceleration), and murmurs are propagated *in the direction* of disturbed or turbulent flow.

Table 11.1. Extra heart sounds

Third heart sound	Fourth heart sound	Opening snap	Ejection sound	Systolic click
Absolute or relative increase in passive inflow volume	Heightened force of atrial systolic contraction into incompliant, usually hypertrophic, ventricle	Abrupt deceleration of atrial blood in mitral sleeve encountering fused leaflets	Abrupt deceleration of ejected blood by fused leaflets; also vigorous opening of outflow valve leaflets into dilated root	Abrupt checking of prolapsing leaflets' systolic excursion by chordal restraint
Valve regurgitation	Aortic and pulmonic stenosis	Mitral or tricuspid stenosis	Aortic and pulmonic stenosis	Mitral prolapse and hypertrophic cardiomyopathy
Normal adolescent, pregnancy, anemia, etc.	Hypertension, systemic or pulmonary		Systemic or pulmonary hypertension	
Dilated or hypertrophic cardiomyopathy	Dilated or hypertrophic cardiomyopathy		Tetralogy of Fallot Marfan, Erdheim	
Ventricular dysfunction			Aortic regurgitation	
Constricted[a] or restricted Ventricle				
Atrial myxoma[b]				

[a] Pericardial constriction and restrictive cardiomyopathy are associated with a "pericardial knock" or a sharp third sound that results from abrupt checking of ventricular filling.

[b] Atrial myxoma may cause a "tumor plop" that results from the plungerlike action of the tumor and the blood pushed by the tumor into the ventricle

The **temporal location** within the cardiac cycle (e.g., systolic or diastolic) narrows the differential diagnosis.

Systolic murmurs, by definition, result from ventricular pumping of blood forward (outflow), backward (atrioventricular valve regurgitation), or sideways (ventricular septal defect). *Diastolic* murmurs occur as a result of disturbed or turbulent ventricular filling either through an atrioventricular valve or from backflow through a regurgitant semilunar valve. *Continuous* murmurs occur as a result of continuous (systolic and diastolic) unidirectional flow from a source with continuously higher pressure (e.g., the aorta) to a recipient chamber with continuously lower pressure (e.g., the pulmonary artery or a right-sided cardiac chamber). They should be distinguished from *to-and-fro* murmurs, which result from bidirectional disturbed or turbulent flow (e.g., aortic stenosis and regurgitation).

The **temporal location** within the subdivision of the cardiac cycle (e.g., midsystolic, holosystolic, early diastolic, middiastolic) further refines the differential diagnostic possibilities.

Outflow murmurs are midsystolic because ventricular ejection begins *after* the first sound and ends *before* retrograde flow in the great artery closes the semilunar valve.

Backflow systolic murmurs (mitral or tricuspid regurgitation) are usually holosystolic, beginning *with* the first sound and continuing *to or through* the second sound. Restrictive (small) ventricular septal defects also produce holosystolic murmurs.

Inflow diastolic murmurs begin *after* the second sound and are therefore middiastolic in onset.

Backflow diastolic murmurs begin *with* the second sound and are therefore early diastolic in onset.

Tables 11.1 and 11.2 summarize the timing of sounds and murmurs associated with most cardiac conditions that produce abnormal

Table 11.2. Abnormalities of the second sound

Persistently split-second sound	Paradoxically split-second sound
Late onset and/or completion of RV systole or early completion of LV systole	**Late onset and/or late completion of LV systole**
Atrial septal defect	LBBB, RV pacemaker
	Aortic stenosis
RBBB	Hypertrophic cardiomyopathy
Mitral regurgitation[a]	
Ventricular septal defect[a]	
Pulmonic stenosis	
Acute elevation of PA pressure (pulmonary embolism)[b]	

LBBB, left bundle branch block; LV, left ventricular; PA, pulmonary arterial; RBBB, right bundle branch block; RV, right ventricular.

[a]The aortic valve may close early as a result of the low resistance alternative path to aortic outflow in these conditions.

[b]Chronic elevation of pulmonary artery pressure leads to near-synchronous closure of aortic and pulmonic valves.

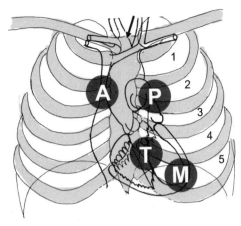

Fig. 11.18. Precordial auscultation areas. *(A)* Aortic area: Second right intercostal space (2RICS). Aortic component of S_2 (A_2); aortic outflow murmurs (aortic stenosis, high outflow in aortic regurgitation, etc.), opening snap of mitral stenosis. *(P)* Pulmonic area (2-3LICS). Pulmonic component of S_2 (P_2); pulmonic outflow murmurs [pulmonic stenosis, atrial septal defect (ASD), anemia, etc.], opening snap of mitral stenosis. *(T)* Tricuspid area (4LICS). Tricuspid closure component of S_1; tricuspid inflow murmurs (tricuspid stenosis, high inflow in tricuspid regurgitation and ASD), tricuspid regurgitation murmur, ventricular septal defect murmur, aortic and pulmonic ejection sounds, opening snap of mitral stenosis, aortic regurgitation murmur. *(M)* Mitral area (apex): mitral closure (S_1), aortic ejection sound, mitral inflow murmurs (mitral stenosis, Austin Flint, high inflow from mitral regurgitation), mitral regurgitation murmur, Gallavardin murmur (of aortic stenosis). Other auscultation areas: Erbs (3-4 LICS): for aortic regurgitation murmur, left subclavian: for patent ductus arteriosus, Harvey's area (3-4 LICS) aortic regurgitation murmur with dilated root.

sounds or murmurs. Figs. 11.18 and 11.19 display *phonocardiograms* in registration with the *ECG* and the *carotid pulse* to assist in determining the **location** of the sonic events within the cardiac cycle.

PRECORDIAL AUSCULTATION AREAS

(A) Aortic area: second right intercostal space (2RICS).

Aortic component of S_2 (A_2)

Aortic outflow murmurs (aortic stenosis, high outflow in aortic regurgitation, etc.)

Opening snap of mitral valve

(P) Pulmonic area: second to third left intercostal space (2-3LICS)

Pulmonic component of S_2 (P_2)

Pulmonic outflow murmurs [pulmonic stenosis, atrial septal defect (ASD), anemia, etc.]

Opening snap of mitral valve

(T) Tricuspid area: (4LICS)

Tricuspid closure component of S_1

Tricuspid inflow murmurs (tricuspid stenosis, high inflow in tricuspid regurgitation, ASD)

Tricuspid regurgitation murmur

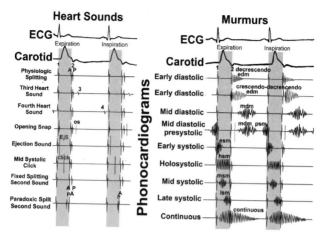

Fig. 11.19. Heart sounds and murmurs. This diagram summarizes **phonocardiographic** depictions of heart sounds and murmurs encountered in bedside cardiac examination. The **carotid pulse** and electrocardiogram (ECG) are displayed for timing within the cardiac cycle, the shaded swaths represent the duration of **systole** in the left heart, and the two cycles represent **expiration** and **inspiration,** respectively. **Inspiration** causes splitting of the two components of the second sound (A and P) in physiologic splitting and fuses them in paradoxic splitting. (EjS, ejection sound; os, opening snap; edm, early diastolic murmur; mdm, middiastolic murmur; psm, presystolic murmur; hsm, holosystolic murmur; msm, midsystolic murmur; lsm, late systolic murmur; esm, ejection systolic murmur.)

Ventricular septal defect murmur
Aortic and pulmonic ejection sounds
Opening snap of mitral stenosis
Aortic regurgitation murmur
(M) Mitral area: (apex)
Mitral closure (S_1)
Aortic ejection sound
Mitral inflow murmurs (mitral stenosis, Austin Flint, high inflow from mitral regurgitation)
Mitral regurgitation murmur
Gallavardin murmur (of aortic stenosis)
Other auscultation areas:
Erbs: (3-4 LICS) for aortic regurgitation murmur
Left subclavian: for patent ductus arteriosus

DIASTOLIC MURMURS

Early diastolic murmurs result from semilunar valve backflow and begin with the second sound (onset of diastole) and extend for variable length into or through all of diastole (holodiastolic); a shorter murmur usually implies a more severe lesion. **Middiastolic murmurs** result from inflow, which begins about 0.12 second after S-2. **Presystolic murmurs** extend into to the first sound. See Table 11.3 for more information on diastolic murmurs.

Table 11.3. Diastolic murmurs

Early diastolic decrescendo	Early diastolic crescendo-decrescendo	Middiastolic (only)	Middiastolic and presystolic
Backflow from semilunar valve	**Backflow from semilunar valve (crescendo from dicrotic waveform)[a]**	**Disturbed inflow through stenotic valve or high-volume inflow through nonstenotic valve**	**Disturbed inflow through stenotic valve or impingement of mitral valve by aortic valve regurgitation**
Aortic regurgitation[b]	Pulmonary regurgitation[c]	Acute severe aortic regurgitation (Austin Flint)[b]	Chronic severe aortic regurgitation (Austin Flint)[b]
Pulmonic regurgitation (Graham Steell)[c]		Mitral or tricuspid[d] stenosis with atrial fibrillation	Mitral and tricuspid[d] stenosis with normal sinus rhythm
		Mitral and tricuspid[d] regurgitation	Mitral stenosis in atrial fibrillation with rapid rate[e]
		L-R shunts: ASD, VSD, PDA	

ASD, atrial septal defect; PDA, patent ductus arteriosus; VSD, ventricular septal defect.
[a]A large dicrotic wave in the pulmonary artery produces an **early crescendo phase.**
[b]Intensity of murmurs related to aortic regurgitation often will increase with **handgrip.**
[c]Murmur usually is caused by **pulmonary hypertension.**
[d]Intensity of murmurs of right heart origin usually will increase with **inspiration.**
[e]**Presystolic crescendo murmurs** can be heard in mitral stenosis with atrial fibrillation during rapid ventricular response (shortened diastoles).

Table 11.4. Systolic murmurs

Early systolic	Midsystolic	Late systolic	Holosystolic
Acute mitral regurgitation	Outflow stenoses: Aortic and pulmonic (valvar, subvalvar supravalvar)	Mitral prolapse	Mitral regurgitation
Mitral regurgitation in dilated CM	High-volume outflow: anemia, pregnancy, atrial septal defect, aortic regurgitation	Hypertrophic CM[a]	Tricuspid regurgitation[b]
Mild-moderate pulmonic stenosis[c]	High-outflow velocity: Hypertrophic CM[a]	Aortic coarctation	Ventricular septal defect
	Dilated aorta or pulmonary artery	Mammary souffle (pregnancy, lactation)	Hypertrophic CM[a]
	Innocent murmur (Still's murmur)	Patent ductus with pulmonary hypertension	Severe pulmonic[c] stenosis

CM, cardiomyopathy.

[a] Hypertrophic cardiomyopathy can be associated with almost all of the types of murmurs listed in the table and, as with **mitral prolapse**, can change markedly with **standing** (longer and louder), **squatting** (shorter and softer), **valsalva strain** (longer and louder), and **post-Premature ventricular contraction** (usually longer and louder).

[b] Murmur intensity of **tricuspid regurgitation** usually will increase with inspiration.

[c] The murmur of **severe pulmonic stenosis** may be **holosystolic** because the murmur begins with the first sound and spills through the aortic component of the second. The murmur usually will increase with inspiration.

TABLE 11.5. Continuous murmurs

Aorta or systemic artery to pulmonary	Pulmonary AV fistulae	Systemic AV fistulae	Constriction or aorta or pulmonary artery	Miscellaneous
Patent ductus arteriosus[a]	Osler-Weber-Rendu	Congenital AV fistulae	Coarctation of aorta	Venous Hum (Innocent)
Bronchial to pulmonary collaterals		Traumatic gunshot or stab wound	Branch pulmonic stenosis or stenoses[a]	Systemic arterial stenoses
Coronary-cameral fistulae		Hemodialysis access		Pulmonary embolism
Blalock-Taussig and Potts shunts				Takayasu's arteritis
Sinus of valsalva rupture into cardiac chamber				Ventricular septal defect with aortic regurgitation[c]
Anomalous origin of left coronary artery[b]				Collateral arteries

AV, atrioventricular.

[a]The murmur of patent ductus arteriosus will be confined to late systole if the diastolic pressure in the pulmonary artery rises to match the aortic as shown in the patient illustrated here.

[b]Anomalous origin of the left coronary artery from the pulmonary artery (**Bland-Garland-White syndrome**) leads to the formation of collateral channels from the right coronary artery to the left, with continuous retrograde flow in the left coronary artery.

[c]**Supracristal** (subpulmonic) **ventricular septal defects** often are associated with **aortic regurgitation**, causing a holosystolic murmur in combination with an early diastolic murmur, which blend together to give the impression of a "continuous murmur."

SYSTOLIC MURMURS

Early systolic murmurs begin with the first heart sound and do not extend to the second. **Midsystolic murmurs** are separate from the first and second sounds and are usually, but not always, associated with ejection through an outflow tract.

Holosystolic murmurs, by definition, start with the first sound and extend to or through the second sound. The term is preferable to "pansystolic," which means *every systole* (as in Pan American), whereas holosystolic means *all of systole*. **Late systolic murmurs** begin after the first sound and extend to or through the second. See Table 11.4 for more information on systolic murmurs.

Note the delayed P-2 and the long, virtually holosystolic murmur in the recording of severe pulmonic stenosis in Fig. 11.19. The right ventricular end-diastolic pressure exceeds the pulmonary artery pressure and (on angiography), initiated forward flow through the stenotic pulmonic valve before the onset of ventricular systole.

CONTINUOUS MURMURS

Continuous murmurs (Table 11.5) extend from systole **through the second sound** into diastole and should not be confused with the **to-and-fro** murmurs of aortic regurgitation in which there is a distinct pause between the systolic (anterograde) and early diastolic (retrograde) flow. In contrast, **continuous murmurs** result from unidirectional flow from a high-pressure source to a lower pressure recipient.

SELECTED READINGS

Carabello BA, Crawford FA: Valvular heart disease (review article). *N Engl J Med* 337:32–41, 1997.

Criley JM, Criley DG, Zalace C: *The physiological origins of heart sounds and murmurs* (CD-ROM). Philadelphia: Lippincott Williams & Wilkins, 1997.

Gorlin R, Gorlin SG: Hydraulic formula for calculation of the stenotic mitral valve, other valves, and central circulatory shunts. *Am Heart J* 41:1–29, 1951.

Otto C, Pearlman A, Gardner C: Hemodynamic progression of mitral stenosis in adults assessed by Doppler echocardiography. *J Am Coll Cardiol* 13:545–550, 1989.

Pellikka P, Nishimura R, Bailey K, et al: The natural history of adults with asymptomatic, hemodynamically significant aortic stenosis. *J Am Coll Cardiol* 15:1012–1017, 1990.

Wood P: An appreciation of mitral stenosis: Part 1. *Br Med J* 1:1051–1064, 1954.

Wood P: An appreciation of mitral stenosis: Part 2. *Br Med J* 1:1113–1124, 1954.

CONGENITAL HEART DISEASE

Many individuals with congenital heart disease survive to adulthood, some without interventions or symptoms, for one or more of the following reasons:

1. The lesions are mild, mitigating significant impairment until adulthood, if ever.
2. The lesions may be severe but are counterbalanced by complementary lesions.
3. Acquired compensations take place in the cardiovascular system.
4. Operative repair or palliation was undertaken previously.

This chapter will provide an overview of congenital heart conditions compatible with adult survival. It is important to remember that most congenital heart defects can be effectively managed, repaired, or palliated with contemporary medical and surgical interventions. A patient with suspected congenital heart disease should undergo an expeditious diagnostic evaluation and, if symptomatic, should be referred to an experienced medical center to determine suitability for intervention. These patients should not be given a "complex congenital heart disease" label and relegated to an "incurable" status because of the apparent severity of the lesions without experienced consultation. Patients with cyanosis, in particular, should have access to tertiary care because of the hazards and complications inherent in conditions where "unfiltered" venous blood has access to the systemic circulation.

EMBRYOLOGY OF THE DEVELOPING HEART

Many congenital heart conditions result from alterations occurring early in fetal development when the heart is evolving from its primordial architecture. Others result from faulty transition from normal intrauterine to a normal neonatal circulatory pattern. A simplified overview of these developmental stages would include the following:

1. *Ductus venosus* (provides oxygenated maternal blood)
2. *Ductus arteriosus* (bypasses lungs)
3. Formation of the atrial and ventricular septa; patency of ostium secundum
4. Spiral septation of the *truncus arteriosus* and interventricular foramen
5. Neonatal closure of the ductus venosus and ductus arteriosus

Oxygenated maternal blood flows through the placenta, umbilical vein, and *ductus venosus* to enter the fetal inferior vena cava (Fig.

12.1) The atrioventricular cushion forms the anchor point for the atrial and ventricular septa, as well as the substrate for development of the septal leaflets of the atrioventricular valves. As the interventricular septum and atrial *septum primum* progress centrally toward the cushion, a communication occurs in the low atrial septum, the *ostium primum*, and permits oxygenated maternal blood to enter the left atrium. By the time the *septum primum* fuses with the cushion, dissolution of the midseptal area has formed the *ostium secundum* through which maternal blood continues to flow to the fetal left atrium. The *septum secundum* then forms a second partial curtain on the right of the *septum primum*. Right-to-left shunting through the *ostium secundum* continues as long as the right atrium has a higher venous return than the left atrium, but the septum primum bulges

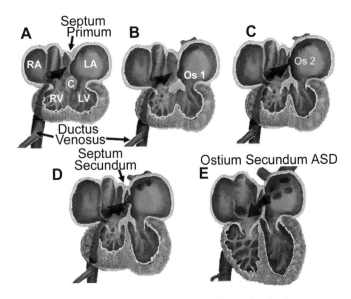

Fig. 12.1. Septation of the heart in the embryo. The cardiac chambers are separated progressively by the formation of the atrial and ventricular septa. **A:** Oxygenated maternal blood (*large curved arrow*) enters the fetal inferior vena cava through the **ductus venosus** and traverses the open communication between the atria. **B:** As the **septum primum** advances toward the atrioventricular cushion (**C**), oxygenated blood traverses the residual **ostium primum** (*Os 1*) defect. **C:** As the septum primum fuses with the cushion, partial dissolution of the midportion of the septum forms the **ostium secundum** (*Os 2*) through which maternal blood flows to the left atrium. **D:** The **septum secundum** grows alongside the septum primum on the right atrial side, forming a one-way flap valve that permits maternal blood to continue to traverse the OS 2 defect into the left atrium. After delivery, pulmonary blood flow increases left atrial pressure and volume, moving the septum primum toward the septum secundum on the right. However, if the secundum defect is too big, or the septum secundum fails to cover the orifice, an **ostium secundum ASD** results, with left-to-right shunting as the fetal right ventricular hypertrophy regresses. The **ductus venosus** shrivels into a ligament when the umbilical cord is clamped.

toward the right in the neonate when pulmonary blood flow increases after delivery and expands the left atrium. A recess in the atrial septum, the *fossa ovalis*, is the site of the fetal ostium secundum after it is covered by the septum secundum. Failure of the developing septa to fuse with the cushion results in so-called "cushion defects," in which atrial and ventricular septal defects (VSDs) are combined with valvar regurgitation. Failure of the *septum secundum* to cover the *ostium secundum* or persistently high right atrial pressure result in persistence of the ostium secundum.

Spiral septation (Fig 12.2) divides the primitive *truncus arteriosus* into an entwined aorta and pulmonary outflow tract and progresses proximally to form the membranous septum closing the interventricular foramen. When septation favors the aorta and fails to close the interventricular septum, there is a small pulmonary outflow tract, large overriding aorta, VSD, and right ventricular hypertrophy (RVH) comprising *Fallot's tetralogy*. Transposition of the great arteries (TGA) results when septation forms a straight double-barrel without entwining, leaving the aorta in line with the right ventricle and the pulmonary artery in line with the left ventricle.

The *ductus arteriosus* (Fig 12.3) provides an alternate pathway for pulmonary arterial blood that is impeded from traversing the high-resistance pulmonary vascular bed. This deoxygenated blood is pumped through the ductus arteriosus into the descending aorta, while oxygenated maternal blood enters the left heart and is pumped to the ascending aorta and brachiocephalic arteries. Shortly after birth, the ductus arteriosus constricts in part because of respiratory oxygenation of the neonatal blood. Neonatal patency of the ductus

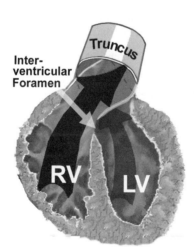

Fig. 12.2. Spiral septation of the primitive truncus arteriosus entwines the aortic and pulmonary outflow tracts, with the aorta behind and to the right and the pulmonary artery in front on the left. The spiral septum progresses caudally to close the interventricular foramen. Tetralogy of Fallot results when the septation is asymmetric, forming a large aorta and small pulmonary outflow tract, with a patent interventricular foramen.

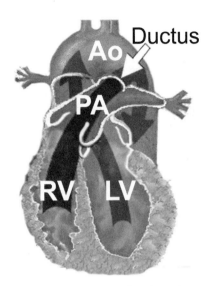

Fig. 12.3. The fetal ductus arteriosus provides a low-resistance pathway for pulmonary artery blood that is inhibited from traversing the high-resistance pulmonary vascular bed. Most of the right ventricular output (*darker arrow*), thus, enters the descending aorta to perfuse the arterial beds downstream with deoxygenated blood. Maternal oxygenated blood (*lighter arrow*) traverses the aortic valve to perfuse the brachiocephalic vascular bed.

arteriosus is favored by prematurity, birth at high altitude, or congenital defects resulting in low arterial oxygen tension (cyanosis). Circulating prostacyclin serves to maintain ductal patency, whereas administration of aspirin or indomethacin may promote closure. The *ligamentum arteriosus*, a fibrous cord remnant of the ductus that anchors the aortic arch to the pulmonary artery, may, by tying the great vessels together, promote aortic transection with rapid deceleration motor vehicle accidents.

When the umbilical cord is clamped during delivery, flow ceases in the umbilical vein and artery, although they remain probe patent for several days after birth and can be used for neonatal cardiac catheterization procedures.

ANATOMIC CLASSIFICATION

A simple *anatomic* classification of congenital cardiovascular problems includes four categories, which may occur alone or in combination. An overview of these categories follows.

1. Defects (communications, shunts)
   a. Atrial septal defect (ASD)
   b. VSD
   c. Patent ductus arteriosus (PDA)
2. Obstructions (stenosis, atresia)
   a. Tricuspid stenosis or atresia
   b. Pulmonic stenosis (PS) or atresia: valvar, subvalvar, or supravalvar
   c. Aortic stenosis, valvar, subvalvar, or supravalvar

3. Transposed vessels
    a. TGA
    b. Anomalous pulmonary venous return
    c. Anomalous systemic venous return
4. Dysplasias (miscellaneous malformations of chambers or valves)
    a. Ebstein's anomaly of tricuspid valve
    b. Cor triatriatum

Defects

Abnormal communications between chambers or great vessels cause shunting of blood, which may be unidirectional or bidirectional depending on downstream compliance or impedance. The direction of flow through defects or communications follows the line of least resistance.

Atrial septal defects (Fig 12.4) result from incomplete septation during fetal development (see Fig. 12.3). Persistence of the *ostium primum* results from failure of the septum primum to fuse with the endocardial cushion and may be associated with mitral and tricuspid regurgitation because of malformation of the septal leaflets of the atrioventricular valves. *Ostium secundum* defects result from failure of the septum secundum to cover the foramen ovale, either because the defect is too large or the septum secundum is undersized. A third type of ASD in the superior portion of the atrial septum is called a *sinus venosus* defect and is associated with pulmonary venous connection of the right superior pulmonary vein to the right atrium (see Fig. 12.4).

An ASD usually will permit flow from the left atrium to the right atrium because the *compliance* of the right ventricle exceeds that of the left ventricle; a normal right ventricle can accommodate more than twice the amount of blood as the left ventricle at the same filling pressure. The pulmonary blood flow may increase to two to four times normal, increasing the size of the pulmonary arteries and the volume in the right atrium and ventricle. If the pulmonary blood flow is increased to more than twice normal and the pulmonary vascular resistance is less than 3 Wood units (mm Hg/L/minute), closure of the defect is indicated and can be performed in some cases by catheter-mounted devices. Open heart surgery is required if the defect is larger than 3 cm^2.

After four to six decades of volume and pressure overload, the right ventricle usually becomes progressively hypertrophic and has a reduced ejection fraction, rendering it less compliant. A chronically enlarged right ventricle that must cope with an increasingly resistant pulmonary vascular bed may fail, reducing its stroke volume and developing a larger residual end-systolic volume. When a bloated right ventricle has a large residual volume, it becomes less compliant in diastole than the left ventricle, and systemic venous blood preferentially may go to the left ventricle. At this "end stage" of the disease, there may be little, if any, benefit from closing the ASD.

Ventricular septal defects are usually *"perimembranous,"* meaning that they are located in or around the membranous septum, although a relatively small percentage occur in the muscular septum (see Fig 12.4). The perimembranous defects may occur in the inflow or outflow portion of the ventricles. Defects in the outflow portion of the right ventricle are termed *supracristal* or *subpulmonic* when they are distal to the *crista supraventricularis*. These defects undermine

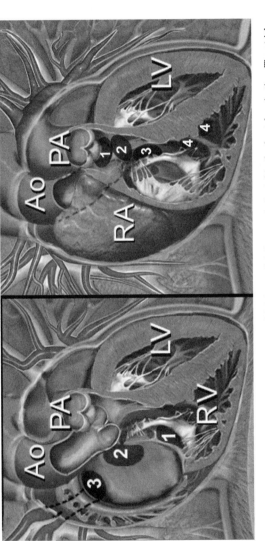

Fig. 12.4.   Locations of atrial (**left**) and ventricular (**right**) septal defects are indicated in the frontal projection. The atrial septal defects (**left panel**) are designated (*1*) ostium primum, (*2*) ostium secundum, and (*3*) sinus venosus. Ostium primum defects usually are associated with atrioventricular valvar regurgitation. Sinus venosus defects are associated with partial anomalous pulmonary venous connections to the right atrium. Perimembranous ventricular septal defects in the **right panel** are designated (*1*) supracristal or subpulmonic, (*2*) subaortic, and (*3*) inlet. Muscular defects (*4*) are often multiple, as shown. Supracristal or subpulmonic defects are associated with prolapse of the adjacent right aortic sinus, which loses its support, causing aortic valve regurgitation into the left and/or right ventricle. The expanding sinus may slide progressively into the right ventricular outflow tract, partially obstructing the orifice of the defect itself, as well as the right ventricular outflow tract.

the support afforded the aortic valve by the subpulmonic ventricular septum and lead to prolapse of the right coronary sinus into the defect and resulting aortic regurgitation. The aortic sinus will partially occlude the septal defect, so the magnitude of the left-to-right shunt from the left ventricle through the defect may be relatively small, but the aortic regurgitation may be directed into the right ventricle. Defects in the subaortic septum are unlikely to be associated with aortic regurgitation. Defects in the inflow portion of the membranous septum may be partially occluded by the tricuspid valve.

Shunts through VSDs also follow the line of least resistance. A small ("restrictive") VSD will allow left-to-right shunting because the left ventricle has a high downstream impedance (the systemic vascular resistance) compared to the pulmonary vascular resistance faced by the right ventricle, so the left ventricular systolic pressure will exceed that of the right ventricle fivefold (100 mm Hg versus 20 mm Hg), permitting an 80-mm Hg pressure drop (gradient) across the defect and unidirectional left-to-right flow (Fig. 12.5, right panel).

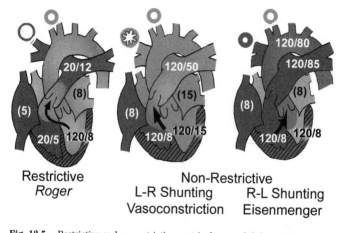

Restrictive
Roger

Non-Restrictive
L-R Shunting   R-L Shunting
Vasoconstriction   Eisenmenger

Fig. 12.5. Restrictive and nonrestrictive ventricular septal defects (VSDs) are compared, with "color coding" indicating the approximate oxygen saturation resulting from the direction and magnitude of the shunt and depictions of the cross-section of resistance arterioles in the systemic and pulmonary circuits. The *maladie de Roger* is a small perimembranous defect that does not significantly alter the hemodynamics or the cardiac chamber size. The left ventricle ejects blood through the defect at high velocity because of the large pressure difference (120 − 20 = 100 mm Hg), creating a loud murmur and a minimal increase in pulmonary blood flow. The pulmonary arterioles are normally thin-walled, yielding normal pulmonary vascular resistance. The **middle panel** depicts a **nonrestrictive VSD with reactive pulmonary vasoconstriction** that serves to diminish otherwise intolerable pulmonary plethora. Although the large defect results in obligatory systemic-level systolic right ventricular and pulmonary arterial pressures, the pulmonary arterioles are actively and reversibly constricted, reducing flow rates through the pulmonary vascular bed. The **Eisenmenger syndrome** depicted on the right has developed "obliterative" changes in the pulmonary arterioles that have caused the pulmonary resistance to exceed systemic resistance, reversing the shunt. The darker shading in the aorta indicates lower oxygen saturation.

A large ("nonrestrictive") VSD will facilitate shunting toward the ventricle whose outflow tract and vascular bed have the least resistance. A nonrestrictive VSD obliges the left and right ventricles to share the same systolic pressure, so there is no pressure gradient across the defect. The systemic baroreceptors set the systemic resistance to an appropriate level to perfuse the brain and, thus, oblige the right ventricle to share systemic systolic pressure. If the pulmonary vascular resistance is lower than systemic, the blood will flow left to right (Fig. 12.5B), and if it is higher (Fig. 12.5C), the shunt will reverse. Cyanosis will result if there is sufficient admixture of venous blood to reduce the arterial saturation to 80% or less. Because the defect has been nonrestrictive since birth, the right ventricle and pulmonary artery always will exhibit systemic-level systolic pressures. For a variable period (years to decades in different subjects), the amount of left-to-right shunting is modulated by reversible pulmonary arteriolar vasoconstriction, but eventually, progressive pulmonary arteriolar thickening and narrowing will obliterate the pulmonary vascular channels and the *Eisenmenger syndrome* ensues. It is thought that the obliterative changes in the pulmonary arteries in the Eisenmenger syndrome are irreversible, but some of the new selective pulmonary arteriolar dilators used to treat primary pulmonary hypertension (endothelin-blocking agents such as prostacyclin and epoprostenol) may prove to be effective and permit closure of these defects,

If a nonrestrictive VSD is combined with PS at valvar and/or subvalvar level, shunting will diminish or reverse, as is the case in tetralogy of Fallot. The direction of shunt flow then will be dependent on the variable resistances encountered downstream from the two communicating ventricles. Because the wide-open VSD dictates that right ventricular (RV) systolic pressure must track with the left, a comparison of tetralogy patients with the most severe and the mildest outflow tract stenosis may have near-identical systemic-level systolic pressures in their right ventricles and near-identical and normal pulmonary arterial pressures (about 20 mm Hg) and, thus, the same magnitude of pressure gradient across their outflow tracts (100 − 20 = 80).

Patent ductus arteriosus flow also will follow the line of least resistance, usually shunting blood from the aorta into the pulmonary vascular bed throughout systole and diastole. A nonrestrictive PDA will oblige the pulmonary artery to share pressures with the aorta, and flow will favor the vascular bed with the least resistance. In fetal life, the ductus arteriosus shunts right to left, diverting venous blood into the descending aorta because the lungs are not inflated and the pulmonary vascular resistance is very high. Following birth, the ductus should constrict in response to changes in oxygen tension and circulating vasoactive substances.

Obstructions

Obstructions can occur at valvar, subvalvar, and supravalvar level and range in severity from mild narrowing to complete blockage of passage, called "atresia" when a valve has no orifice. The aortic and pulmonic valves are affected most commonly; the tricuspid and mitral valves valve rarely are affected. A *bicuspid aortic valve*, which may be stenotic, regurgitant, or functioning normally, is thought to be present in about 2% of live births, more commonly in males than females. Left ventricular outflow obstruction also may occur below (upstream of) the aortic valve, downstream of the valve in the ascending aorta, or by a coarctation at the junction of the aortic arch and descending aorta. Similarly, RV outflow may be impeded by obstructions below the infundibulum by anomalous muscle bundles ("two-chamber right ventricle"), at valvar and/or infundibular level, or downstream of the valve in single or multiple sites in the pulmonary arteries.

Outflow tract stenoses promote ventricular hypertrophy of the involved ventricle and to a lesser extent the contralateral ventricle. Hypertrophy diminishes compliance of the involved chamber, elevates the upstream atrial pressure, and increases the reliance on active atrial systolic transport (more powerful atrial contractions). Elevation of right atrial pressure, secondary to RVH, may promote right-to-left shunting through the foramen ovale. Another deleterious byproduct of hypertrophy involving the right ventricle is the development of infundibular hypertrophy, which can cause a functional constriction of the outflow tract. A "suicide ventricle" may result, in which relief of the valvar stenosis downstream by balloon or operative intervention causes sphincteric closure of the outflow tract.

Complete interruption of the distal aortic arch by coarctation surprisingly may allow survival to adulthood as a result of compensatory development of collateral channels. In the case of total obstruction at the level of an aortic coarctation, multiple collateral arterial channels arise from the brachiocephalic arteries and travel through chest wall and intercostal arteries to rejoin the aorta downstream. Although the proximal aortic pressure is usually hypertensive, the distal aortic pressure may be systemic in magnitude (more than 100 mm Hg), albeit blunted in upstroke and pulse pressure. Because aortic coarctation frequently is associated with a bicuspid aortic valve, the increased impedance imposed by the coarctation may promote aortic valvar regurgitation.

Pulmonic atresia (complete obliteration of RV outflow at valvar or subvalvar level) requires shunting at atrial or ventricular level to offload the venous blood into the systemic circuit and the development of systemic-pulmonary collateral vessels that feed the pulmonary artery beyond the total obstruction and permit oxygenation thereof. Persistence of fetal ductus arteriosus patency under these circumstances may provide near-normal growth and function. Tricuspid atresia almost invariably is combined with hypoplasia (underdevelopment) of the right ventricle, a VSD, and pulmonic stenosis or atresia. These individuals offload the right atrium through an ASD and oxygenate the venous blood by way of systemic-pulmonary collateral vessels or a PAD.

Transposed Vessels

Transposition of great arteries provides "obligatory" shunting of blood. When the aorta arises from the right ventricle and the pulmonary artery arises from the left ventricle in TGA, the "wrong blood" is circulated, with desaturated blood in the aorta and oxygenated blood in the pulmonary artery. In pure form, TGA would be lethal in infancy, but if combined with ASD, VSD, or PDA, admixture of the bloodstreams occurs and permits survival. A unique form of TGA, called *corrected transposition of the great arteries* or *C-TGA*, results from a congenital ventricular inversion that counteracts the arterial transposition, so that "two wrongs make a right" and remarkably trouble-free function may result. The ventricle that gives rise to the aorta is a morphologic right ventricle, but it receives left atrial blood, whereas the morphologic left ventricle receives right atrial blood. The atrioventricular valves are endocardial ventricular structures, so the mitral valve stays with the left ventricle, which in turn receives right atrial blood. The tricuspid valve serving the morphologic right ventricle may not have the structural integrity to withstand systemic pressure needs or may be malformed in an Ebsteinlike fashion. Patients with C-TGA may present with a clinical picture of "mitral regurgitation" and surprise the unsuspecting cardiologist or surgeon who embarks on a diagnostic workup or operative repair.

A more common and often well-tolerated category of inappropriate connection is *anomalous venous return*, including pulmonary veins that directly enter the right atrium or systemic veins and systemic veins that enter the left atrium. The shunting is obligatory because the veins bring back blood to the "wrong place" and must continue to do so regardless of downstream conditions. As noted earlier, *sinus venosus atrial septal defects* are associated with *partial anomalous venous return* of the right upper lobe pulmonary veins (see Fig. 12.4). When anomalous right pulmonary veins connect with the inferior vena cava, the venous channel, often visible on a chest x-ray, resembles a curved Arabic sword and therefore is called the *scimitar syndrome*. *Total anomalous pulmonary venous return* occasionally permits survival to adulthood and can be recognized by the "snowman" silhouette of the chest x-ray, with the head of the snowman formed by the pulmonary venous blood entering the innominate veins via a vertical vein and from there into the superior vena cava. The left atrium receives desaturated blood from the inferior vena cava via the foramen ovale, whereas the highly saturated superior vena caval blood enters the right atrium and ventricle, greatly enlarging these chambers to form the "body" of the snowman.

Dysplasias

The remaining category, dysplasias, includes conditions as diverse as Ebstein's anomaly of the tricuspid valve, tricuspid atresia, and cor triatriatum.

The malformed *Ebstein* tricuspid valve has the septal and posterior leaflet attachments displaced downward into the right ventricle, with compensatory elongation of the anterior leaflet, commonly causing tricuspid regurgitation and/or stenosis. The right ventricle is partially replaced by the "atrialized ventricle" incorporated within the displaced tricuspid valve and may be thin-walled and dysplastic. The dilated right atrium becomes a nidus of arrhythmias, and the frequent association (about 20%) of a Wolff-Parkinson-White (WPW) bypass tract adds to the likelihood of symptomatic and even life-threatening arrhythmias. The foramen ovale is often patent, permitting right-to-left shunting away from the dysplastic right ventricle. Despite all of these potential problems, survival to asymptomatic adulthood is not unusual, and the initial presentation often is precipitated by the onset of atrial fibrillation or detection of an enlarged cardiac silhouette on chest x-ray.

Tricuspid atresia (absence of a patent orifice from the right atrium into the right ventricle, with hypoplasia of the ventricle) causes the systemic venous blood to divert through the foramen ovale into the left heart. If there is a VSD, some blood has access to the pulmonary arteries through the underdeveloped right ventricle. Alternative routes to the pulmonary arteries include a PDA and/or systemic-pulmonary collateral arterial channels. Cyanosis is invariably present because of the low pulmonary blood flow.

Cor triatriatum is an abnormal septation of the left atrium resulting in a high-pressure pulmonary venous inflow chamber and a mitral valve outflow chamber emulating the pathophysiology of mitral stenosis and often presenting as severe pulmonary hypertension.

Combinations of Defects

Combinations of the previous categories may add to the burden imposed by the individual components or, in some cases, provide beneficial compensation. A subpulmonic (supracristal) membranous VSD fails to provide structural support for the aortic valve, leading to prolapse of the right sinus of Valsalva that partially occludes the defect (beneficial), but the aortic regurgitation adds to the hemodynamic burden on the left and/or right ventricle. However, PS combined with a VSD serves to "protect" the pulmonary vascular bed from the excessive flow and pressure that would have resulted from an isolated large VSD. A PDA confers benefit to any condition in which there is inadequate pulmonary blood flow in a low-pressure pulmonary circuit (e.g., tricuspid atresia). TGA is lethal in isolation, and defects of the atrial and ventricular septa or persistence of the ductus arteriosus will permit life-supporting access of oxygenated blood to the systemic arteries.

CYANOSIS

Another classification of diverse inborn abnormalities defines *cyanotic* conditions in a separate category from acyanotic defects. *Central cyanosis* (blue tongue, lips, and mucous membranes, usually accompanied by clubbing of the terminal digits) requires that oxygen-depleted erythrocytes in the venous blood have access to the systemic arteries in sufficient quantity to yield more than 3.5 gm/L of unsaturated hemoglobin in arterial blood. For example, if the hemoglobin content is 20 gm/L and the arterial saturation is 75%, 25% or 4 g of hemoglobin is unsaturated and cyanosis will be evident. However, if the subject is anemic, with only 10 g of hemoglobin, only 2.5 g of hemoglobin will be desaturated if the arterial saturation is 75%. Because most adults with cyanotic heart disease have polycythemia, anemia rarely will mask cyanosis after infancy.

For desaturated blood to enter the systemic circulation, there must either be an *obligatory access* pathway or a combination of a communication and downstream impedance. Obligatory access categories would include pulmonary arteriovenous fistulae, systemic veins that directly enter the left atrium, or TGA in which the right ventricle is obliged to pump its venous blood into the aorta.

The other category, *communication plus downstream impedance*, is more common than obligatory access in adults with cyanotic congenital heart disease. An ASD will shunt right to left if the tricuspid valve is diseased or atretic so that systemic venous blood follows the line of least resistance into the left atrium and the systemic circulation (Table 12.1). Similarly, if the right ventricle is hypertrophic and/or failing, or the right ventricle is impeded by downstream pathology (PS or pulmonary hypertension), blood will flow right to left

Table 12.1. Shunt determination in congenital heart disease

Site of communication	Site of downstream impedance		
	Tricuspid valve	Right ventricular	Pulmonary arterial tree
Atrial septal defect	Tricuspid stenosis or atresia	Pulmonary stenosis or atresia or right ventricular hypertrophy and/or failure	Peripheral pulmonary branch stenosis or arteriolar constriction
Ventricular septal defect single ventricle		Pulmonary stenosis or atresia or anomalous muscle bundle	Arteriolar constriction or obliteration (pulmonary hypertension)
Patient ductus arteriosus Aortic-pulmonary window			Arteriolar constriction or obliteration (pulmonary hypertension)

Obligatory admixtures include transposition of great arteries, anomalous systemic vein drainage, and pulmonary arteriovenous fistulae.

and may produce cyanosis. It is important to note that an ASD absent the downstream impediments noted in the table will facilitate left-to-right flow because of the increased *compliance* of the right ventricle as compared with the thicker-walled left ventricle.

If the communication is at *ventricular level*, an anomalous muscle bundle in the subinfundibular area, infundibular or valvar PS, or pulmonary arteriolar vasoconstriction or obliterative changes of pulmonary hypertension will facilitate right-to-left shunting.

A simple rule that applies to most patients with cyanotic heart disease is that the presence of a *prominent systolic "outflow murmur"* usually implies that there is a high likelihood of success with a palliative procedure or definitive repair. However, the absence of a systolic murmur, or the presence of only a diastolic murmur, carries a low likelihood of surgical improvement. A continuous murmur in a cyanotic patient provides some optimism. The reason behind these somewhat simplistic scenarios is that systolic murmurs usually are generated by ventricular pumping through a narrow channel into a low-resistance circuit; in a patient with cyanosis, this type of murmur would imply PS and a low pulmonary vascular resistance.

Shunting through a large, nonrestrictive VSD will not produce a murmur *per se* because the flow through the large communication is not sufficiently high in velocity and it is not "turbulent." If the impedance is caused by pulmonary arteriolar obliteration with resulting pulmonary hypertension, there will be no systolic murmur and there may be a diastolic murmur of pulmonary valvar regurgitation. The latter scenario would represent the Eisenmenger syndrome, considered inoperable by today's standards, whereas the patient with the systolic murmur could undergo a definitive operation that will close the VSD and relieve or bypass the PS.

Continuous murmurs in an individual with cyanosis imply unidirectional systolic and diastolic flow from a high-pressure circuit (usually a systemic artery) to a low-pressure recipient chamber, usually the pulmonary artery. Systemic-to-pulmonary-artery collateral channels facilitate survival in patients with cyanosis with severe obstruction or atresia (complete closure) of the RV outflow and actually may provide enough flow to form a pulmonary arterial tree that can be incorporated into a definitive operative repair. More often, these collateral vessels are multiple, arising from many locations along the aortic arch and descending aorta, and lead to one or more lobar arteries that may or may not be in continuity with central pulmonary arteries. In the latter instance, they may have to be joined up with the central arteries in staged operations to fabricate an effective pulmonary arterial tree.

CLINICAL RECOGNITION OF CONGENITAL HEART DISEASES

Congenital heart conditions may emulate the physical findings of valvar heart disease, but the astute observer armed with an accurate history and well-performed examination supplemented with an electrocardiogram (ECG) and chest x-ray should be able to reach an appropriate diagnosis or, at the very least, an appropriate differential diagnosis. The salient features that aid in recognition of the more common lesions follows in alphabetic order. It should be noted that actual recordings of heart sounds and murmurs described are available on the CD-ROM listed in the appended bibliography.

Atrial septal defect in a young individual (younger than 40 years) causes an increase in pulmonary artery flow that may be two to four times normal, increasing RV inflow and outflow and delaying closure of the pulmonic valve. Flow across the septal defect itself is silent, but enhanced pulmonary outflow is associated with a midsystolic murmur and persistent splitting of the second heart sound in the pulmonic area, and increased inflow volume may cause a middiastolic murmur in the tricuspid area. The first heart sound is often "split" as well, as a result of asynchronous closure of the atrioventricular valves, or alternatively, an ejection sound generated in the dilated pulmonary artery. The ECG usually demonstrates a delay in RV depolarization, with an rSR′ "incomplete right bundle branch block" (RBBB) pattern. Clues favoring an *ostium primum* defect are the presence of a murmur of mitral and/or tricuspid regurgitation and left-axis deviation in the frontal plane ECG. The chest x-ray reveals enlarged pulmonary arteries and right heart chambers, whereas a pronounced "hilar dance" is seen on fluoroscopy.

Bicuspid aortic valve may present as stenosis, regurgitation, a combined lesion, or a normally functioning aortic valve. An auscultatory feature common to all is an aortic ejection sound that emulates a "split first heart sound" best heard upstream of the valve, at the apex, or along the left sternal border. Detailed descriptions of the pulses and murmurs can be found in Chapter 4.

Ebstein's anomaly of the tricuspid valve in an adult may or may not be associated with cyanosis (resulting from shunting via the foramen ovale) and often produces a cacophony of auscultatory events: splitting of the first and second sounds, third sound, and a low pitched systolic murmur of tricuspid regurgitation. The second component of the split first sound is the "sail sound" resulting from delayed closing excursion of the greatly elongated anterior tricuspid leaflet, and the second sound's split results from the RBBB. The ECG usually demonstrates tall, broad P waves, P-R prolongation, and a distorted RBBB QRS complex over the right ventricle that resembles a splintered tree trunk with multiple upward shards. In the presence of WPW, anterograde atrioventricular conduction may proceed down the bypass tract and obscure the unique RBBB pattern. The cardiac silhouette often is enlarged on chest x-ray and may simulate a water-bottle heart of pericardial effusion because of dilation of the right atrium and the outflow tract of the right ventricle, combined with a small pulmonary artery and relatively avascular lung fields.

Patent ductus arteriosus, in the absence of pulmonary hypertension, usually presents a diagnostic picture of a wide arterial pulse pressure and a continuous murmur in the left subclavian area radiating down the left sternal border. At the far end of the spectrum, when there is a large (nonrestrictive) ductus with equalization of aortic and pulmonary artery pressures, a classical presentation called *differential cyanosis* makes it possible to make an accurate diagnosis by mere inspection of the digits. The toes, downstream from the right-to-left shunting ductus, will be clubbed and cyanotic, whereas the fingernail beds will be normal and pink. In this latter presentation, there is no murmur from the ductus *per se* and only a murmur of pulmonic valve regurgitation. In between these extremes is a spectrum of abbreviated murmurs, some confined to late systole only. When the ductus is restrictive, the left ventricle does most of the work, pumping out the shunted blood in addition to the blood sent from the right ventricle. An increased blood volume is presented to the left atrium and ventricle and is reflected in enlargement of these chambers on ECG and x-ray.

Pulmonic stenosis usually results from fusion of the pulmonic valve cusps, forming a systolic dome with a central orifice. The early systolic upward thrust of the deformed valve is impeded by its limited elasticity, causing a sharp ejection sound when the blood pushing the dome upward is halted abruptly. This extra sound closely follows the first sound, or it may fuse with the first sound during inspiration, and initiates a long, harsh midsystolic murmur. The length of the murmur is a rough guide to the severity of the obstruction, and the murmur may seem to be holosystolic when it spills past the aortic closure sound, especially when the delayed pulmonic valve closure sound is not heard. The hypertrophic right ventricle resists passive filling and requires a powerful "atrial kick" to fill adequately. Augmented atrial contractions are associated with prominent a waves in the jugular venous pulse and a fourth heart sound along the lower left sternal border and left midprecordium. The ECG usually reflects RVH, with the height of the R wave in V-1 serving as a guide to the RV pressure. The chest x-ray usually shows a small heart with a dilated main and left pulmonary artery (poststenotic dilation) and may exhibit right atrial enlargement when the obstruction is severe.

Tetralogy of Fallot (Fig. 12.6) covers a broad spectrum of mild to severe outflow tract obstructions in association with a stereotypic large, nonrestrictive VSD. Some individuals with moderate PS are "pink," whereas those with severe stenosis or atresia may be profoundly cyanotic; all share the same systemic level RV pressures and normal pulmonary artery pressure. The difference in systemic

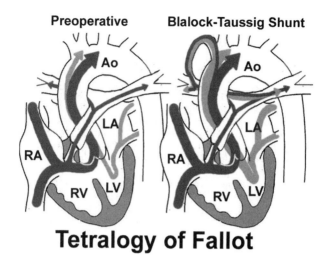

Preoperative   **Blalock-Taussig Shunt**

Tetralogy of Fallot

Fig. 12.6. Tetralogy of Fallot with Blalock-Taussig shunt. The defects consist of a nonrestrictive ventricular septal defect, right ventricular outflow obstruction, and an "overriding aorta" with resulting right ventricular hypertrophy. Preoperatively, right ventricular outflow impedance diverts most of its outflow (*dark arrow*) to the aorta where it blends in with scanty outflow of oxygenated blood (*light arrow*) returning from the lungs. The Blalock-Taussig shunt (subclavian artery to pulmonary artery anastomosis) increases pulmonary blood flow and, thus, increases the quantity of oxygenated blood entering the aorta, increasing its saturation.

oxygenation thus is dependent on the amount of pulmonary blood flow that is able to traverse the RV outflow tract. The more severe the stenosis, the shorter and softer the outflow murmur, which may seem paradoxic but can be explained by the presence of an alternate outlet for the right ventricle—the "overriding aorta." The first heart sound may seem to be accentuated, but this is caused by a loud ejection sound occurring with ventricular ejection into a dilated aortic root. Flow through a large VSD is of insufficient velocity to generate a murmur, so murmurs heard in patients with Fallot's tetralogy are generated by high velocity flow through the outflow tract, or continuous murmurs may be heard if there are systemic-to-pulmonary artery collateral channels or a prior Blalock-Taussig anastomosis (see *Operations* later in this chapter). The chest radiograph usually demonstrates the *Coeur en sabot* (bootlike heart) with a concave instep resulting from the small pulmonary artery and an upturned toe from the hypertrophic right ventricle. The ECG invariably exhibits RVH.

Ventricular septal defects often present a diagnostic clinical picture of a palpable murmur (thrill) in an otherwise healthy, asymptomatic individual. When the defect is small (*maladie de Roger*, see Fig. 12.5), the murmur is holosystolic and quite loud because of the high velocity flow through the small hole, and the second sound may be persistently split because the aortic valve closes early having offloaded some of its stroke volume into the right ventricle.

Flow and velocity through larger, nonrestrictive defects are comparable in magnitude to normal aortic or pulmonic outflow and therefore do not generate a murmur in the defect *per se*. The pressures in both ventricles are equal by definition. However, these large defects, when associated with large left-to-right shunts as shown in the middle panel in Fig. 12.5, will produce high-velocity flow through the pulmonary outflow tract, which generates a midsystolic murmur and a middiastolic flow rumble emanating from the large volume traversing the mitral valve. At the extreme end of the spectrum, a nonrestrictive VSD with reversal of flow (Eisenmenger syndrome) may have no murmur or only manifest an early diastolic murmur of pulmonic regurgitation. Depending on the additional work performed by the ventricles, the ECG may be normal; show left atrial and ventricular enlargement/hypertrophy; or, in the case of pulmonary hypertension, show RVH. The spectrum of chest x-rays manifests a small heart at either end (both Roger and Eisenmenger) because of the small amount of intracardiac shunting, whereas the larger defects with significant shunting cause enlargement of the left atrium and ventricle and radiographic evidence of increased pulmonary arterial flow.

OPERATIONS IN CONGENITAL HEART DISEASE

Operations to relieve or correct congenital heart defects have a long and distinguished history. Some bear the names of the innovators, and some evolved from trial and error by many investigators. Dr. Robert Gross performed the first operation on a patient with congenital heart disease (aortic coarctation) in 1938, and Alfred Blalock performed the first operative procedure on a patient with tetralogy of Fallot in 1944. Open heart surgery using cardiopulmonary bypass was not performed widely before the mid 1950s, so the earliest procedures were performed with the heart beating and the circulation intact, and others were done under profound hypothermia. All of the closed heart procedures listed later in this chapter, with the exception of the Blalock-Hanlon and Potts procedures, still are performed today. It should be acknowledged that the late Mr. Vivien Thomas, a gifted surgical technician working for Dr. Blalock in his animal research laboratory, was largely responsible for developing the two palliative procedures listed here bearing Dr. Blalock's name.

Palliative procedures are designed to aid, but not correct, congenital heart defects. For example, patients with tetralogy of Fallot are cyanotic because of decreased pulmonary blood flow resulting from RV outflow obstruction and right-to-left shunting through a VSD from right ventricle to aorta (see Fig. 12.6). The Blalock-Taussig procedure does not decrease the amount of blue blood entering the aorta but, by increasing pulmonary blood flow, will increase the amount of oxygenated blood returning to the left heart. The increase in pulmonary venous return will increase the amount of oxygenated blood ejected into the aorta by the left ventricle. The mixed aortic blood thus will contain an increase in oxygen content, cyanosis will be lessened or relieved, and exercise tolerance will be increased. Rather than using the subclavian artery, prosthetic graft material now is used for the Blalock-Taussig operation.

"Closed Heart" Procedures

1938–1950

Resection of aortic coarctation (Robert Gross, 1938)
Blalock-Taussig (Thomas): subclavian-pulmonary anastomosis for tetralogy
Blalock-Hanlon (Thomas): creation of ASD for transposition
Brock: transventricular pulmonary valvotomy (valvotome inserted through RV wall)
Potts: aortic arch–left pulmonary artery anastomosis
Ligation and division of patent ductus

1950–1965

Glenn: superior vena caval-pulmonary artery anastomosis for tricuspid atresia
Rashkind: catheter-balloon septostomy for creation of ASD for transposition
Waterston-Cooley: ascending aorta to right pulmonary artery graft for increasing pulmonary blood flow
Pulmonary artery banding to reduce pulmonary blood flow and pressure in VSD

"Open Heart" Procedures

Closure of ASDs and VSDs
Definitive correction of tetralogy of Fallot: closure of VSD, outflow tract patch
Mustard, Senning: atrial baffle to reroute ventricular inflow in complete transposition

1965–present

Rastelli: outflow tract conduit for pulmonary atresia and tetralogy of Fallot
Fontan: right atrial or vena caval conduit for tricuspid atresia
"Switch": aortic and pulmonary artery switched for complete transposition

Many adult patients with congenital heart disease have had palliative surgical procedures that have allowed them to survive to adulthood to then undergo more definitive procedures. For example, infants or young children with large (nonrestrictive) VSDs often undergo *pulmonary artery banding* to protect the pulmonary vascular bed from the mandatory exposure to systemic pressure and thus become an iatrogenic "pink tetralogy" equivalent. Other procedures are designed to be performed in stages (e.g., placement of a *Blalock-Taussig* shunt to increase the size of the underdeveloped pulmonary arteries for a later definitive repair). The *Glenn* and *Fontan* procedures often are combined in treatment of patients with tricuspid atresia. The superior vena caval return is directed to the pulmonary arteries by an end-to-side anastomosis with the right pulmonary artery, whereas the inferior vena caval blood is routed to the main pulmonary artery.

CATHETER-BASED CORRECTIVE PROCEDURES

Interventional catheter-based procedures currently are being used in some centers to perform pulmonary and aortic valvotomy, dilate aortic coarctation, close the ductus arteriosus, and occlude ASDs. These procedures have the potential advantage of precluding major open heart surgery, but many are still in the experimental development stages and are not yet able to reliably close large defects.

SELECTED READINGS

Brickner ME, Hillis LD, Lange RA: Congenital heart disease in adults (review article in 2 parts). *New Engl J Med* 342:257–263, 334–342, 2000.

Criley JM, Criley DG, Zalace C: *The physiological origins of heart sounds and murmurs* (CD-ROM). Philadelphia: Lippincott Williams and Wilkins, 1997.

Criley JM, French WJ: Cardiac catheterization. In: Roberts WC, ed. *Adult congenital heart disease.* Philadelphia: F.A. Davis, 1987.

Perloff JK: *The clinical recognition of congenital heart disease.* Philadelphia: W.B. Saunders, 2003.

THE CARDIOMYOPATHIES

DEFINITION AND CLASSIFICATION

The cardiomyopathies are defined as diseases of the myocardium associated with cardiac dysfunction. They have been classified into four groups: (a) dilated cardiomyopathy, (b) hypertrophic cardiomyopathy, (c) restrictive cardiomyopathy, and (d) arrhythmogenic right ventricular cardiomyopathy (1). Previously, the cardiomyopathies were defined as "heart muscle disease of unknown cause" and were differentiated from heart muscle disease of known cause. They now are classified by the dominant pathophysiology or, if possible, by etiologic or pathogenetic factors.

DILATED CARDIOMYOPATHY

The dilated cardiomyopathy group is characterized by poor myocardial systolic function. Left ventricular (LV), and often right ventricular (RV), contractility is diminished, leading to decreased cardiac output and increased end-systolic and end-diastolic ventricular volumes and pressures (2). Cardiomegaly, resulting more from dilatation than from hypertrophy, invariably is present. There is evidence to suggest that reduced ability of the sarcoplasmic reticulum to accumulate calcium plays a major role in the altered excitation–contraction coupling in patients with dilated cardiomyopathy (3). The reported annual incidence of the idiopathic form in the United States is between 5 to 8 cases per 100,000 population (2,4) and is the cause of congestive heart failure (CHF) in approximately 25% of all cases of CHF (5). Approximately 35% are believed to be familial (6).

Etiologies include:

- Idiopathic
- Familial/genetic
- Viral and/or immune
- Alcoholic/toxic
- Association with a recognized cardiovascular disease (e.g., hypertension, ischemic heart disease)

Clinical Profile

Patients most commonly present with signs and symptoms of CHF, with symptoms of left-sided failure predominating (see Chapter 10). In addition, it is not uncommon for the patient to present with signs of a myocardial, cerebral, renal, or mesenteric infarction or a pulseless, blue extremity resulting from an embolus from a mural thrombus. Sudden death is frequent in patients with a dilated cardiomyopathy and is most commonly the result of ventricular arrhythmias or conduction system disease (2).

Murmurs frequently are heard during cardiac auscultation and are not themselves indicative of primary valvular disease. A holosystolic mitral or tricuspid regurgitation murmur is very common and is the result of ventricular dilatation and resultant lateral displacement of the papillary muscles, which inhibits leaflet coaptation. Annular dilatation also may occur and serve as the major mechanism for functional mitral regurgitation. Occasionally, an apical "diastolic rumble" also may be heard and results from increased early diastolic atrioventricular flow, mitral regurgitation, or a loud summation gallop.

The chest x-ray most commonly shows cardiomegaly and evidence of pulmonary venous and arterial hypertension. The electrocardiogram (ECG) is almost always abnormal. In addition to evidence of ventricular and atrial enlargement, Q or QS waves and poor R wave progression across the anterior precordial leads frequently are seen. Atrioventricular nodal and intraventricular conduction defects, particularly left bundle branch block, and arrhythmias, particularly atrial fibrillation and premature ventricular depolarizations, are common associated findings. The characteristic echocardiographic findings (see Chapter 4) in a patient with a congestive cardiomyopathy reflect poor contractile function: decreased ejection fraction, decreased velocity of circumferential fiber shortening, increased end-systolic and end-diastolic volumes, chamber enlargement, and regurgitant murmurs.

Management

The goal of therapy is to alleviate the symptomatic manifestations of CHF (see Chapter 10). Additional interventions, in the case of cardiomyopathy with known etiology, will be dictated by the underlying disease, such as complete abstinence in the case of alcoholic cardiomyopathy. The true natural history of the disease is difficult to determine because asymptomatic cardiomegaly may precede clinical manifestations for months to years. Recent data suggest that the 5-year mortality is approximately 20% (2). Death may result from progressive heart failure or from ventricular arrhythmias that accompany LV dysfunction (see Chapter 15). Dilated cardiomyopathy is currently the most common reason for cardiac transplantation. Novel therapies have been described and include biventricular or multisite cardiac pacemakers (7,8).

HYPERTROPHIC CARDIOMYOPATHY

Hypertrophic cardiomyopathy is characterized by an increased ventricular muscle mass without associated increase in cavity size and asymmetric hypertrophy of the septum (9). The disorder is most commonly familial (the majority have autosomal dominant transmission), and mutations in sarcomere contractile proteins have been demonstrated (10). This disorder also has been called hypertrophic obstructive cardiomyopathy, idiopathic hypertrophic subaortic stenosis, and muscular subaortic stenosis, to name a few.

Hemodynamically, hypertrophic cardiomyopathy is characterized by poor diastolic function of the left ventricle as a result of reduced compliance. The decrease in compliance is reflected in an increased LV end-diastolic pressure and impedance to diastolic filling. Systolic function is maintained (normal cardiac output, ejection fraction, and end-diastolic volume). A systolic pressure gradient between the body of the left ventricle and the outflow tract may be recorded in some patients at rest or following provocation (i.e., exercise, Valsalva maneuver, or isoproterenol infusion) (Fig. 13.1). Proposed explanations for this gradient include: (a) dynamic outflow obstruction by the hypertrophied septum; (b) outflow obstruction by the anterior leaflet

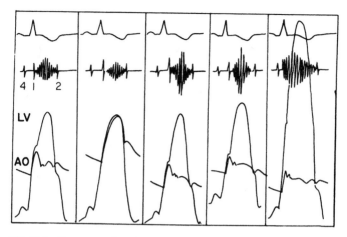

Fig. 13.1.   Pressure gradients in hypertrophic cardiomyopathy (HCM). Variable pressure gradients between the left ventricular cavity (*LV*) and the aorta (*AO*) may be recorded during cardiac catheterization of a patient with HCM. AO and LV pressure recordings and a phonocardiogram demonstrate characteristic hemodynamic and auscultatory findings in HCM. The LV–AO pressure gradient may be present at rest (control) as shown here, may appear spontaneously during the course of the hemodynamic study, or may manifest itself only after provocation. Interventions that decrease ventricular filling (Valsalva maneuver), decrease arterial resistance (vasodilators such as amyl nitrate), or increase the force of ventricular contraction (isoproterenol or postectopic beat) may provoke the appearance of a gradient and systolic murmur not present at rest or enhance an existing LV–AO gradient and systolic murmur as shown here. Increasing the impedance to LV ejection using a vasopressor agent will decrease the magnitude of the gradient. Provocation of a pressure gradient in a patient without other evidence of HCM should not be considered diagnostic of HCM because such a gradient can be produced in normal hearts and in patients with other cardiac conditions.

of the mitral valve during systole; and (c) forceful, exaggerated LV contraction with late systolic isometric contraction. The variability of the gradient and the fact that the left ventricle ejects nearly its entire volume during the first half of systole suggests that true obstruction or impediment to outflow does not occur. The presence of symptoms and the higher apparent death rate in symptomatic patients without pressure gradients render the significance of the pressure gradient unclear (11).

Clinical Profile

Dyspnea on exertion, chest pain that may be anginal in character, palpitations, and/or syncope are the major symptoms in patients with hypertrophic cardiomyopathy. A family history of sudden death or "heart failure" is not uncommon. This disease may present as sudden death, particularly in younger patients with a history of syncope or a family history of sudden death (12).

Physical examination reveals large dominant a waves in the jugular venous pulse and a jerky carotid pulse or "pulsus bisferiens." A sustained late systolic LV impulse preceded by a presystolic thrust is noted on palpation of the precordium. A variable mid- to late-systolic murmur and a fourth heart sound may be heard at the apex and left sternal border. The intensity of the systolic murmur is increased by standing and during the strain phase of the Valsalva maneuver.

The chest x-ray is usually normal. Left ventricular and left atrial hypertrophy are frequently but not always noted on the ECG. Small Q waves in leads V4 through V6 and an R/S ratio in V1 greater than 0.2 are suggestive of hypertrophic cardiomyopathy. Less frequently, prominent Q waves in II, III, and aVF are seen and are presumed to result from hypertrophy of the upper septum.

On the ECG, an increase in the thickness of the interventricular septum with a lesser increase in the thickness of the LV posterior basal wall is seen [septum to posterior wall thickness ratio of greater than 1.3—a reflection of asymmetric septal hypertrophy (ASH)]. Additional echocardiographic features include decreased systolic thickening of the septum, systolic anterior motion (SAM) of the anterior leaflet of the mitral valve, decreased E to F slope of the mitral valve, a normal or reduced LV end-diastolic dimension, and mid-systolic closure of the aortic valve (see Chapter 4). It should be noted that ASH on the ECG is not pathognomonic of hypertrophic cardiomyopathy and has been observed in a number of other situations, including systemic arterial hypertension with valvular aortic stenosis, in healthy athletes, following insertion of prosthetic aortic valves, after inferior myocardial infarction, and in hypothyroid heart disease.

Management

The clinical course of patients with hypertrophic cardiomyopathy is variable and not clearly related to the measured systolic pressure gradient. Overall, hypertrophic cardiomyopathy confers an annual mortality rate of about 1% (11). Subsets of patients with a higher mortality have defined (10,12). Beta-adrenergic blockade remains the mainstay of therapy and is most useful in alleviating the chest pain associated with this disease. The primary rationale for β-blockade therapy is based on the premise that prevention of exercise tachycardia aids in ventricular filling and reduces the oxygen demands of the ventricle. Additional benefits are the antiarrhythmic effects of beta blockers and the possible blocking of the "hypertrophying" influence of circulating catecholamines. Calcium-blocking agents (i.e., verapamil) also have been used in selected patients and have been found to alleviate symptoms. The rationale for their use is based on their demonstrated effects on myocardial contractility (a decrease in contractility improves the O_2 supply/demand ratio) (11,13). However, verapamil may cause serious hemodynamic complications and should be used cautiously. Myectomy for symptomatic patients unresponsive to medical therapy has been performed for more than three decades and may provide symptomatic benefit. Other novel therapies, including dual-chamber pacing and alcohol ablation of the first septal perforator, also have been shown to be beneficial in symptomatic patients who have not responded to medical therapy (13,14).

RESTRICTIVE CARDIOMYOPATHY

The restrictive cardiomyopathy group is characterized by restricted filling and reduced diastolic volume of either or both ventricles with normal or nearly normal systolic function and wall thickness. Interstitial fibrosis may be present. Strict echocardiographic diagnostic criteria include dilated atria with nonhypertrophied and nondilated ventricles (15,16). The major hemodynamic fault is a decrease in ventricular compliance, which produces a distinctive early diastolic "dip and plateau" configuration of RV and LV pressures. However, the LV end-diastolic pressure characteristically is higher than RV end-diastolic pressure and serves to distinguish a restrictive cardiomyopathy from constrictive pericarditis, which it may mimic (see Chapter 14). Ventricular end-diastolic volume is usually normal or decreased. Cardiac output may be normal or decreased, depending on the extent of replacement of contractile myocardium and the limitation to ventricular filling. A restrictive cardiomyopathy may be present in the absence of demonstrable systemic disease or cause (idiopathic) or it may occur in association with other diseases (e.g., amyloidosis, endomyocardial disease with or without eosinophilia).

Clinical Profile

Patients may present with signs and symptoms of CHF that is of diastolic origin (see Chapter 10). Physical findings may mimic those of constrictive pericarditis in that a rapid "y" descent of the jugular venous pulse, Kussmaul's sign, and pulsus paradoxus can be noted in patients with restrictive cardiomyopathies. Cardiac auscultation usually reveals a third and fourth heart sound, and murmurs of mitral and tricuspid regurgitation may be heard. Chest x-ray usually shows a normal or slightly enlarged cardiac silhouette. The ECG may be normal. Intraventricular conduction delay and arrhythmias (ventricular and supraventricular) are not uncommon. ECG may demonstrate symmetric wall thickening with variable degrees of chamber enlargement. Diffuse hypokinesis also may be noted.

Management

The natural history of the idiopathic form is variable (15). Initial management should be undertaken to alleviate the symptoms of CHF.

ARRHYTHMOGENIC RIGHT VENTRICULAR CARDIOMYOPATHY

Arrhythmogenic right ventricular cardiomyopathy is characterized by progressive fibro-fatty replacement of the RV myocardium. Standardized diagnostic criteria have been proposed and are based on the presence of major and minor criteria encompassing ECG, arrhythmic, morphofunctional, histopathologic, and genetic factors (17). The disease begins as a focal regional process followed by global RV involvement. The septum and left heart typically are spared. It is most commonly of familial origin with autosomal dominant inheritance and incomplete penetrance (18,19).

SPECIFIC CARDIOMYOPATHIES

The term *specific cardiomyopathies* now is used to describe heart muscle disease that is associated with specific cardiac or systemic disorders. They may present with the characteristic features of a dilated or restrictive cardiomyopathy or have features of both. Included within this group are the following:

- Ischemic cardiomyopathy
- Valvular cardiomyopathy

- Hypertensive cardiomyopathy
- Inflammatory cardiomyopathy: usually defined as myocarditis associated with cardiac dysfunction. Myocarditis is diagnosed histologically by established methods. Idiopathic, autoimmune, and infectious forms have been described. An infectious etiology is common, and pathogens include human immunodeficiency virus, enterovirus, adenovirus, and cytomegalovirus (20,21).
- Metabolic cardiomyopathy: included in this group are the cardiomyopathies associated with hyperthyroidism and acromegaly; familial storage diseases and infiltrations (e.g., hemochromatosis, glycogen storage disease, Hurler syndrome); nutritional disorders (e.g., beri-beri); and amyloidosis (primary, secondary, senile, or hereditary) (22,23).
- General systemic disease: includes primarily those disorders broadly classified as connective tissue or collagen–vascular disorders (e.g., systemic lupus erythematosus, scleroderma, polyarteritis nodosa). Infiltrative and granulomatous disease also would fall into this category (e.g., sarcoidosis, leukemia, lymphoma) (24,25).
- Muscular dystrophies and neuromuscular disorders
- Sensitivity and toxic reactions: alcohol, anthracyclines, cocaine (26,27)
- Peripartum cardiomyopathy (28)

REFERENCES

1. Report of the 1995 World Health Organization/International Society and Federation of Cardiology Task Force on the Definition and Classification of Cardiomyopathies. *Circulation* 93:841, 1996.
2. Dec GW, Fuster V: Idiopathic dilated cardiomyopathy. *N Engl J Med* 331:1564, 1994.
3. Meyer M, Schillinger W, Pieske B, et al: Alterations of sarcoplasmic reticulum proteins in failing human dilated cardiomyopathy. *Circulation* 92:778, 1995.
4. Manolio TA, Baughman KL, Rodeheffer R, et al: Prevalence and etiology of idiopathic dilated cardiomyopathy (Summary of a National Heart, Lung, and Blood Institute Workshop). *Am J Cardiol* 69:1458, 1992.
5. Brown CA, O'Connell JB: Myocarditis and idiopathic dilated cardiomyopathy. *Am J Med* 99:309, 1995.
6. Franz WM, Muller OJ, Katus HA: Cardiomyopathies: from genetic to the prospect of treatment. *Lancet* 358:1627, 2001.
7. Auricchio A, StellBrink C, Sack S, et al: The Pacing Therapies for Congestive Heart Failure (PATH-CHF) study: rationale, design, and endpoints of a prospective randomized multicenter study. *Am J Cardiol* 83:130D, 1999.
8. Gras D, Mabo P, Tang T, et al: Multisite pacing as a supplemental treatment of congestive heart failure: preliminary results of the Medtronic Inc. InSync Study. *Pacing Clin Electrophysiol* 21:2249, 1998.
9. Wigle ED, Rakowski H, Kimball BP, et al: Hypertrophic cardiomyopathy. Clinical spectrum and treatment. *Circulation* 92:1680, 1995.
10. Roberts R, Sigwart U: New concepts in hypertrophic cardiomyopathies, Part I. *Circulation* 104:2113: 2001.
11. Maron BJ: Hypertropic cardiomyopathy. A systematic review. *JAMA* 287:1308, 2002.
12. Elliot PM, Poloniecki J, Dickie S, et al: Sudden death in hypertrophic

cardiomyopathy: identification of high risk patients. *J Am Coll Cardiol* 36:2212, 2000.

13. Roberts R, Sigwart U: New concepts in hypertrophic cardiomyopathies, Part II. *Circulation* 104:2249, 2001.

14. Maron BJ: Role of alcohol in septal ablation in treatment of obstructive hypertrophic cardiomyopathy. *Lancet* 355:425, 2000.

15. Kushwaha SS, Fallon JT, Fuster V: Restrictive cardiomyopathy. *N Engl J Med* 336:267, 1997.

16. Ammash NM, Seward JB, Bailey KR, et al: Clinical profile and outcome of idiopathic restrictive cardiomyopathy. *Circulation* 101:2490, 2000.

17. Corrado D, Basso C, Nava A, et al: Arrhythmogenic right ventricular cardiomyopathy: current diagnostic and management strategies. *Cardiol Rev* 9:259, 2001.

18. Fontaine G, Fontaliran F, Frank R: Arrhythmogenic right ventricular cardiomyopathies. Clinical forms and main differential diagnoses. *Circulation* 97:1532, 1998.

19. Nava A, Bauce B, Basso C, et al: Clinical profile and long-term follow-up of 37 families with arrhythmogenic right ventricular cardiomyopathy. *J Am Coll Cardiol* 36:2226, 2000.

20. Pisani B, Taylor DO, Mason JW: Inflammatory myocardial diseases and cardiomyopathies. *Am J Med* 102:459, 1997.

21. Barbaro G, Di Lorenzo G, Grisorio B, et al: Incidence of dilated cardiomyopathy and detection of HIV in myocardial cells of HIV-positive patients. *N Engl J Med* 339:1093, 1998.

22. Andrews NC: Disorders of iron metabolism. *N Engl J Med* 341:1986, 1999.

23. Falk RH, Comenzo RL, Skinner M: The systemic amyloidoses. *N Engl J Med* 337:898, 1997.

24. Moder KG, Miller TD, Tazelaar HD: Cardiac involvement in systemic lupus erythematosus. *Mayo Clin Proc* 74:275, 1999.

25. Newman LS, Rose CS, Maier LA: Sarcoidosis. *N Engl J Med* 336:1224, 1997.

26. Pai VB, Nahata MC: Cardiotoxicity of chemotherapeutic agents: incidence, treatment, and prevention. *Drug Safety* 22:263, 2000.

27. Mouhaffel AH, Madu EC, Satmary WA, et al: Cardiovascular complications of cocaine. *Chest* 107:1426, 1995.

28. Pearson GD, Veille JC, Rahimtoola S, et al: Peripartum cardiomyopathy. *JAMA* 283:1183, 2000.

PERICARDIAL HEART DISEASE

The pericardium consists of a serous or loose fibrous membrane (visceral pericardium), beneath which lies the myocardium, and a dense collagenous sac (parietal pericardium), which surrounds the heart. Under normal conditions, up to 50 mL of fluid may be present in the space between the visceral and parietal pericardium. The pericardium supports the heart and limits its movement within the mediastinum, serves as a barrier to the spread of infection from the lungs and pleural (if sudden cardiac dilatation occurs), and may modify the ventricular pressure-volume (compliance) relationship as preload is increased (1,2).

Because its layers are serosal surfaces (lined with mesothelial cells) and because of its proximity and attachments to other structures (pleura, diaphragm, sternum, and myocardium), the pericardium may be involved in a number of systemic or localized disease processes. The clinical presentations of pericardial disease are variable and are dependent not only on the pericardium's response to an injury (exudation of fluid, fibrin, or inflammatory cells; granuloma formation; fibrous proliferation; or calcification) but also on how the response affects cardiac function.

The following discussion highlights the clinical presentation and evaluation of acute pericarditis, cardiac tamponade, and constrictive pericarditis.

ACUTE PERICARDITIS

Symptoms and Signs

The vast majority of patients with acute pericarditis will complain of retrosternal or precordial chest pain. The pain is most often, but not always, "pleuritic" in character (worsened with deep inspiration, movement, or lying down) and relieved by sitting up, leaning forward, and taking shallow inspirations. Because the pain may be aggravated by inspiration, the patient may complain of shortness of breath. Additional symptoms most often will be determined by the underlying etiology.

A pericardial friction rub is the most common and important physical finding in pericarditis. It is most often triphasic in character, consisting of a systolic component during ventricular systole, an early diastolic component occurring during the early phase of ventricular filling, and a presystolic component synchronous with atrial systole. The friction rub is less commonly biphasic—a systolic component with either an early diastolic or presystolic component.

A single component or monophasic rub is rare (less than 20% of cases) and is usually systolic. The friction rub is best heard at the cardiac apex with the patient sitting up or in the hands-and-knees position. It may be transient, and its presence does not preclude the presence of a large pericardial effusion.

Chest X-Ray

A routine chest x-ray may be of value in acute pericarditis but not necessarily in diagnosis because heart size may be normal with a small pericardial effusion. The presence of a pericardial friction rub in association with pleuropulmonary or mediastinal abnormalities may assist in establishing an etiology (e.g., neoplastic or infectious).

Electrocardiogram

The electrocardiogram (ECG) may be diagnostic, especially if followed over time (3). In the acute phase (stage 1), the ST segment vector is directed anteriorly, inferiorly, and leftward, causing ST segment elevation (reflecting subepicardial injury) in the precordial leads, especially in V5 and V6 and in leads I and II (Fig. 1.4 in Chapter 1). ST segment elevation in V6 is usually greater than 25% of the T wave amplitude (using the PR interval as baseline, measure the ST amplitude at the J point and the T wave amplitude at the peak of the T wave). An isoelectric or depressed ST segment commonly is seen in V1. PR segment depression may be noted in leads II, aVF, and V4-V6. In stage 2, the ST segment begins returning to the isoelectric line and T wave amplitude decreases. T wave inversion in those leads previously showing ST segment elevation is noted during stage 3. At this time, the ST segment is isoelectric. Stage 4 is characterized by resolution of the ECG abnormalities. Additional ECG abnormalities may be noted during pericarditis and include atrial arrhythmias (usually insignificant) and, if a large effusion is present, low-voltage QRS complexes and electrical alternans. The latter phenomena are the result of the "insulating" effect of the pericardial fluid and the pendulum motion of the heart within the pericardium at a frequency one-half of the heart rate.

Etiology

Common causes of pericarditis/pericardial effusion include the following:

- Idiopathic: commonly proceeded by a febrile illness or "viral syndrome." In most cases, the etiology is not established.
- Infections

Viral: Coxsackie virus (especially group B), echovirus, adenovirus, mumps virus, influenza virus, and Epstein-Barr virus. Human immunodeficiency virus (HIV) is becoming an increasingly recognized cause of pericarditis (4). Viral pericarditis frequently is associated with a myocarditis and cardiac enzyme elevation; in this instance, the term myopericarditis is used.
Bacterial: usually the result of spread from a contiguous myocardial abscess or pleuropulmonary focus (pneumonia or empyema) or after thoracic surgery or trauma. *Staphylococcus aureus* and *Streptococcus pneumoniae* are the most common organisms (5,6). Infection is often polymicrobial, and anaerobic organisms are more common if the focus of origin is a mediastinitis secondary to an orofacial or dental infection. Mycobacteria should be considered in populations at risk. Pericarditis may occur during acute rheumatic fever.
Other infectious agents: mycoplasma, histoplasma, coccidioidomycosis, nocardia, actinomycosis, Q fever, Lyme disease
Connective tissue disease: scleroderma, systemic lupus, mixed connective tissue disease, rheumatoid arthritis, polymyositis/dermatomyositis (7)
- **Malignancy:** most commonly metastatic from breast or lung; however, lymphoma, leukemia, and melanoma have a high incidence

of metastasis to the pericardium. Adenocarcinoma of unknown origin also may present as pericarditis or cardiac tamponade (8).

- **Uremia:** usually treatable by dialysis or more frequent dialysis in those already undergoing dialysis (9)
- **Drug-induced:** "lupus syndrome" resulting from procainamide, hydralazine, isoniazid, or diphenylhydantoin. The anthracycline antineoplastic agents, such as doxorubicin, may cause pericarditis in addition to the more common myocardial toxicity.
- **Postmyocardial (Q wave) infarction (Dressler's syndrome)** (10)
- **Postpericardiotomy:** incidence as high as 30% within 2 to 4 weeks after open-heart surgery, often associated with pulmonary infiltrate and/or pleural effusion. It is probably of immunologic origin and different than the acute pericarditis that may occur within the first week after an ST segment elevation myocardial infarction (STEMI) (11).
- **Mediastinal radiation therapy**
- **Myxedema**
- **Sarcoidosis**

Laboratory Assessment

In addition to careful history and physical examination, the following laboratory studies may be of value in establishing an etiologic diagnosis:

- Complete blood count and differential: may suggest infection or leukemia
- Erythrocyte sedimentation rate (ESR): usually elevated but not specific for pericarditis or its etiology. ESR may be useful in following course and assessing response to therapy if pericarditis results from an inflammatory process (infection, autoimmune disorder).
- Blood urea nitrogen and creatinine
- Blood cultures
- Serology: acute- and convalescent-phase viral titers, antinuclear antibody, double-stranded (DNA), RA latex, HIV, toxoplasma, and mycoplasma titers
- Tuberculosis (TB) skin test and sputum for acid-fast staining and TB culture
- Cardiac enzymes or serum markers: often elevated in acute viral pericarditis (12,13). The occurrence of ST segment elevation and increased serum markers may mimic STEMI
- ECG
- Chest X-ray
- Echocardiography: to confirm the presence of pericardial fluid; to rule out a contiguous cardiac process (endocarditis, myocardial abscess); and to assess for cardiac compromise (14)
- Pericardiocentesis: indicated in suspected cardiac tamponade and occasionally indicated as a diagnostic procedure, especially if infection or malignancy is suspected

Noninvasive evaluation of patients with pericarditis will yield a specific etiology in only about 15% of cases (15). Pericardiocentesis findings increase the likelihood of a specific diagnosis by about another 10%. If pericarditis and pericardial effusion are recurrent and life threatening, pericardioscopy and pericardial biopsy may be useful (16).

Therapy

Therapy is directed most appropriately at the underlying etiology if a treatable cause can be defined. Chest pain may be alleviated with the use of salicylates or nonsteroidal antiinflammatory drugs. Corticosteroid therapy for several days may be necessary to treat severe pain. Patients with viral myopericarditis should be placed on bed rest and frequently assessed for signs and symptoms of declining left ventricular (LV) function. Echocardiography may be helpful in differentiating depressed myocardial contractility from cardiac tamponade or constriction. Corticosteroids have been instilled directly into the pericardial space to treat uremic pericarditis. Instillation of antineoplastic agents or sclerosing agents into the pericardial space has been used in malignant causes of pericarditis.

It is not unusual for the patient to have one or more relapses of acute symptoms weeks or months after apparent resolution. If these episodes continue to recur, a trial of corticosteroid therapy may be more effective than other antiinflammatory drugs. Colchicine has been shown to be an effective agent in small, uncontrolled clinical trials (17). Rarely, pericardiectomy is indicated to relieve recurrent symptoms or as prophylaxis against constrictive pericarditis or cardiac tamponade (18).

CARDIAC TAMPONADE

Intrapericardial pressure is normally subatmospheric. An increase in the quantity of intrapericardial fluid, whatever the cause, results in an increase in the intrapericardial pressure. The initial portion of the pericardial pressure-volume curve is relatively flat (i.e., relatively large increases in intrapericardial volume produce small changes in intrapericardial pressure). The curve becomes steeper as the fibrous and relatively inelastic parietal pericardium is "stretched." Eventually, continued fluid accumulation will increase the intrapericardial pressure to a level that exceeds the normal filling pressure of the ventricles (19). When this occurs, ventricular filling is restricted, and cardiac tamponade is present. The slope of the pressure-volume curve of the pericardial sac and the point at which cardiac tamponade occurs is dependent on the following:

- **The rate of fluid accumulation:** with slow accumulation, large volumes of fluid can be accommodated more readily as a result of gradual stretching of the pericardium.
- **Pericardial compliance:** a previously diseased and thickened pericardium is likely to be less distensible.
- **Intravascular volume:** tamponade will inhibit cardiac output to a greater extent during hypovolemia.

The pathophysiology of cardiac tamponade is complex, yet it explains a number of physical and hemodynamic findings. Pulsus paradoxus is one of the most consistent and important clinical features of cardiac tamponade. An understanding of its genesis may be helpful in understanding the physiology of tamponade.

Pulsus Paradoxus

As originally described in constrictive pericarditis, a paradoxic arterial pulse is said to be present when the cardiac rhythm is regular, and there are apparent "dropped beats" in the peripheral pulse during inspiration. Manometrically, pulsus paradoxus is present when there is a greater than 10-mm Hg decrease in systolic blood pressure during inspiration in the supine position. A few mm Hg of inspiratory decrease in arterial pressure is normal.

Pulsus paradoxus results from the inspiratory decrease in LV filling, caused by the dominance of augmented right heart filling (during inspiration) in the confined intrapericardial space. Inspiration creates a negative intrathoracic pressure that causes the left heart filling pressure to decrease. As the pulmonary vasculature becomes more compliant and the left atrium and its tributaries are subjected to a negative pressure, the overfilled extrathoracic systemic venous reservoir provides a more constant pressure head for right heart filling. Thus, the right heart dominates the limited intrapericardial cardiovascular space during inspiration and this augmented filling is translated into increased right heart output, which, in turn, causes an increase in left heart filling pressure as inspiration ends and expiration begins (20).

Figure 14.1 demonstrates the phasic swings in left heart filling pressure (pulmonary capillary wedge) and the relatively constant right atrial pressure, resulting in inspiratory inhibition of left heart filling and a marked decrease in arterial pulse amplitude—the paradoxic pulse. During apnea, there is an equilibration of atrial pressures, with "equal sharing" of the limited intrapericardial space and a steady arterial pressure.

Pulsus paradoxus is not diagnostic of cardiac tamponade and it may be noted in the following:

- Constrictive pericarditis
- Restrictive cardiomyopathy
- Shock

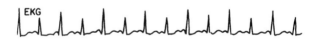

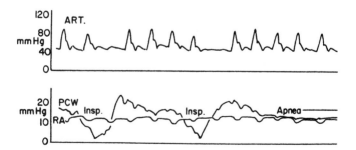

Fig. 14.1. Pulsus paradoxus. From the description of the mechanism of pulsus paradoxus, it should be apparent that ventricular filling in tamponade (and constrictive pericarditis) is dependent on systemic venous pressure (21).

- Pulmonary embolism
- Asthma, or severe obstructive airway disease
- Tension pneumothorax

Pulsus paradoxus may be absent in tamponade in the following settings (19):

- Hypovolemia
- Chronic LV dysfunction manifested by elevated LV diastolic pressure
- Atrial septal defect
- Pulmonary arterial obstruction
- Severe aortic regurgitation

Etiology

The most common causes of nontraumatic cardiac tamponade and their approximate frequency are as follows:

- Malignant disease—55%
- Idiopathic pericarditis—15%
- Uremia—15%
- Bacterial or mycobacterial infection—5%
- Anticoagulant therapy—5%
- Connective tissue disease—5%

Signs and Symptoms

The symptoms associated with cardiac tamponade are nonspecific. The patient most commonly will complain of intolerance to minimal activity and dyspnea. Congestive failure might be diagnosed and inappropriate and potentially dangerous therapy (diuresis) may be instituted if a careful history and attention to salient physical findings are ignored.

Physical Examination

Physical examination commonly reveals a decreased systolic blood pressure with a narrow pulse pressure and pulsus paradoxus. The absence of pulsus paradoxus of more than 15 mm Hg suggests that a pericardial effusion is not hemodynamically significant. A value of more than 25 mm Hg usually separates true tamponade from lesser degrees of cardiac filling impairment (20). Exceptions when an abnormal pulsus may not be present in the setting of tamponade were noted earlier in this chapter. The neck veins are distended, and examination of jugular venous pulsations reveals a rapid "x" descent and attenuated or absent "y" descent. Tachycardia, a compensatory mechanism to maintain cardiac output, usually is present. The apical impulse is indistinct, and the lateral border of cardiac dullness is displaced laterally. Cardiac auscultation commonly demonstrates "distant" heart sounds. Pulmonary rales are uncommon, but a pleural effusion may be present. There may be right-upper-quadrant tenderness as a result of hepatic engorgement.

Chest X-Ray

Chest x-ray may or may not demonstrate enlargement of the cardiac shadow, depending on the volume of intrapericardial fluid. The rapid accumulation of a relatively small amount of pericardial fluid may produce tamponade with minimal enlargement of the cardiac silhouette. On the lateral chest x-ray, an epicardial fat pad line may be seen within the cardiac silhouette. The pulmonary vasculature usually appears normal. Additional chest x-ray findings will be dependent on the etiology, such as mediastinal adenopathy, a lung mass, infiltrate, or the like.

Electrocardiogram

The ECG may demonstrate low-voltage QRS complexes, ST segment elevation, and PR segment depression characteristic of pericarditis or electrical alternans (beat-to-beat variation in P, R, and T wave amplitude). Alternans is seen in only 10% to 20% of cases of tamponade, and 50% to 60% of these cases are neoplastic in origin.

Echocardiography

In addition to pericardial fluid, the following echocardiographic and Doppler echo findings have been described in cardiac tamponade (22):

- Right atrial compression
- Right ventricular (RV) diastolic collapse
- Abnormal variations in ventricular dimension during respiration
- Abnormal variation in atrioventricular valve flow velocities with respiration
- Distended inferior vena cava without inspiratory collapse
- "Swinging" heart

Cardiac Catheterization

If cardiac catheterization is performed, equalization of right atrial, RV, pulmonary artery diastolic, pulmonary capillary wedge or left atrial, and LV end-diastolic pressures will be recorded during suspended respiration (Fig. 14.1). The intracardiac diastolic pressure will approximate intrapericardial pressure. A "dip and plateau" configuration of ventricular pressure, characteristic of constrictive pericarditis and restrictive cardiomyopathy, is not seen.

Treatment

Volume expansion with normal saline usually will increase cardiac output and blood pressure but is, at best, only a temporary measure. Pericardiocentesis may improve dramatically the hemodynamic status of the compromised patient.

Pericardiocentesis is a lifesaving procedure in patients with tamponade, but the procedure is potentially hazardous and should be performed with considerable care and under optimal circumstances. The potential hazards of cardiac perforation and coronary artery laceration can be minimized, and the therapeutic and diagnostic yield can be enhanced by appropriate planning and attention to detail (23).

Whenever possible, pressure from a pulmonary artery or right atrial catheter should be monitored before, during, and after pericardiocentesis. The presence of tamponade may be confirmed by a prompt decrease in central venous pressure attendant with pericardial fluid aspiration, and the recurrence of tamponade can be detected by an elevation of right heart pressures toward prepericardiocentesis levels.

Pericardiocentesis should be performed in the cardiac catheterization laboratory whenever circumstances permit. The availability of fluoroscopy, a defibrillator, and adequate laboratory facilities (e.g., hematocrit centrifuge) and the ease of ECG and pressure monitoring and recording in such a setting enhance the safety and diagnostic yield. Pericardiocentesis is best performed with the aid of two-dimensional echocardiography to help guide the needle away from vital structures, but it can be done without imaging if echocardiography is not readily available and severe hemodynamic compromise is present.

The subxiphoid approach with the patient sitting at a 45-degree angle is the preferred technique. A 16- to 18-gauge spinal needle is inserted between the xiphoid process and the left costal margin at a 30 to 45-degree angle to the skin. Alternatively, a catheter over a needle (Seldinger technique) can be used and a pig-tail can be catheter inserted and left in place for repeated aspiration if reaccumulation of fluid is expected. The needle is directed toward the left shoulder. The V lead of an ECG monitor electrode can be attached to the needle to detect epicardial contact (ST segment elevation on the V lead recording) and prevent ventricular puncture. As much fluid as possible should be aspirated, and samples should be sent for appropriate studies.

As noted earlier, if there is tamponade, monitoring of right heart pressures will confirm the diagnosis because withdrawal of fluid will cause a prompt decrease in filling pressure. If there is no decrease in venous pressure despite fluid removal, the diagnosis of tamponade is in doubt.

CONSTRICTIVE PERICARDITIS

Constrictive pericarditis is clinically and pathologically distinct from acute pericarditis. Following pericardial injury, a chronic reparative process characterized by fibrous thickening of the layers of the pericardium may occur. When this process advances to the point where diastolic filling of the normally distensible cardiac chambers is prevented by a nondistensible, thickened pericardium, "constriction" is said to be present.

Etiology

By its nature, constrictive pericarditis is most commonly a chronic process and the end result of a remote and/or occult episode of acute pericarditis or pericardial injury. Common causes include the following:

- Previous open-heart surgery
- Idiopathic
- Mediastinal radiation
- Bacterial or tuberculous pericarditis
- Renal failure

In nearly 50% of cases, a specific etiology is never determined. Such cases usually are ascribed to a previous, clinically inapparent viral pericarditis (24,25).

Signs and Symptoms

The patient with constrictive pericarditis most commonly presents with symptoms that mimic congestive heart failure; edema and ascites are often more pronounced than orthopnea and dyspnea. Careful physical examination may provide the initial clues to the presence of constrictive pericarditis. Pulsus paradoxus may or may not be present. Although the neck veins are distended, the lungs are clear, the heart is not enlarged, and the precordium is not overactive. Examination of the jugular venous pulsations reveals a rapid "y" descent. Kussmaul's sign, inspiratory increase in venous pressure, may be noted. During cardiac auscultation, an early diastolic sound, a pericardial knock 60–120 msec after the second heart sound, may be heard. A pericardial knock occurs later than an opening snap and slightly earlier than an S3, which it may mimic. Hepatosplenomegaly may be present along with ascites.

Chest X-Ray

The chest x-ray most commonly shows a normal or slightly enlarged cardiac silhouette and clear lung fields with normal pulmonary vasculature. Pericardial calcification may be seen in approximately 50% of patients with constrictive pericarditis and is best seen on a lateral chest x-ray.

Electrocardiogram

The ECG shows no diagnostic features.

Echocardiography

Echocardiography and chest computed tomography (CT) occasionally demonstrate pericardial thickening. Echocardiographic septal motion may be abnormal, and the LV wall shows abrupt cessation of outward motion during early diastole. The pattern of transmitral flow variation observed with Doppler echo is comparable to that observed in cardiac tamponade. However, a prominent "y" descent is often is observed on hepatic vein or superior vena cava Doppler study (26).

Computed Tomography and Magnetic Resonance Imaging

Both CT imaging and magnetic resonance imaging of the heart have been shown to be of diagnostic value in suspected constrictive pericarditis (27).

Cardiac Catheterization

Cardiac catheterization and hemodynamic assessment are the most important diagnostic studies. Typical hemodynamic features include the following:

1. Rapid "x" and "y" descent in the right atrial pressure trace
2. Early diastolic pressure "dip and plateau" configuration in the right ventricle (Fig. 14.2)
3. Equalization of increased diastolic pressures in the right atrium, right ventricle, left ventricle, and pulmonary artery
4. Elevated RV and pulmonary arterial pressures

These hemodynamic findings are by no means diagnostic of constrictive pericarditis. Similar pressures may be noted in patients with restrictive cardiomyopathy. Left heart catheterization may serve to differentiate the two (see Chapter 13). In addition, characteristic Doppler echocardiographic abnormalities also may serve to differentiate the two (28,29).

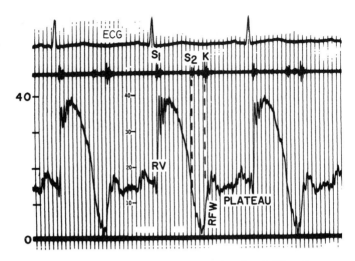

Fig. 14.2.   Constrictive pericarditis. The characteristic diastole "dip and plateau" or "square wave" configuration of right ventricular (*RV*) pressure in constrictive pericarditis is demonstrated. A similar configuration was noted in the left ventricle. At the onset of diastole, inflow into the ventricles from the distended atria is rapid, producing an abrupt increase in intraventricular pressure corresponding to the rapid filling wave (*RFW*) shown in the figure. Later, diastolic inflow is inhibited as the expanding ventricles encounter noncompliant pericardium. Early equalization of atrial and ventricular pressures and the near cessation of diastolic inflow result in a high-pressure plateau of equal magnitude in all cardiac chambers. A simultaneous phonocardiogram demonstrates the presence of a diastolic knock (*K*) occurring approximately 0.12 seconds after the second heart sound (*S2*). This sound is heard during the rapid-filling phase of diastole as ventricular filling suddenly is inhibited by the constricting pericardium (time lines = 0.04 seconds).

Therapy

Surgical pericardial stripping generally is effective in symptomatic individuals.

REFERENCES

1. Oakley CM: Myocarditis, pericarditis, and other pericardial diseases. *Heart* 84:449, 2000.
2. Spodick DH: Pericardial disease. In: Braunwald E, Zipes DP, Libby P, eds. *Heart disease: a textbook of cardiovascular medicine*, 6th ed. Philadelphia: WB Saunders Co., p. 1823, 2002.
3. Niemann JT: The cardiomyopathies, myocarditis, and pericardial heart disease. In: Tintinalli JE, Kelen GD, Stapczynski JS, eds. *Emergency medicine: a comprehensive study guide*, 5th ed. St. Louis: McGraw Hill, p. 387, 2000.
4. Krishnaswamy G, Chi DS, Kelly JL, et al.: The cardiovascular and metabolic complications of HIV infection. *Cardiol Rev* 8:260, 2000.
5. Go C, Asnis DS, Saltzman H: Pneumococcal pericarditis since 1980. *Clin Infect Dis* 27:1338, 1998.
6. Brook I, Frazier EH: Microbiology of acute purulent pericarditis. A

12-year experience in a military hospital. *Arch Intern Med* 156:1857, 1996.

7. Langley RL, Treadwell EL: Cardiac tamponade and pericardial disorders in connective tissue diseases: case report and literature review. *JAMA* 86:149, 1994.

8. Keefe DL: Cardiovascular emergencies in cancer patients. *Semin Oncol* 27:244, 2000.

9. Gunukula SR, Spodick DH: Pericardial disease in renal patients. *Semin Nephrol* 21:52: 2001.

10. di Caserta OP: Pericardial involvement in acute myocardial infarction in the post-thrombolytic era: clinical meaning and value. *Clin Cardiol* 20:327, 1997.

11. Prince SE, Cunha BA: Postpericardiotomy syndrome. *Heart Lung* 26:165, 1997.

12. Bonnefoy E, Godon P, Kirkorian G, et al: Serum cardiac troponin I and ST-segment elevation in patients with acute pericarditis. *Eur Heart J* 21;832, 2000.

13. Brandt RR, Filzmaier K, Hanrath P: Circulating cardiac troponin I in acute pericarditis. *Am J Cardiol* 87:1326, 2001.

14. Chandraratna PA: Echocardiography and Doppler ultrasound in the evaluation of pericardial disease. *Circulation* 84(Suppl I):I-303, 1991.

15. Zayas R, Anguita M, Torres F, et al: Incidence of specific etiology and role of methods for specific etiologic diagnosis of primary acute pericarditis. *Am J Cardiol* 75:378, 1995.

16. Nugue O, Millaire A, Porte H, et al: Pericardioscopy in the etiologic diagnosis of pericardial effusion in 141 consecutive patients. *Circulation* 94:1645, 1996.

17. Adler Y, Finkelstein Y, Guindo J, et al: Colchicine treatment for recurrent pericarditis. A decade of experience. *Circulation* 97:2183, 1998.

18. Sagrista-Sauleda J, Angel J, Permanyer-Miralda G, et al.: Long-term follow-up of idiopathic chronic pericardial effusion. *N Engl J Med* 341:2052, 1999.

19. Folwer NO: Cardiac tamponade. A clinical or an echocardiographic diagnosis? *Circulation* 87:1738, 1993.

20. Curtiss EI, Reddy PS, Uretsky BF, et al.: Pulsus paradoxus: definition and relation to the severity of cardiac tamponade. *Am Heart J* 115: 391, 1988.

21. Cogwell TL, Bernath GA, Wann, et al: Effects of intravascular volume state on the value of pulsus paradoxus and right ventricular diastolic collapse in predicting cardiac tamponade. *Circulation* 72:1076, 1985.

22. Zhang S, Kerins DM, Byrd BF 3rd: Doppler echocardiography in cardiac tamponade and constrictive pericarditis. *Echocardiography* 11: 507, 1994.

23. Spodick DH: The technique of pericardiocentesis. When to perform it and how to minimize complications. *J Crit Illn* 10:807, 1995.

24. Myers RB, Spodick DH: Constrictive pericarditis: clinical and pathologic characteristics. *Am Heart J* 138 (2Pt1):219, 1999.

25. Ling LH, Oh JK, Schaff HV, et al: Constrictive pericarditis in the modern era: evolving clinical spectrum and impact on outcome after pericardiectomy. *Circulation* 100:1380, 1999.

26. Kronzon I, Tunick PA, Freedberg RS: Transesophageal echocardiography in pericardial disease and tamponade. *Echocardiography* 11: 493, 1994.

27. Breen JF: Imaging of the pericardium. *J Thorac Imaging* 16:47, 2001.

28. Hancock EW: Differential diagnosis of restrictive cardiomyopathy and constrictive pericarditis. *Heart* 86:343, 2001.
29. Rajagopalan N, Garcia MJ, Rodriquez L, et al: Comparison of new Doppler echocardiographic methods to differentiate constrictive pericardial heart disease and restrictive cardiomyopathy. *Am J Cardiol* 87:86, 2001.

SUDDEN CARDIAC DEATH

DEFINITION AND INCIDENCE

Sudden cardiac death (SCD) is best defined as the unexpected natural death from a cardiac cause within a short period, generally 1 hour or less from the onset of symptoms, in a person without any prior condition that would appear fatal (1). SCD is the leading cause of death in the United States, claiming approximately 350,000 victims annually. Approximately 30% of victims have no prior symptoms of heart disease, and SCD is often the first indication of clinical heart disease. Although the absolute number of cases of SCD has decreased in parallel with the reduction of overall cardiovascular mortality in the United States, the proportion of all cardiovascular deaths as a result of SCD has remained relatively constant at 50%. SCD most commonly occurs in the out-of-hospital setting and is associated with 80% to 90% mortality.

ETIOLOGY

The most common causes of SCD among descendants aged 35 years or older and their relative frequencies as determined by International Classification of Diseases—9 codes include the following (2):

- Coronary artery disease (CAD) (acute and chronic ischemic heart disease)—65%
- Cardiomyopathy and arrhythmias—9%
- Heart failure—7%
- Hypertensive heart disease—5%
- Carditis and valvular heart disease—2%
- Pulmonary heart disease—1%
- Cardiovascular disease, unspecified—12%

PATHOPHYSIOLOGY

Severe atherosclerotic CAD (i.e., more than 70% occlusion of one or more of the three major epicardial vessels) is found in the majority of victims of SCD. The extent and degree of involvement is typically greater than that encountered in patients presenting with acute myocardial infarction (AMI) or angina pectoris as their first symptom of CAD. Despite the severity of CAD, only about 30% of victims will have pathologic evidence of an acute thrombotic coronary occlusion or enzymatic evidence of AMI (in those victims who are resuscitated successfully). However, 70% to 80% will have evidence of prior infarction, myocardial fibrosis (scar), and depressed left ventricular (LV) function (3,4).

This myocardial substrate of obstructive CAD, chronic ischemia, and myocardial fibrosis is a predisposition to arrhythmias (5). Ambulatory monitoring has demonstrated that ventricular tachyarrhythmias most commonly precede or cause SCD. Ventricular fibrillation

(VF) typically is preceded by frequent premature ventricular contractions (PVCs) or monomorphic or polymorphic ventricular tachycardia. Bradyarrhythmias are less common (10% to 20% of monitored cases). Various "triggers" acting on the myocardial substrate have been described and include acute ischemia, electrolytic abnormalities (hypokalemia and hypomagnesemia), autonomic influences, circulating catecholamines, and cardioactive drugs that have proarrhythmia effects.

RISK OF SUDDEN CARDIAC DEATH

It has been estimated that the risk of SCD in the unselected adult population is two per 1,000 persons per year. Therefore, screening of unselected patients is impractical. Based on the pathophysiology of SCD, it has been more practical to focus on patient groups with known heart disease and attempt risk stratification. Risk is best represented in relative terms and can be estimated as follows in terms of average annual risk (6):

- Sudden death survivors (SCD not associated with AMI)—10% to 30% average annual risk
- Dilated cardiomyopathy—10%
- First year post-myocardial infarction (MI)—5%
- Hypertrophic cardiomyopathy—1% to 3%
- Long QT syndrome—1% to 3%
- U.S. adult population—0.22%

APPROACHES TO THE PROBLEM OF SUDDEN CARDIAC DEATH (7)

The Patient with Structural Heart Disease Who Has Survived Sudden Cardiac Death

In the absence of an acute infarction, the SCD recurrence rate may be as high as 50% at 2 years. In patients who have been resuscitated from SCD, an aggressive assessment and management program should be pursued. However, the extent of evaluation and interventions should be guided logically by the likelihood of a meaningful functional recovery (7).

Transient abnormalities that may have facilitated or "triggered" the development of a sustained and hemodynamically unstable rhythm should be investigated. Such abnormalities would include, but are not limited to, serum electrolyte abnormalities, drug toxicity (particularly digoxin antiarrhythmics with proarrhythmic effects), or pacemaker malfunction in patients with permanent pacemakers. However, patients with VF or tachycardia associated with "transient correctable causes" that were included in the AVID (Antiarrhythmics Versus Implantable Defibrillators) trial had a mortality rate of nearly 18% within approximately 18 months of follow-up. This risk was similar to the general group of VF arrest survivors (8).

Echocardiography should be performed to assess the presence of other cardiac causes of SCD other than CAD, particularly valvular heart disease and hypertrophic cardiomyopathy. Echocardiography also will allow a determination of wall motion and ejection fraction. Radionuclide angiography also can be performed to evaluate ventricular function.

Cardiac catheterization should be performed to evaluate coronary anatomy and the extent of disease. Significant stenosis of the left main coronary artery, severe multivessel CAD, or a ventricular aneurysm detected at catheterization may dictate early surgical intervention. Several studies suggest that coronary revascularization may provide antiarrhythmic benefits (9). However, revascularization alone provides incomplete protection from recurrent SCD in this high-risk group (10).

Three large, randomized, multicenter trials addressed the use of an implantable cardioverter defibrillator (ICD) versus antiarrhythmic drug therapy in secondary prevention of SCD (8,11,12). Taken together, these studies demonstrate that ICD therapy is superior to the "best" antiarrhythmic drug therapy (amiodarone, metoprolol, sotalol, or propafenone was used in most trials) in patients with structural heart disease and sustained ventricular arrhythmias (13). The greatest benefit was observed in patients with the lowest ejection fractions. ICDs are the current therapy of choice for the secondary prevention of SCD in patients with preexisting structural heart disease (14). Although such patients usually also are treated with antiarrhythmics, there is no clear benefit on outcome of adding electrophysiologically guided antiarrhythmic drug selection (i.e., suppression of inducible sustained ventricular arrhythmias) (15).

The Patient Who Has Sustained a Myocardial Infarction

The incidence of SCD in patients with known CAD and prior MI is 10 to 100 times that of the general population. Of those patients with SCD resulting from coronary disease, about 50% will have a prior history of coronary disease.

In the prerecanalization (thrombolytic therapy or percutaneous coronary intervention) era, if SCD (VF) occurred during the course of an AMI (within 48 hours of the event) and the patient survived, the risk of SCD recurrence after discharge was no greater than that in the general post-MI population whose early course was not complicated by VF or tachycardia (16). In patients who receive thrombolytic therapy, primary VF within the first 48 hours does not increase the risk of SCD after discharge (17).

In the absence of contraindications, all patients who are post-MI should be receiving beta blockers. These drugs have both antiarrhythmic and antiischemic properties and have been shown in numerous large-scale studies to improve long-term survival (3 or more years) after AMI. These studies are reviewed in Chapter 9. In practice, this group of drugs is underutilized. Additional beneficial interventions in this group include lifestyle modification, serum cholesterol lowering, and daily aspirin therapy.

Data from the Coronary Artery Surgery Study (CASS) indicate that revascularization is beneficial in preventing SCD. Patients in high-risk subgroups with three-vessel disease and depressed LV function appear to derive the greatest benefit (9).

In contrast to beta blocker trials, many studies evaluating the routine use of other conventional antiarrhythmic drugs in post-MI patients with ventricular arrhythmias have yielded negative results. These trials have been subjected to meta-analysis methods that demonstrate a worse outcome or no difference in outcome for treatment groups, with the exception of amiodarone, when compared to groups who did not receive treatment or who received placebo (13). Currently, there are no data to support the routine use of conventional antiarrhythmic drug therapy for PVC suppression in asymptomatic patients after MI. The lack of a beneficial effect most likely is the result of proarrhythmic effects of the treatment drugs.

Amiodarone has been shown in several studies to be efficacious in preventing SCD in post-MI patients (18,19). These studies differ with respect to comparative study groups and the inclusion of patients at high or moderate risk of SCD or those who are asymptomatic. In the BASIS (Basel Antiarrhythmic Study of Infarct Survival) investigation, post-MI patients with frequent and complex but asymptomatic ventricular ectopy during Holter monitoring were randomized to individualized conventional antiarrhythmic therapy, empiric amiodarone (200 mg/day), or no antiarrhythmic therapy. At 1 year, the probability of survival was significantly greater in the amiodarone group when compared to the control group. A significant reduction in arrhythmic events also was observed in the amiodarone group. Significant benefits were not observed in the conventional treatment group (20). Patients treated with amiodarone who had preserved LV function (ejection fraction more than 40%) derived greater mortality benefit than those with ejection fraction of less than 40% (21). Similar differences between patients treated with amiodarone and post-MI patients with asymptomatic high-grade ventricular ectopy treated with placebo were observed in the CAMIAT (Canadian Amiodarone Myocardial Infarction Arrhythmia Trial) investigation (10% all-cause mortality at 2 years in the amiodarone group versus 21% in the placebo group) (22). Comparatively low doses of amiodarone have been used in amiodarone postinfarction trials, yet noncardiac toxicity remains a problem.

ICDs in selected post-MI patients also may decrease the risk of SCD. In patients who are post-MI with an ejection fraction of less than 30% and who have complex ventricular ectopy, prophylactic ICD therapy has been shown to decrease mortality over more than 2 years of follow-up when compared to antiarrhythmic drugs, including amiodarone and beta blockers, when given empirically or guided by programmed stimulation results (13,23).

The Patient Without Structural Heart Disease Who Has Survived Sudden Cardiac Death

Only about 5% of survivors of SCD are found to have no structural heart disease. These patients generally fall into one of three groups:

1. Congenital or acquired long QT syndrome (24)—management consists of discontinuing all drugs known to prolong the QT interval (25), pacing, use of beta blockers, and ICD therapy (14).
2. The Brugada syndrome (26)—recognized by right bundle branch conduction pattern, ST segment elevation in the anterior precordial leads, and a history of sustained ventricular arrhythmias or SCD. ICD therapy is recommended (14).
3. Idiopathic VF—usually diagnosed in the absence of both structural heart disease and long QT interval syndromes. ICD therapy is recommended.

REFERENCES

1. Zipes DP, Wellens HJJ: Sudden cardiac death. *Circulation* 98:2334, 1998.
2. Zheng Z, Croft JB, Giles WH, et al: Sudden cardiac death in the United States, 1989 to 1998. *Circulation* 104:2158, 2001.

3. Farb A, Tang AL, Burke AP, et al: Sudden coronary death. Frequency of active coronary lesions, inactive coronary lesions, and myocardial infarction. *Circulation* 92:1701, 1995.
4. Farb A, Burke AP, Tang AL, et al: Coronary plaque erosion without rupture into a lipid core. A frequent cause of coronary thrombosis in sudden coronary death. *Circulation* 93:1354, 1996.
5. Peters NS, Wit AL: Myocardial architecture and ventricular arrhythmogenesis. *Circulation* 97:1746, 1998.
6. Gilman JK, Naccarelli GV: Sudden cardiac death. *Curr Probl Cardiol* 17:695, 1992.
7. Callans DJ: Management of the patient who has been resuscitated from sudden cardiac death. *Circulation* 205:2704, 2002.
8. Anderson JL, Hallstrom AP, Epstein AE, et al: Design and results of the Antiarrhythmics versus Implantable Defibrillators Registry. *Circulation* 99:1692, 1999.
9. Holmes DR Jr, Davis KB, Mock MB, et al: The effect of medical and surgical treatment on subsequent sudden cardiac death in patients with coronary artery disease. A report from the coronary artery surgery study. *Circulation* 73:1254, 1986.
10. O'Rourke RA: Role of myocardial revascularization in sudden cardiac death. *Circulation* 85(Suppl I):I-112, 1992.
11. Connolly SJ, Gent M, Roberts RS, et al: Canadian Implantable Defibrillator Study (CIDS): a randomized trial of the Implantable cardioverter defibrillator against amiodarone. *Circulation* 101:1287, 2000.
12. Kuck KH, Cappato R, Siebels J, et al: Randomized comparison of antiarrhythmic drug therapy with implantable defibrillators in patients resuscitated from cardiac arrest: the cardiac arrest study Hamburg (CASH). *Circulation* 102:748, 2000.
13. Heidenreich PA, Keeffe B, McDonald KM, et al: Overview of randomized trials of antiarrhythmic drugs and devices for the prevention of sudden cardiac death. *Am Heart J* 144:422, 2002.
14. Gregoratos G, Abrams J, Epstein AE, et al: ACC/AHA/NASPE 2002 guideline update for implantation of cardiac pacemakers and antiarrhythmic devices: a report of the American College of Cardiology/ American Heart Association Task Force on Practice Guidelines. Available at www.acc.org.
15. Lee KL, Hafley G, Fisher JD, et al: Effect of Implantable defibrillators on arrhythmic events and mortality in the Multicenter Unsustained Tachycardia Trial. *Circulation* 106:233, 2002.
16. Tofler GH, Stone PH, Muller JE, et al: Prognosis after cardiac arrest due to ventricular tachycardia or ventricular fibrillation associated with acute myocardial infarction (the MILIS Study). *Am J Cardiol* 60:755, 1987.
17. Newby KH, Thompson T, Stebbins A, et al: Sustained ventricular arrhythmias in patients receiving thrombolytic therapy: incidence and outcomes. *Circulation* 98:2567, 1998.
18. Podrid PJ: Amiodarone: reevaluation of an old drug. *Ann Intern Med* 122:689, 1995.
19. Zamerbski DG, Nolan PE Jr, Slack MK, et al: Empiric long-term amiodarone prophylaxis following myocardial infarction. A meta-analysis. *Arch Intern Med* 153:2661, 1993.
20. Burkart F, Pfisterer M, Kiowski W, et al: Effect of antiarrhythmic therapy on mortality in survivors of myocardial infarction with asymptomatic complex ventricular arrhythmias: Basel Antiarrhythmic Study of Infarct Survival (BASIS). *J Am Coll Cardiol* 16:1711, 1990.

21. Pfisterer M, Kiowski W, Burckhardt D, et al: Beneficial effect of amiodarone on cardiac mortality in patients with asymptomatic complex ventricular arrhythmias after acute myocardial infarction and preserved but not impaired left ventricular function. *Am J Cardiol* 69: 1399, 1992.

22. Cairns JA, Connolly SJ, Gent M, et al: Post-myocardial infarction mortality in patients with ventricular premature depolarizations. Canadian Amiodarone Myocardial Infarction Arrhythmia Trial Pilot Study. *Circulation* 84:550, 1991.

23. Moss AJ, Zareba W, Hall J, et al: Prophylactic implantation of a defibrillator in patients with myocardial infarction and reduced ejection fraction. *N Engl J Med* 346:877, 2002.

24. Spooner PM, Albert C, Benjamin EJ, et al: Sudden cardiac death, genes, and arrhythmogenesis. Consideration of new population and mechanistic approaches from a National Heart, Lung, and Blood Institute Workshop, Part I. *Circulation* 103:2361, 2001. Part II. *Circulation* 103:2447, 2001.

25. Tan HL, Hou CJY, Lauer MR, et al: Electrophysiologic mechanisms of the long QT interval syndromes and torsade de pointes. *Ann Intern Med* 122:701, 1995.

26. Naccarelli GV, Antzelevitch C: The Brugada syndrome: clinical, genetic, cellular, and molecular abnormalities. *Am J Med* 110:573, 2001.

CARDIAC PACEMAKERS

Electrical devices for the heart have changed rapidly over recent years, with both increasing complexity and miniaturization. A basic knowledge of their purposes and modes of operation allows for simple clinical evaluation at time of implantation or follow-up evaluation. This chapter will discuss temporary and permanent pacemakers.

TEMPORARY PACEMAKERS

With the availability of effective external, transcutaneous pacemakers and a better understanding of the natural history of conduction system disease, the use of transvenous temporary pacemakers has declined. Indications for their use still include transient bradyarrhythmia or clinical situations with a high risk of transient bradyarrhythmia. Whenever possible, a patient with an inadequate rhythm without a defined reversible cause should be considered for early or immediate permanent pacing to avoid the risks and costs of temporary pacing.

Transient bradyarrhythmias most often are seen in drug toxicity. Digitalis excess can be treated effectively with antibody therapy, but may require temporary pacing until the onset of antibody effects. Beta blockers and calcium channel blockers, especially verapamil and diltiazem, either alone or in combination, can induce symptomatic sinus bradycardia or atrioventricular (AV) block requiring temporary pacing. The class IA antiarrhythmics also may produce AV block.

Prophylactic temporary pacing is indicated in acute myocardial infarction where development of AV and bundle branch block increases the risk of complete AV block. Table 16.1 summarizes these situations where the risk of developing symptomatic complete AV block may be significant (more than 20%). Most of these patients have large anterior infarctions, and outcome is related more to left ventricular function than the need for pacing. Inferior infarctions may develop AV block above the His bundle. With a stable, narrow QRS junctional rhythm, these patients rarely require pacing. Other situations, such as asymptomatic bifascicular block and asymptomatic Wenckebach type 1 AV block, are not considered indications for prophylactic pacing.

Temporary pacing is indicated in a few other special circumstances. Bradycardia-dependent arrhythmia such as torsade de pointes in the setting of sinus bradycardia and long QT interval may be managed with temporary transvenous pacing. Overdrive pacing of the right atrium may be used to terminate an AV reentrant rhythm unresponsive to drug therapy.

Approaches to Temporary Pacing

Transvenous temporary pacing remains the standard approach for prolonged patient support, with external pacing suitable only for

Table 16.1.   Indications for prophylactic pacing in acute myocardial infarction

Indicated	Not indicated	Controversial
Mobitz II AV block	1° AV block	New LBBB
Complete AV block	Mobitz I AV block	New RBBB in IMI
New RBBB in AMI	Old LBBB	
RBBB + LAFB	Old RBBB	
RBBB + LPFB		
LBBB +1° AV block		
Symptomatic bradycardia		

AMI, anterior myocardial infarction; AV, artrioventricular; IMI, inferior myocardial infarction; LAFB, left anterior fascicular block; LBBB, left bundle branch block; LPFB, left posterior fascicular block; RBBB, right bundle branch block.

standby or brief capture of the heart. The transthoracic route no longer is used.

Very emergent transvenous pacing can be accomplished from the right internal jugular vein with blind or electrocardiogram-guided placement into the right ventricle. When the patient's condition allows, more controlled conditions with full sterility and fluoroscopic guidance are preferred. In the subclavian vein approach, the wire can be secured well to the chest wall and subsequent patient mobility is less restricted. The femoral vein approach still is used, but leg movement can displace the wire.

Many pacing catheters (pacing leads) are available and usually are bipolar with both anode and cathode near the wire tip. The pacing lead for temporary pacing may have a fixed curve or inflatable balloon on the tip, similar to a flow-directed pulmonary artery catheter, to facilitate placement in the right ventricle. Complications vary with the site and include bleeding, ventricular arrhythmias, thrombosis, pneumothorax, inadvertent arterial puncture, and infection. Cardiac perforation with tamponade is a rare problem.

Once positioned, the catheter is tied to the skin and sterile dressing is placed. Usually, a connecting cable is used, with the distal wire connected to the negative pole. All connections need to be checked daily with a "tug test" because some connections screw tightly clockwise and seem opposite to normal hardware. Rate and output adjustment are straightforward, with daily check of capture threshold. The output is set at two to three times threshold. The sensitivity "dial" is most sensitive to the far right and least sensitive to the far left. To the extreme left is no sensing, or asynchronous pacing.

PERMANENT PACEMAKERS

Indications for Permanent Pacing

Guidelines for implantation of cardiac pacemakers have been standardized and are updated when new evidence of benefit becomes available. Common indications for permanent pacing are enumerated in Table 16.2.

Pacemaker Types

The four most common permanent pacemakers are listed in Table 16.3. A letter code, initially established in 1974 and since revised as technology has advanced, standardizes nomenclature for the pacemaker type or pacing mode. Although there are five positions in the code, the fifth position rarely is used. Most commonly, only the first three letters of the code are used. Table 16.4 includes an explanation of the first four positions and potential abbreviations in each category.

Using Table 16.4, one should be able to understand the features of any pacing mode. For example, an AAIR is capable of atrial pacing and atrial sensing, is inhibited by intrinsic atrial activity, and has rate-adaptive capability; a VDD pacemaker is capable of pacing the ventricle and sensing both atrial and ventricular intrinsic activity and responds by inhibiting ventricular pacing in the presence of intrinsic ventricular activity and triggering a paced ventricular beat response to a sensed atrial. Fig. 16.1 is a typical algorithm for the selection of an optimal pacing system for an individual patient.

PACEMAKER FACTS

- Magnetic resonance imaging (MRI) is contraindicated for patients with pacemakers because MRI can cause inhibition of the pacemaker.
- During radiofrequency ablation in patients with a pacemaker, a programmer should be available during the procedure because

Table 16.2. Indications for permanent pacing

I. Definite indications
   A. Symptomatic rhythms
      - Second- or third-degree heart blocks
      - Sinus bradycardia
      - Tachycardia–bradycardia syndrome
      - Bundle branch block with prolonged H-V interval and no other cause of symptoms
      - Recurrent syncope with demonstration of carotid sinus hypersensitivity
   B. Asymptomatic rhythms
      - Mobitz II block with demonstration of block below the his bundle
      - Third-degree block within His-Purkinje system
      - Alternating bundle branch block
      - Bifasicular block with H-V >100 msec
II. Pacing is not indicated.
      - Asymptomatic sinus mode dysfunction
      - Asymptomatic block in the atrioventricular node (1° or 2° Mobitz I)
      - Asymptomatic bifasicular block in the absence of evidence of unstable His-Purkinje conduction

Table 16.3.   Common permanent pacemakers

Code	Indication	Advantages	Disadvantages
VVI	Intermittent backup pacing inactive patient	Simplicity, limited cost	Fixed rate, loss of atrial transport, potential pacemaker syndrome
VVIR	Atrial fibrillation	Rate responsiveness	Requires appropriate programming
DDD	Complete heart block	Atrial tracking restores normal physiology	If sick sinus develops no rate responsiveness, requires two leads and more programming
DDDR	Sinus node dysfunction, atrioventricular block, and need for guaranteed rate responsiveness	Universal pacemaker, all options available by programming	Complexity, expense, programming, and follow-up

Table 16.4.   Pacemaker codes

Position category	I Chamber(s) paced	II Chamber(s) sensed	III Modes of responses	IV Programmable functions
Letters used	A=Atrium V=Ventricle D=Dual	A=Atrium V=Ventricle D=Dual O=None	I=Inhibited T=Triggered O-Asynchronous	P=Programmable (rate and/or output) M=Multiprogrammable R=Rate adaptive

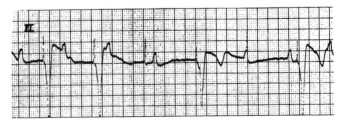

Fig. 16.1.   Selection of pacing mode.

radiofrequency energy can result in reprogramming of a pace-maker.

- External defibrillation can result in reprogramming of a permanent pacemaker, transient elevation in pacing/sensing threshold, circuitry damage, or localized myocardial necrosis if the energy is transmitted through the leads.
- Class IC antiarrhythmic drugs are the only ones that result in significant elevation in pacing and/or sensing threshold.
- Hyperkalemia is the most common metabolic disturbance to increase pacing thresholds.
- Currently used microwave ovens no longer interfere with pacemaker function. However, cellular phones may alter programmed pacing parameters if held near the pacemaker pulse generator.

PACEMAKER PROBLEMS AND COMPLICATIONS

Infection

Infection complicates 2% to 5% of pacemaker insertions. This complication includes wound infection, a deep-seeded infection of the "pocket" created for the pulse generator, bacteremia, and infection of the pacing lead. Infectious complications typically occur within 30 days of implantation. Clinical findings include pain, superficial cellulitis, and swelling at the site of the pulse generator. The majority of infections are the result of *Staphylococcus aureus* or *S. epidermidis*, and approximately 20% to 25% of patients with an apparent local infection have positive blood cultures.

Thrombophlebitis and Thrombosis

Thrombosis and thrombophlebitis are encountered in 30% to 50% of patients following permanent pacemaker insertion. These complications typically are seen within less than 60 days of implantation.

However, only 1% to 3% of patients develop symptoms as a result of extensive collateralization in the upper extremity. Typical symptoms include edema, pain, and venous engorgement of the arm ipsilateral to the side of pacemaker lead insertion. The superior vena cava syndrome and pulmonary embolism have been reported following pacemaker insertion, but they are rare. Duplex ultrasonography, conventional venography, or contrast computed tomography of the affected arm are effective in diagnosis. Usual therapy includes intravenous heparin and long-term warfarin use. Thrombolytic therapy may be efficacious if undertaken within 10 days of symptom onset.

The Pacemaker Syndrome

In the 1970s, it became evident that after ventricular pacemaker placement, some patients became more symptomatic, developing fatigue, dyspnea, and limited exercise output, even to the point of heart failure. This came to be known as the pacemaker syndrome, and occurs in 7% to 20% of patients with VVI pacemakers. In VVI pacing, the AV synchrony is lost. Losing atrial transport and filling of the ventricles in late diastole may decrease cardiac output 20% to 40%, especially in noncompliant stiff ventricle. If retrograde ventriculoatrial conduction occurs with retrograde P waves after the ventricular paced event, the atria contracting on closed AV valves and sending blood backward during early diastole. This may further decrease cardiac output and cause symptomatic cannon waves. The pacemaker syndrome has been resolved with dual-chamber pacing. The atrial lead usually is placed in a high right atrial appendage. Current pacemakers can be programmed effectively for the optimum atrial and ventricular sensing and pacing and AV interval.

In the 1980s, the first ventricular rate-adaptive pacemaker became available; later in the decade, the dual-chamber rate-adaptive pacemaker also became available. In patients with chronotropic incompetence, rate-adaptive pacing is important to provide adequate heart rate response to exercise. The pacing system might be VVIR, DDDR, DDDIR, or AAIR, depending on the presence of associated AV nodal conduction disease and atrial arrhythmia. Up to 40% to 50% of patients with complete heart block have sinus-node dysfunction. Because conduction disease can be progressive, it is important to make certain that patients with complete AV block undergo some evaluation of sinus-node function to determine if rate-adaptive pacing will provide additional benefit.

Pacemaker Malfunction

Pacemaker malfunction can be classified broadly as failure to pace or failure to sense. True electrical malfunction is relatively uncommon. Abrupt failure of the pacemaker generator (battery) is rarely a cause of pacemaker malfunction because of the long life of current lithium batteries (typically more than 7 years) and the frequent follow-up visits afforded patients with pacemakers. Battery depletion usually is detected long before cessation of pacing occurs. The use of tined or "screw-in" pacemaker leads typically prevents lead displacement from the atrial and/or ventricular endocardium. Most instances of suspected malfunction usually are related to programming problems or errors (e.g., undersensing or oversensing of spontaneous electrical activity) that can be corrected noninvasively with current technology. True life-threatening pacemaker emergencies rarely are encountered now.

SUGGESTED READING

Gregoratos G, Adams J, Epstein AE, et al: ACC/AHA/NASPE 2002 guideline update for implantation of cardiac pacemakers and antiarrhythmic devices. *J Am Coll Cardiol* 40:1703, 2002.

Kusumoto FM, Goldschlager N: Cardiac pacing. *N Engl J Med* 334:89, 1996.

Kusumoto FM, Goldschlager N: Device therapy for cardiac arrhythmias. *JAMA* 287:1848, 2002.

Kusumoto FM, Goldschlager NF: *Cardiac pacing for the clinician.* Baltimore: Lippincott Williams & Wilkins, 2000.

CARDIAC SURGERY

Surgery for Ischemic Heart Disease

Coronary artery bypass grafting (CABG) remains the most common cardiac surgical procedure performed in the United States, with more than 500,000 operations completed in 2000. Although there has been a trend toward operating on sicker and more elderly patients, results continue to improve, with overall mortality rates less than 3%. Advanced age continues to be the risk factor most consistently related to increased mortality.

There is a trend toward increasing the use of arterial grafts, which have better long-term patency rates when compared with saphenous vein bypass grafts. It has been recognized for many years that the left internal mammary is the optimum coronary artery bypass conduit, with a patency rate of more than 90% at 10-year follow-up (1). Furthermore, the use of the left internal mammary artery to the left anterior descending (LAD) correlates with improved long-term survival over patients with vein grafts to the heart (2). There is continued increasing use of bilateral internal mammary artery revascularization. The radial artery frequently subject to arterial spasm, but it can be used as a graft that is readily available, is easily obtained, and has better long-term patency than saphenous vein grafts (3). Although not quite as good as the internal mammary artery, the radial artery patency rates at 5 years is 85% (4). The right gastroepiploic artery also has been grafted successfully to arteries on the diaphragmatic surface of the heart (5).

Minimally invasive techniques for CABG are generating an enormous amount of interest in both the medical and lay literature. These techniques allow surgeons to perform single and sometimes multiple coronary bypass operations through small anterior thoracotomy incisions instead of the traditional median sternotomy. With the minimally invasive direct coronary artery bypass (MIDCAB) procedure, the left internal mammary artery is anastomosed to the LAD with the heart beating, thus avoiding the risks of cardiopulmonary bypass and cardiac arrest (6,7). Whereas advantages include shortened hospital stays with the potential for less morbidity and earlier return to normal activity, there is concern that long-term patency rates of these technically more difficult anastomoses will be inferior to those performed with the heart arrested. Furthermore, the MIDCAB procedure tends to be limited to patients with single- or two-vessel disease.

Advances in surgical technique and instrumentation such as stabilizers now allow most coronary artery bypass operations to be performed on a beating heart without the need for cardiopulmonary bypass (8). Off-pump coronary bypass surgery has many advantages (Table 17.1). The higher-risk patients stand to benefit the most (9).

Minimally invasive endoscopic vein harvesting has become the new standard of care in the CABG procedure. It has the benefits of reduced pain, smaller incisions, low wound complications, and accelerated ambulation.

**Table 17.1.   Advantages of
off-pump coronary artery bypass**

Avoidance of cardiopulmonary bypass complications
Less systemic inflammatory response
Decreased heparin requirement
Less blood loss
Shorter operations
No global ischemia
Less hypotension
Less central nervous system and cognitive impairment

Coronary bypass grafting still is performed with cardiopulmonary bypass in some subsets of patients. Young patients (younger than age 55) with low cerebrovascular accident rates where maximum patency is a prime concern, unstable patients, and patients with small diffusely diseased arteries are still candidates for standard cardiopulmonary bypass techniques.

Hybrid procedures involve integrated coronary revascularization using MIDCAP to the LAD combined with percutaneous interventions of the other vessels. This secures the left internal mammary artery to the LAD and is safe and effective. Despite some obvious advantages, hybrid procedures represent only a small minority of cases.

SURGERY FOR CHRONIC CONGESTIVE HEART FAILURE

Surgery for patients with end-stage congestive heart failure currently is limited to heart transplantation, frequently after a period of left ventricular assistance with a mechanical device. The number of heart transplants performed in the United States each year is limited to approximately 2,000 because of the shortage of donor organs. Improved resuscitative techniques have the potential to expand the donor heart pool. As results with cardiac transplantation continue to improve with advances in immunosuppressive therapy and follow-up care, the selection criteria for donors and recipients are being relaxed. Patients older than age 60 have been shown to have similar early mortality and length of hospitalization as younger groups. Five-year survival ranges from 71% in older patients to 82% in younger patients (10). Hypercholesterolemia affects 60% to 80% of recipients and may contribute to coronary vasculopathy. Transplant atherosclerosis is responsible for many late deaths. HMG-CoA (3-hydroxy-3-methyl-glutaryl-CoA) reductase inhibitors reduce the level of cholesterol and appear to have the added advantage of decreasing the incidence of cardiac rejection (11). New devices have been used to provide hemodynamic support to the increasing number of patients awaiting cardiac transplantation. Left ventricular assist systems have significantly reduced pretransplantation mortality by improving renal and hepatic function and physical capacity (12).

New options are available to patients with ischemic cardiomyopathy when large anterior or posterior wall segments are noncontractile. Development of surgical ventricular restoration (SVR) procedures has achieved survival advantages (80% at 5 years) compared to medical therapy at acceptable operative mortality (approximately

12%) (13). These techniques alter the sphere-shaped ventricle and restore it to an elliptic shape and, thus, decrease wall stress. Revascularization plus ventricular restoration appears to be a promising approach.

SURGERY FOR VALVULAR HEART DISEASE

Progress continues to be made in the field of cardiac-valve surgery. The advantage of durability of mechanical valves has to be weighed against the risks of anticoagulation therapy and problems with thromboembolism. No current mechanical prosthesis is ideal, and all require chronic anticoagulation. Current generation mechanical valves offer low profile and superior hemodynamics over the older, caged-ball prostheses (Starr-Edwards, Smeloff-Cutter valves). The Medtronic-Hall valve is a pivoting-disk mechanical prosthesis that is extremely low profile. The St. Jude and Carbomedics valves are hinged, bileaflet valves that are popular among cardiac surgeons because of their excellent hemodynamics and ease of implantation (14).

Cryopreserved aortic homografts offer durability in younger patients without the need for anticoagulation. They require special techniques for procurement, storage, and implantation. They particularly are applicable for patients with native or prosthetic valve endocarditis (15).

The Ross procedure is particularly effective in young patients with aortic valve disease. This technique involves replacing the patient's diseased aortic valve with his or her own pulmonic valve and reimplanting the coronary arteries. The pulmonary valve then is replaced with a pulmonary homograft. The Ross procedure offers superior longevity over bioprostheses in younger patients, as well as the advantage of not requiring anticoagulation (16).

Bioprostheses continue to be the valve replacements of choice in older patients, especially those older than age 70. Three popular bioprostheses are available in the United States: The Hancock and Carpentier-Edwards valves, which are both porcine bioprostheses, and the Baxter pericardial valve, which is constructed from bovine pericardium. Bioprostheses are not composed of living tissue; they are a combination of chemically treated biologic tissues and artificial material. In general, these valves have a low incidence of thromboembolism, especially in the aortic position. Many patients can go without anticoagulation, but anticoagulation still is advisable for patients with atrial fibrillation, atrial clots, or previous thromboembolism. The primary concern of bioprosthetic valves is valve durability. They are susceptible to primary valve failure as a result of calcification and structural deterioration, which tends to be accelerated in patients under the age of 40. Improvements in valve design and calcification-retardant techniques will prove to increase valve durability (17).

Mitral valve repair offers significant advantages over valve replacement in many patients with mitral valve disease. Surgical approaches that preserve the mitral apparatus result in substantial improvement in left ventricular function compared to replacement procedures in which the subvalvular apparatus is disrupted. Ideal patients for mitral valve repair are those with noncalcified valves and mitral regurgitation. Valve repair can include partial resection of leaflets; lengthening, shortening, transposition, or replacement of chorda tendineae; and placement of valvuloplasty rings to decrease the size of the mitral annulus (18). Transesophageal echocardiography (TEE) is the best tool to assess the competency of the repair in the operating room. TEE is also valuable to study the aortic root and gives morphologic data of the aortic annulus, sinus of Valsalva, and sinotubular junction. Echocardiographic normal bicuspid or tricuspid aortic valves are candidates for repair, such as cases of dilated aortic roots or patients with a bicuspid valve and prolapse of a single cusp.

In 1996, minimally invasive valve surgery began with new technology using smaller incisions, mandatory use of TEE, newer perfusion techniques, and modifications of repair and replacement techniques (19). Operative mortality is equal to or less than conventional open sternotomy cases, and the safety of the procedure has been established. Added benefits are shorter length of stay in the intensive care unit, less cost, less blood transfusions, and less atrial fibrillation. Candidates for this procedure include patients with isolated aortic, mitral, or tricuspid disease. Extremely ill (Class IV) patients with valvular disease such as a ruptured papillary muscle should undergo a standard sternotomy. Patients with severe chest wall abnormalities, as well as patients who cannot have a TEE probe placed should not have minimally invasive procedures.

As endoscopic cardiac surgery has gone from the realm of speculation to a clinical reality, robotics in cardiac surgery has emerged. Computer control systems and robotic manipulators likely will have a revolutionary impact in cardiac surgery, resulting in significant expansion of surgical ability and reduction in morbidity (20).

SURGERY FOR CONGENITAL HEART DISEASE

Approximately 20,000 operations of the heart and circulation in patients with congenital heart disease are performed each year in the United States. Nearly 80% of the first-year survivors live to reach adulthood (21). The trend in cardiac surgery for congenital heart disease has gone from palliative to staged anatomic correction to single-stage total repair. As a testament to the value of improved techniques and focused long-term follow-up care, it is estimated that there currently are more than 1 million people with adult congenital heart disease in the United States.

REFERENCES

1. Torelli G, Mantovani V, Maugeri R, et al: Comparison between single and double internal mammary artery grafts: results over ten years. *Ital Heart J* 2(6):423, 2001.
2. Dewar LRS, Jamieson WRE, Jenusz MR, et al: Unilateral versus bilateral internal mammary revascularization: survival and event-free performance. *Circulation* 92(Suppl II):II-8, 1995.
3. Fremes SE, Christakis GT, Del Rizzo DF, et al: The technique of radial artery bypass grafting and early clinical results. *J Card Surg* 10:537, 1995.
4. Acar C, Ramsheyi A, Pagny JV, et al: The radial artery for coronary artery bypass grafting: clinical and angiographic results at five years. *J Thorac Cardiovas Surg* 116:981, 1998.
5. Pyon J, Brown P, Pearson M, et al: Right gastroepiploic to coronary artery bypass. The first decade of use. *Circulation* 92(Suppl II):II-45, 1995.

6. Benetti FJ, Ballester C: Use of thoracoscopy and minimal thoracotomy in mammary-coronary bypass to left anterior descending artery without extracorporeal circulation. *J Cardiovasc Surg* 36:195, 1995.

7. Borst C, Jansen EWL, Tulleken CAF, et al: Coronary artery bypass grafting without cardiopulmonary bypass and without interruption of native coronary flow using a novel anastomosis site restraining device ("Octopus"). *J Am Coll Cardiol* 27:1356, 1996.

8. Mack MJ: Coronary surgery: off-pump and port access. *Surg Clin North Am* 80(5):1575, 2000.

9. Plomondon ME, Cleveland JC Jr, Ludwig ST, et al: Off-pump coronary artery bypass is associated with improved risk-adjusted outcomes. *Ann Thorac Surg* 72(1):114, 2001.

10. Bergin P, Rabinov M, Esmore D: Cardiac transplantation in patients over 60 years. *Transplant Proc* 27:2150, 1995.

11. Kobashigawa JA, Katznelson S, Laks H, et al: Effect of pravastatin on outcomes after cardiac transplantation. *N Engl J Med* 333:621, 1995.

12. Frazier OH, Rose EA, McCarthy P, et al: Improved mortality and rehabilitation of transplant candidates treated with long-term implantable left ventricular assist system. *Ann Surg* 222:327, 1995.

13. Beyersdorf F, Doenst T, Athanasuleas C, et al: The beating open heart for rebuilding ventricular geometry during surgical anterior resection. *Semin Thorac Cardiovasc Surg* 13(1):42, 2001.

14. Carlson D, Stephensen LW: Mechanical cardiac valves: current status. *Cardiol Clin* 3:439, 1995.

15. Kirklin JK, Kirklin JW, Pacifico AD: Homograft replacement of the aortic valve. *Cardiol Clin* 3:329, 1995.

16. Reddy VM, Rajasingke HA, McElhinney DB, et al: Extending the limits of the Ross procedure. *Ann Thorac Surg* 60(Suppl VI):VI-600, 1995.

17. Pupello DF, Bessone LN, Hibo SP, et al: Bioprosthetic valve longevity in the elderly: an 18 year longitudinal study. *Ann Thorac Surg* 60: 270, 1995.

18. Kumar AS: Chordal replacement or repair. *Ann Thorac Surg* 71(6): 2084, 2001.

19. Lytle BW: Minimally invasive cardiac surgery. *J Thorac Cardiovas Surg* 111(3):554, 1996.

20. Mohr FW, Falk V, Diegler A, et al: Computer enhanced "robotic" cardiac surgery: experience in 148 patients. *J Thorac Cardiovasc Surg* 121(5):842, 2001.

21. Moller JH, Taubert KA, Allen HD, et al: Cardiovascular health and disease in children: current status. *Circulation* 89:923, 1994.

CARDIAC DRUG THERAPY

This chapter is intended to provide a summary and ready-reference source for information regarding common drugs mentioned or discussed in some detail in the preceding chapters. The focus of this chapter is on the medications used to treat the more common problems encountered in cardiovascular medicine: ischemic heart disease, congestive heart failure (CHF), and arrhythmias.

ANTIARRHYTHMIC DRUGS

Several classifications have been proposed for drugs used for the treatment of cardiac arrhythmias. These classifications are based on the premise that drugs with similar electrophysiologic properties also have similar therapeutic effects, as well as toxicities. In practice, the choice of drugs is based largely on the results of controlled trials and clinical experience (Table 18.1). Such studies have demonstrated that, although drugs may have similar properties when tested in the experimental laboratory, they may have different effects in the clinical population (Table 18.2). The most common classification of antiarrhythmic drugs is the modified Vaughan-Williams Classification as noted in the following section (1).

Modified Vaughan-Williams Classification of Antiarrhythmic Drugs

Class IA

Class IA drugs depress or slow the rapid upstroke of the action potential (phase 1) and decrease conduction velocity (sodium channel blockade effect) and prolong repolarization (phase 3) (potassium channel blockade). Examples include quinidine, procainamide, and disopyramide.

Class IB

Class IB drugs have slow action potential upstroke in abnormal tissue and facilitate repolarization. These drugs have little effect on normal myocardial tissue. Examples include lidocaine, mexiletine, tocainide, and moricizine.

Class IC

Class IC drugs markedly slow phase 1 of action potential and decrease conduction velocity, but they exert little effect on phase 3 (repolarization). Examples include propafenone, flecainide, and moricizine. (Moricizine has both IB and IC properties.)

Class II

Class II drugs block adrenergic receptors. Examples include propranolol, metoprolol, atenolol, and others.

Class III

Class III drugs primarily slow repolarization (phase 3). Examples include sotalol, amiodarone, ibutilide, and dofetilide.

Table 18.1.   Drugs of choice for common arrhythmias

Arrhythmia	Drug of choice	Alternatives
Atrial fibrillation or flutter	Diltiazem, verapamil, or beta-blocker for urgent ventricular rate control	Ilbutilide for conversion, digoxin, beta-blockers, calcium channel blockers, amiodarone for long-term management
Atrioventricular nodal reentrant supraventricular	Adenosine, verapamil, or diltiazem for conversion	Esmolol, other beta-blocker, or digoxin for conversion
Tachyarrhythmias Premature ventricular contractions	None indicated for the asymptomatic patient	
Sustained ventricular tachycardia	Lidocaine or amiodarone for acute therapy	Procainamide
Ventricular fibrillation	Direct current cardioversion	Drug therapy is for prevention of recurrence and is the same as for sustained ventricular arrhythmias
Torsade de pointes	Magnesium sulfate	Isoproterenol, pacing

Class IV

Class IV drugs block calcium channels. Examples include verapamil, diltiazem, nifedipine, and others.

General Comments

Class I

Advances in antiarrhythmic devices and ablation therapy have revolutionized the treatment of many arrhythmias. In addition, new knowledge derived from molecular, structural, and translational biology is likely to result in new therapeutic opinions for arrhythmia management (2). The popularity and clinical use of the class I agents had been based largely on their perceived effectiveness in the management of ventricular arrhythmias and prevention of sudden cardiac death (SCD). However, several clinical trials indicate that many drugs within this class worsen outcome when compared to no treatment or placebo therapy in patients with ventricular arrhythmias at risk for SCD (3). Similarly, the widespread use of quinidine as adjunctive therapy for long-term rate control or maintenance of sinus rhythm after cardioversion of atrial fibrillation has been shown to worsen long-term outcome (4). Several drugs within this class (e.g.,

Table 18.2. Antiarrhythmic drugs

Drug	Usual dose	Comments
Adenosine	IV: 6 mg rapid bolus; if no effect, 2 doses of 12 mg at 2 min intervals	Side effects brief; ventricular escape rhythm common
Amiodarone	IV: 150 mg over 10 min Infusion: 360 mg over 6 hr maintenance: 540 mg over 18 hrs PO: low dose 200 mg qd	Higher PO doses needed for ventricular arrhythmias
Diltiazem	IV: 0.25 mg/kg over 2 min, repeat at 0.35 mg/kg in 15–30 min if needed Infusion: 5–15 mg/hr	
Esmolol	See text	
Flecainide	PO: 50–200 mg bid	PO loading dose required
Ibutilide	IV: 1 mg over 10 min, repeat once in 10 min if needed	Torsade in 8%
Lidocaine	See text	Central nervous system side effects
Magnesium	IV: 1–2 g over 5–10 min	May give up to 5 mg
Metoprolol	IV: 5 mg q 5 min to total dose 15 mg	Preferred in acute myocardial infarction
Procainamide	IV: up to 17 mg/kg at 20 mg/min Infusion: 2–4 mg/min PO: 50–100 mg/kg/day	Hypotension may occur with IV loading
Propafenone	PO: 150–300 mg q 8 hrs	
Propranolol	IV: 1–5 mg total (1 mg/min) PO: varies with formulation	
Sotalol	PO: 80–160 mg bid	Higher doses needed for effect on repolarization
Verapamil	IV: 5–10 mg over 1–3 min, repeat in 15–30 min if needed PO: varies with formulation	Hypotension resulting from vasodilatation; consider pretreatment with calcium

IV, intravenously; PO, per Os (by mouth).

procainamide, propafenone, and flecainide) remain in use, largely for the urgent or long-term management of atrial fibrillation (5).

Procainamide most commonly is used in the acute management of arrhythmias, particularly rate control in patients with atrial fibrillation with a rapid ventricular response rate and symptomatic ventricular arrhythmias unresponsive to lidocaine or amiodarone. Because hypotension can occur with rapid intravenous (IV) loading doses, the loading dose (up to 17 mg/kg) should be given at a rate of 20 mg/minute or less. The therapeutic serum concentration is 4 to 10 µg/mL. Long-term use is associated with a lupuslike syndrome in approximately 30% of patients, and many patients will develop antinuclear antibodies within 3 to 6 months of starting the drug. N-acetyl procainamide (NAPA) is an active metabolite and may be increased in patients with renal failure.

Propafenone has beta-blocking effects in addition to its Class IC electrophysiologic effects (6). Both propafenone and flecainide have been shown to be effective in preventing recurrent episodes of paroxysmal atrial fibrillation and atrioventricular (AV) nodal reentrant tachyarrhythmias (5).

Prophylactic lidocaine no longer is recommended in the management of acute myocardial infarction (AMI). A meta-analysis of available literature, in fact, has suggested that it may be detrimental in this setting (7). It is likewise no longer recommended for the treatment of asymptomatic ventricular arrhythmias. Current protocols recommend its use only for the treatment of hemodynamically significant ventricular tachycardia and prevention of recurrent ventricular fibrillation (8). Lidocaine is given as a loading dose—usually 1 mg/kg given over 2 minutes, then 0.5 mg/kg over 2 minutes every 8 to 10 minutes for 3 doses, if needed, for arrhythmia suppression. An infusion (1 to 4 mg/minute) is required to maintain therapeutic serum levels (1.5 to 5 µg/mL). The loading dose should be decreased in patients with heart failure or liver dysfunction and in those older than 70 years of age.

Class II Agents

Beta blockers are effective in slowing the ventricular response rate in atrial fibrillation, converting reentrant supraventricular tachyarrhythmias, and suppressing ventricular arrhythmias. Sotalol is a nonselective beta blocker that also prolongs the QT interval (9), a property of Class III drugs. Propranolol, acebutolol, sotalol, and esmolol are approved for the treatment of arrhythmias. Esmolol is a short-acting IV agent with an elimination half-life of approximately 9 minutes and is particularly useful in patients at risk for the common complications of beta blockade because adverse effects are typically brief in duration (less than 30 minutes). Chronic treatment with propranolol, metoprolol, or timolol following myocardial infarction (MI) decreases 1-year mortality (see Chapter 9).

Class III Agents

Amiodarone has been shown to be more effective than Class IA agents for the treatment of ventricular arrhythmias (3). However, adverse effects, the most serious of which are proarrhythmia, pulmonary fibrosis, and thyroid dysfunction, can occur with doses commonly used to suppress ventricular ectopy. Low doses have been shown to be effective in suppressing paroxysmal supraventricular arrhythmias and converting new-onset atrial fibrillation (10). This drug also has recently been shown to be effective when given intravenously to suppress sustained ventricular tachycardia and prevent recurrent ventricular fibrillation (8,11). Amiodarone can increase the serum concentrations of digoxin, diltiazem, quinidine, procainamide, flecainide, and beta blockers. Sotalol is approved only for use in the management of ventricular arrhythmias but has been shown to be effective in the prevention and termination of atrial fibrillation.

Class IV Agents

Verapamil and diltiazem can be given intravenously and are effective in terminating reentrant supraventricular tachyarrhythmias as well as controlling the ventricular response rate in atrial fibrillation (5). IV use can be complicated by hypotension and bradycardia, particularly in patients receiving beta blockers or other calcium channel blockers. These drugs should be avoided in patients with wide QRS complex tachyarrhythmias when it is unclear if the rhythm is of ventricular origin or the result of aberrant conduction of a supraventricular rhythm. Chronic oral therapy with these drugs may be useful in preventing reentrant supraventricular tachycardias. Chronic therapy may raise serum digoxin levels.

ANGIOTENSIN CONVERTING ENZYME INHIBITORS

Angiotensin converting enzyme (ACE) inhibitors are used primarily in the management of chronic CHF and systemic hypertension and in the treatment of post-MI patients. Data convincingly indicate that ACE inhibitors reduce mortality and morbidity in all grades of CHF and are superior to direct-acting vasodilators. They also improve survival and reduce the risk of major cardiovascular events in patients with impaired left ventricular function or heart failure after MI. Other trials show that ACE inhibitors reduce the risk of MI (12–14).

There are currently ten ACE inhibitors marketed in the United States. The major differences between drugs are in zinc ligand portion of the drug, whether the parent drug (prodrug) is converted to an active metabolite, and cost. Captopril has a sulfhydryl ligand, and fosinopril has a phosphodyl ligand; the remainder have a carboxyl ligand. All except captopril and lisinopril are prodrugs. Prodrugs have a longer onset of peak action and a longer duration of action. The sulfhydryl group is felt to be responsible for a higher incidence of side effects. Table 18.3 lists common doses, comparative costs, and target doses shown to be effective in improving mortality in patients with CHF (15) or in patients following an AMI (16).

These drugs share common adverse effects including (a) dry cough; (b) rash or, rarely, angioedema; (c) hypotension and worsening of renal function with volume or salt depletion or concomitant use of diuretics; (d) hyperkalemia in patients with renal dysfunction, especially diabetics, and in those receiving potassium supplements or potassium-sparing diuretics; (e) loss of taste; and (f) acute renal failure in patients with bilateral renal artery stenosis.

ANGIOTENSIN II RECEPTOR BLOCKERS

The ACE inhibitors prevent conversion of angiotensin I to angiotensin II, but angiotensin II may continue to be formed through alternative pathways. Angiotensin II receptor blockers (ARBs) block the

Table 18.3. Angiotensin converting enzyme (ACE) inhibitors

Drug	Daily dosage	Cost ($)	Target dose
Benazepril (Lotensin)	Initial: 10 mg Usual: 20–40 mg qd or bid	26	
Captopril (generic)	Initial: 25 mg bid or tid Usual: 25–150 mg bid or tid	8	50 mg tid 6.25–50 mg bid[a]
Enalapril (generic)	Initial: 5 mg Usual: 10–40 mg qd or divided	20	10 mg bid
Fosinopril (Monopril)	Initial: 10 mg Usual: 20–40 mg qd or bid	29	
Lisinopril (Zestril or Prinivil)	Initial: 10 mg Usual: 20–40 mg qd	28	2.5–10 mg qd[a]
Moexipril (Univasc)	Initial: 10 mg Usual: 7.5–30 mg qd or divided	21	
Quinapril (Accupril)	Initial: 10 mg Usual: 20–80 mg qd or divided	31	
Ramipril (Altace)	Initial: 2.5 mg Usual: 2.5–20 mg qd or divided	26	5 mg bid 2.5–5 mg bid[a]

Cost, average cost to the patient for 30 days' treatment with the lowest dose (17).
Target dose, doses associated with increased survival in congestive heart failure clinical trials:
[a] Target dose for patients who are post-myocardial infarction.

renin-angiotensin-aldosterone system by preventing angiotensin II binding to angiotensin II type-1 receptors. ACE inhibitors block the breakdown of bradykinin, which may contribute to the drugs' antihypertensive and cardiorenal protective effects but also may cause the angioedema seen with ACE inhibitor therapy. The angiotensin-receptor blockers do not block bradykinin breakdown, and they do not significantly alter prostaglandin metabolism (18).

As of 2002, seven ARBs have been approved for use in the United States. All ARBs are more effective than placebo, some calcium channel blockers, and some beta blockers in lowering blood pressure in patients with mild-to-moderate hypertension. The utility of ARBs in the management of CHF remains uncertain. The ELITE-2 (Evaluation of Losartan In The Elderly) study, comparing losartan and captopril,

Table 18.4.   Angiotensin II receptor blockers

Drug	Usual daily dose (mg qd)	Cost ($)
Candesartan (Atacand)	16–32	43
Eprosartan (Tevetan)	600–800	41
Irbesartan (Avapro)	150–300	46
Losartan (Cozaar)	50–100	45
Olmesartan medoxomil (Benicar)	20–40	39
Telmisartan (Micardis)	40–80	45
Valsartan (Diovan)	80–320	44

Cost for 30 days' treatment based on lowest usual daily dosage (22). The initial dose of irbesartan and losartan should be reduced if the patient also is taking a diuretic.

demonstrated similar mortality in the study group of elderly patients (18). The Val-HeFT (Valsartan Heart Failure) trial, in which valsartan or placebo was added to standard therapy and which included ACE inhibitors and beta blockers in some patients, demonstrated that valsartan significantly reduced the combined endpoint of mortality and morbidity and improved clinical signs and symptoms in patients with heart failure when added to standard therapy. However, there was an adverse effect on mortality and morbidity in the subgroup also receiving an ACE inhibitor or beta blocker (19). Several trials are in progress to evaluate the long-term effects of ARBs in patients with CHF, early effects in patients with AMI, and renal preservation in patients with diabetic nephritic syndrome (18,20).

The ARBs are generally better tolerated than the ACE inhibitors. The incidence of cough is less frequent with ARBs, and these agents are an alternative when the adverse effects of ACE inhibitor therapy require discontinuation. Angioedema has been reported with ARBs, often in patients in whom this complication occurred with ACE inhibitors (21) (Table 18.4).

BETA-ADRENERGIC BLOCKING AGENTS

Beta-adrenergic blocking agents differ primarily in their selectivity for β-1 receptors and intrinsic sympathomimetic activity (ISA) (receptor stimulation by virtue of molecular structure). Agents that are "cardioselective" have a greater effect on cardiac (β-1) adrenoreceptors than on β-2 adrenergic receptors of the bronchi and blood vessels. Selectivity is dose-dependent, and these drugs become less selective as dosage is increased and even in low doses can cause bronchospasm in patients with asthma. Selectivity is an advantage for diabetics because selective beta blockers are less likely to mask the symptoms of hypoglycemia, to delay recovery from hypoglycemia, or to cause severe hypertension when hypoglycemia leads to increased circulating catecholamines. Agents with ISA produce less of a decrease in heart rate at rest and may be preferred for patients who develop symptomatic bradycardia with other beta blockers. They have not, however, been shown to lower mortality after MI. These agents also do not increase serum triglyceride concentrations or decrease high-density lipoprotein (HDL) cholesterol levels as noted with other beta blockers.

The bioavailability, protein binding, lipid solubility, and metabolism of these drugs vary widely. Drugs that are primarily metabolized by the liver are subjected to a "first pass" phenomenon, which has a substantial impact on bioavailability. For drugs with more than 90% hepatic metabolism (e.g., labetalol, metoprolol, propranolol), the bioavailability of an oral dose of drug ranges from 10% to 50%. Drugs metabolized by the liver have shorter half-lives than drugs excreted primarily by the kidney. This is important in the management of patients with renal or hepatic dysfunction, for whom dosages of beta blockers may have to be adjusted, especially because the pharmacodynamic effects of beta blockers are longer than their pharmacologic half-lives. Table 18.5 summarizes the β-1 selectivity and ISA for commonly used beta blockers and includes usual doses (23).

Labetalol also has α-adrenoreceptor-blocking properties, which makes it particularly useful in the management of selected cardiovascular emergencies (e.g., hypertensive crisis, acute aortic dissection) when given intravenously. The usual IV dose is 20 mg, then 40 to 80 mg every 10 minutes until the desired effect on blood pressure and heart rate are achieved or a total dose of 300 mg is given.

Table 18.5. β-Adrenergic blocking agents

Drug	Relative β-1 selectivity	Intrinsic sympathomimetic activity	Dose	Cost (
Acebutolol (generic)	+	+	200–1,200 mg in 1 or 2 doses	21
Atenolol (generic)	+	0	25–100 mg in 1 or 2 doses	9
Betaxalol (generic)	+	0	5–40 mg qd	25
Carvedilol	0	0	12.5–50 mg in 2 doses	92
Labetalol (generic)	0	0	200–1,200 mg in 2 doses	25
Metoprolol (generic)	+	0	50–200 mg in 1 or 2 doses	8
Toprol XL			LA 50–400 mg qd	20
Nadolol (generic)	0	0	20–240 mg qd	18
Pindolol (generic)	0	+	10–60 mg in 2 doses	22
Propranolol (generic)	0	0	40–240 in 2 doses	8
			LA 60–240 qd	28
Sotalol	0	0	80–160 mg bid	
Timolol (generic)	0	0	10–40 mg in 2 doses	16

Cost, average cost to the patient for 30 days' treatment with lowest dosage (23).

The most frequent or severe side effects associated with these drugs are (a) fatigue, (b) decreased exercise tolerance, (c) precipitation of CHF in patients with marginal left ventricular function, (d) bronchospasm in patients with asthma, (e) bradycardia and heart block, (f) impotence, (g) acute mental disorders including acute delirium, (h) changes in triglyceride and HDL cholesterol levels, and (i) exacerbation of angina and acute infarction with sudden withdrawal or cessation of therapy.

Atenolol, metoprolol, and timolol have been shown to decrease short- and long-term mortality in AMI. IV and oral dosing are discussed in Chapter 9.

CALCIUM CHANNEL BLOCKING AGENTS

Calcium channel blocking drugs cause selective inhibition of transmembrane flux of calcium in excitable tissue. Their ability to block calcium-mediated electromechanical coupling in contractile tissue reduces the contractile activity of heart (decreasing myocardial oxygen demand) and also produces arterial dilatation in both the coronary (increased myocardial oxygen supply) and peripheral vascular bed (decreased afterload). Their inhibition of transmembrane cellular flow of calcium during the slow inward current of cardiac action potentials decreases sinus-node automaticity and slows both sinoatrial and atrioventricular conduction, thereby increasing refractoriness. This wide range of effects has led to the use of these drugs in the management of chronic angina pectoris, cardiac arrhythmias (particularly AV-nodal reentrant tachyarrhythmias), and hypertension.

These agents are most commonly classified based on structure. However, there appears to be little or no simple structure-activity relationship for the different classes of drugs.

Structural classification involves the following:

Benzothiazepine derivative—diltiazem
Dihydropyridine derivative—nifedipine, nicardipine, isradipine, nisodipine, nimodipine, and felodipine
Phenylalkylamine derivative—verapamil
Other—bepridil

Five other classifications have been proposed. The most useful would be one based on tissue specificity because it would correlate most closely with clinical indications for use. Table 18.6 represents

Table 18.6.   Pharmacologic effects of calcium antagonists

Drug	Systemic vasodilatation	Negative inotropic effects	Negative dromotropic effects	Vasodilatory side effects
Diltiazem	+	+	+	+
Nifedipine	+++	+	0	+++
Verapamil	+	+++	++	+
Felodipine	++	+	+	++
Nicardipine	++	0	0	++
Nisoldipine	++	0	0	++
Isradipine	++	0	0	++

Table 18.7.   Calcium blockers

Drug	Usual daily dose	Cost ($)
Diltiazem (generic, extended release)	120–360 mg in 2 doses	40
Verapamil (generic)	120–480 mg in 2 or 3 doses	22
Extended release	120–480 mg in 1 or 2 doses	24
Amlodipine (Norvasc)	2.5–10 mg in 1 dose	40
Felodipine (Plendil)	2.5–10 mg in 1 dose	32
Isradipine (DynaCirc)	5–10 mg in 1 or 2 doses	46
Nicardipine (generic)	60–120 mg in 3 doses	32
Nifedipine-extended release (generic)	30–90 mg in 1 dose	37
Nisoldipine (Sular)	20–60 mg in 1 dose	30

Cost, average cost to the patient for 30 days' treatment with the lowest dose.

a simplified version of pharmacologic or physiologic classification. Selected drugs, usual daily adult dose, and costs are shown in Table 18.7.

Frequent or severe adverse effects of these agents include (a) dizziness, (b) headache, (c) bradycardia and AV block, (d) precipitation of heart failure in patients with marginal left ventricular function, (e) peripheral edema, and (f) flushing. Verapamil and diltiazem can increase serum digoxin concentration and precipitate digoxin toxicity.

Calcium channel blockers should be avoided in patients who have had a Q wave infarction because they have been shown to worsen 1-year mortality when compared to placebo.

ORAL NITRATES

Oral nitrates have an established history in the management of stable and unstable angina pectoris. Despite this extensive history, there is no evidence that nitrates improve mortality as a result of ischemic heart disease. However, they have been shown to improve exercise tolerance and the quality of life in patients with coronary artery disease.

Recent advances in nitrate therapy have included a better understanding of the phenomenon of nitrate tolerance and the introduction of extended-release preparations. The usual maintenance dose of isosorbide dinitrate is 30 mg tid for the immediate-release preparation and 40 mg bid for the extended-release preparation. Isosorbide mononitrate is the major active metabolite of isosorbide dinitrate and is available in an immediate-release preparation (20 mg bid) or an extended-release preparation (120 mg qd) (25).

All nitrates cause rapid development of tolerance, but a dosing interval of tid versus qid and a drug-free overnight interval can largely reverse the tolerance that develops during the day. Transdermal nitroglycerin preparations, although initially greeted with enthusiasm, are being replaced by extended-release oral preparations. However, they can be effective if they are removed for 10 to 12 hours daily.

Table 18.8.   Nitrate pharmacokinetics and common dosing schedules

Drug	Usual dose (mg)	Action onset (min)	Duration of action
Sublingual	0.3–0.8	2–5	20–30 min
NTG	2.5–10.0	5–20	45–120 min
ISDN			
Oral	6.5–19.5 bid/tid	20–45	2–6 hrs
NTG-SR	10–60 bid/tid	15–45	2–6 hrs
ISDN	20 bid	30–60	3–6 hrs
ISMN	40–60 bid	60–90	10–14 hrs
ISDN-SR	60–120 qd	60–90	10–14 hrs
ISMN-SR			
NTG	0.5–2.0 inches tid	15–60	3–8 hrs
Ointment (2%)	10–20 mg	30–60	8–12 hrs
Patch			

NTG, nitroglycerin; ISDN, isosorbide dinitrite; ISMN, isosorbide mononitrate; SR, sustained release.

Patients who have frequent angina or angina at night during the nitrate-free period should be treated with a second drug such as a beta blocker or a calcium channel blocker (Table 18.8).

REFERENCES

1. Kowey PR: Pharmacological effects of antiarrhythmics drugs. *Arch Intern Med* 158:325, 1998.
2. Members of the Sicilian Gambit: New approaches to antiarrhythmic therapy, Part I. Emerging therapeutic applications of the cell biology of cardiac arrhythmias. *Circulation* 104:2865, 2001. Part II: *Circulation* 104:2990, 2001.
3. Heidenrich PA, Keeffe B, McDonald KM, et al: Overview of randomized trials of antiarrhythmic drugs and devices for the prevention of sudden cardiac death. *Am Heart J* 144:422, 2002.
4. Flaker GC, Blackshear JL, McBride R, et al: Antiarrhythmic drug therapy and cardiac mortality in atrial fibrillation. *J Am Coll Cardiol* 20:527, 1992.
5. Fuster V, Ryden LE, Asinger RW, et al: ACC/AHA/ESC guidelines for the management of patients with atrial fibrillation. *J Am Coll Cardiol* 38:1231, 2001.
6. Khan IA: Single oral loading dose of propafenone for pharmacological cardioversion of recent-onset atrial fibrillation. *J Am Coll Cardiol* 37:542, 2001.
7. Antman EM, Lau J, Kupelnick B, et al: A comparison of results of meta-analyses of randomized control trials and recommendations of clinical experts. Treatments of myocardial infarction. *JAMA* 268:240, 1992.
8. The American Heart Association in Collaboration with the International Liaison Committee on Resuscitation (ILOR): Guidelines 2000 for Cardiopulmonary Resuscitation and Emergency Cardiovascular Care: adult advanced cardiac life support. *Circulation* 102:I-1, 2000.
9. Hohnloser SH, Woosley RL: Sotalol. *N Engl J Med* 331:31, 1994.

10. Kerin NZ, Faitel K, Naini M: The efficacy of intravenous amiodarone for the conversion of chronic atrial fibrillation. *Arch Intern Med* 156: 49, 1996.
11. Naccarelli GV, Jalal S: Intravenous amiodarone. Another option in the acute management of sustained ventricular tachyarrhythmias. *Circulation* 92:3154, 1995.
12. McMurray J, Pfeffer MA: New therapeutic options in congestive heart failure: Part I. *Circulation* 105:2099, 2002. Part II: *Circulation* 105: 2223, 2002.
13. Konstam MA, Mann DL: Contemporary medical options for treating patients with heart failure. *Circulation* 205:2244, 2002.
14. Sleight P: Angiotensin II and trials of cardiovascular outcomes. *Am J Cardiol* 89(2A): 11A, 2002.
15. Cohn JN: The management of chronic heart failure. *N Engl J Med* 335:490, 1996.
16. Latini R, Maggioni AP, Flather M, et al: ACE inhibitor use in patients with myocardial infarction. Summary of evidence from clinical trials. *Circulation* 92:3132, 1995.
17. Drugs for hypertension. *Med Lett Drugs Ther* 43:17, 2001.
18. Grossman E, Messerli FH, Neutel JM: Angiotensin II receptor blockers. Equal or preferred substitutes of ACE inhibitors? *Arch Intern Med* 160:1905, 2000.
19. Cohn JN, Tognoni C: A randomized trial of the angiotensin-receptor blocker valsartan in chronic heart failure. *N Engl J Med* 345:1667, 2001.
20. Pfeffer MA, McMurray J, Leizorovicz A, et al: Valsartan in acute myocardial infarction trial (VALIANT): rationale and design. *Am Heart J* 240:727, 2000.
21. Abdi R, Dong VM, Lee CJ, et al: Angiotensin II receptor blocker-associated angioedema: on the heels of ACE inhibitor angioedema. *Pharmacotherapy* 22:1173, 2002.
22. Olmesartan (benicar) for hypertension. *Med Lett Drugs Ther* 44:69, 2002.
23. Which beta-blocker? *Med Lett Drugs Ther* 43:9, 2001.
24. Fihn SD, Williams SV, Daley J, et al: Guidelines for the management of patients with chronic stable angina: treatment. *Ann Intern Med* 135:616, 2001.
25. Extended-release isosorbide mononitrate for angina. *Med Lett Drugs Ther* 36:13, 1994.

Index